Workbook for

Radiation Protection in Medical Radiography

Workbook for

Radiation Protection in Medical Radiography

Eighth Edition

Mary Alice Statkiewicz Sherer, AS, RT(R), FASRT

ELSEVIER

ELSEVIER

3251 Riverport Lane
St. Louis, Missouri 63043

WORKBOOK FOR RADIATION PROTECTION IN MEDICAL
RADIOGRAPHY, EIGHTH EDITION

ISBN: 978-0-323-55509-8

Content Strategist: Sonya Seigafuse
Content Development Manager: Lisa Newton
Senior Content Development Specialist: Laura Selkirk
Publishing Services Manager: Deepthi Unni
Project Manager: Radhika Sivalingam
Cover Designer: Muthukumaran Thangaraj

Printed in the United States of America

Last digit is the print number: 9   8   7   6   5   4

Working together
to grow libraries in
developing countries

www.elsevier.com • www.bookaid.org

Contents

Acknowledgments

This free standing workbook has been designed to accompany the eighth edition of *Radiation Protection in Medical Radiography*. Each of the 15 chapters in the workbook contains a variety of exercises, including matching of terms or phrases with their definitions, multiple choice questions, true or false statements, fill-in-the-blank statements, labeling of diagrams or missing information in boxes or charts, short answer questions, general discussion questions, and a chapter post test. Use of the workbook in conjunction with the textbook will provide a challenging experience for the learner. It will reinforce learning and help students remember important concepts and material covered in each chapter of the book. The answers for all the exercises are located in the back of the workbook. Using both the textbook and workbook simultaneously will be of significant value in helping the radiography student prepare for credentialing examinations such as the American Registry of Radiologic Technologists certification examination for full-scope radiographers. Limited-scope x-ray students preparing for credentialing examinations administered through individual state licensing boards can also use the textbook in conjunction with the workbook to prepare for their state licensing examinations.

To be of significant value, a workbook must be designed to accompany a textbook that has both adequate and significant technical information in the specific subject matter. The new eighth edition of *Radiation Protection in Medical Radiography* is a compilation of updated, new, and standard information developed with the assistance of three exceptional and highly knowledgeable collaborating authors who have given their time and expertise to make the new edition the best it can be. It is with great pride and sincere gratitude that I acknowledge and thank Paula J. Visconti, PhD, DABR; E. Russell Ritenour, PhD, DABR, FAAPM, FACR; and Kelli Welch Haynes, MSRS, RT(R) for all their contributions to the new edition of the textbook. In addition, a very special thank you is given to E. Russell Ritenour for his participation in developing selective material for the workbook and for reviewing various chapter exercises. Dr. Ritenour's recommendations for this new edition of the workbook have been most valuable.

Sincere gratitude for effective communication, hard work, and ongoing support is given to the highly competent and wonderful staff of Elsevier, Inc. Special acknowledgment and thanks are given to Executive Content Strategist Sonya Seigafuse, Senior Content Development Specialist Laura Selkirk, Project Manager Manchu Mohan, and Project Manager Radhika Sivalingam. Thanks is also given to the anonymous reviewer who provided recommendations to improve some statements in various exercises throughout this book. I appreciate everything they have done to bring this workbook to publication.

Finally, I want to thank my three sons, Joseph F. Statkiewicz, Christopher R. Statkiewicz, and Terry R. Sherer, Jr., for the consistent love, support, and encouragement they have given me during the development of the textbook and this ancillary. Also, not to be forgotten are my two little shih tzus, Dexter and Roxie, who were always by my side while I worked on this entire project.

Mary Alice Statkiewicz Sherer, AS, RT(R), FASRT

1 Introduction to Radiation Protection

Chapter 1 provides an introduction to radiation protection that includes discussion of the use of ionizing radiation in the healing arts, beginning with the discovery of x-rays in 1895. The following topics are also covered in this chapter: fundamental properties of x-rays; team concept in the medical field; control of radiant energy; goals and concepts of radiation protection, including an introduction to radiation quantities and units of measure; justification and responsibility for imaging procedures; and the as low as reasonably achievable (ALARA) principle. Other topics covered include patient protection and patient education, which take into consideration the risk of imaging procedures versus the potential benefit of such procedures; use of background equivalent radiation time (BERT) to inform patients of the amount of radiation they will receive during a specific x-ray procedure; increased radiation sensitivity in children; the Alliance for Radiation Safety in Pediatric Radiology; the Image Gently and Image Wisely campaigns; monitoring and reporting radiation dose; the Nationwide Evaluation of X-ray Trends (NEXT) project; and reference values and protocols for dose alerts.

CHAPTER HIGHLIGHTS

- Radiation is the transfer of kinetic energy from one location to another.
- X-rays have several unique properties.
- X-rays are a form of ionizing radiation.
- Ionizing radiation has both a beneficial and a destructive potential.
- A team approach to patient care is an organized collaborative approach that can also have the benefit of increased radiation safety for patients and directly involved members of the imaging team.
- Radiant energy can be controlled by using the knowledge of radiation-induced hazards that has been gained over many years and by employing effective methods to limit or eliminate those hazards.
- Radiologic technologists and radiologists should adhere to good radiology practices that minimize the possibility of causing damage to healthy biologic tissue.
- The goals of modern radiation protection programs are twofold: to protect persons from both short-term and long-term effects of radiation.
- To safeguard patients, personnel, and the general public from unnecessary exposure to ionizing radiation, effective radiation protection measures should always be employed when diagnostic imaging procedures are performed.

- Healthy normal biologic tissue of animals and humans can be damaged by exposure to ionizing radiation; therefore it is necessary to safeguard against unnecessary exposure to ionizing radiation.
- The realized benefits of exposing patients to ionizing radiation should far outweigh any slight chance of inducing radiogenic cancer or any genetic defects.
- Referring physicians should justify the need for every radiation procedure and accept basic responsibility for protecting the patient from nonuseful ionizing radiation.
- Radiographers should select the smallest radiation exposure that produces the best radiographic results and should avoid errors that result in repeated radiographic exposures.
- Radiation exposure should always be kept ALARA to minimize the probability of any potential damage to people.
- The three basic principles of radiation are time, distance, and shielding.
- Imaging facilities must have an effective radiation safety program in place that provides patient protection and patient education.
- A significant understanding of biologic effects of ionizing radiation, improved designs of medical x-ray equipment, and more stringent radiation safety standards have greatly reduced the risk from imaging procedures for both patients and radiographers.
- BERT is used to compare the amount of radiation a patient receives from a radiologic procedure with natural background radiation received over a specific period.
- Children are significantly more radiation sensitive than are adults, and exposure to radiation early in life, at levels found in computed tomography (CT) and even lower, leads to a measurable increase in cancer incidence as these individuals age into their 50s and 60s.
- The goal of the Alliance for Radiation Safety in Pediatric Imaging is to increase awareness of the need to reduce radiation dose for pediatric patients, especially in CT imaging.
- The Image Gently campaign advocates lowering patient dose by "child sizing" the kV and mA x-ray machine settings, scanning only the indicated areas, and removing multiphase scans from pediatric protocols.
- The objectives of the Image Wisely campaign are lowering the amount of radiation used in medically necessary imaging studies and eliminating unnecessary procedures for adults.
- In CT and in interventional procedures, various added measures related to patient dose recording are becoming the norm. The Food and Drug Administration

Copyright © 2018, Elsevier Inc. All rights reserved.

(FDA) mandates that measures of dose in CT be available as part of the record of each examination. The Joint Commission requires monitoring of patient dose in CT and in interventional procedures, and there are indications of it also moving toward requirements for all modalities in radiology.

- Reference values for patient dose are usually based on large-scale surveys of actual measurement of x-ray machines in hospitals.
- Alert levels are sometimes used when patient dose is predicted to or has actually substantially exceeded preset dose levels.

Exercise 1: Matching

Match the following terms with their definitions or associated phrases.

1. __P__ ALARA

2. __X__ Distance

3. __F__ Risk
4. __C__ Millisievert (mSv)

5. __K__ BERT

6. __A__ Radiation protection

7. __H__ The Alliance for Radiation Safety in Pediatric Imaging
8. __Y__ Optimization for radiation protection

9. __G__ Radiation-induced cancer

10. __B__ Diagnostic efficacy

11. __I__ Radiation safety officer (RSO)

12. __E__ Appropriate and effective communication

13. __T__ Radiation phobia

14. __D__ Adverse biologic effects
15. __N__ The NEXT program

16. __J__ milligray (mGy)
17. __O__ The Joint Commission

18. __R__ Creation of free radicals
19. __N__ 1895

20. __U__ Radiologic technologists

A. Effective measures employed by radiation workers to safeguard patients, personnel, and the general public from unnecessary exposure to ionizing radiation

B. The degree to which the diagnostic study accurately reveals the presence or absence of disease in a patient

C. A subunit of the sievert equal to 1/1000 of a sievert

D. Damage to living tissue of animals and humans exposed to radiation

E. Makes patients feel that they are active participants in their own health care

F. In the medical industry with reference to the radiation sciences, the possibility of inducing adverse biologic effects such as injury to the skin or induction of cancer or a genetic defect after irradiation

G. A disease process that does not have a fixed threshold

H. A partnership of medical societies whose overall common purpose is to reduce the radiation dose for pediatric patients

I. Individual in a hospital setting expressly charged by the administration to be directly responsible for the execution, enforcement, and maintenance of the ALARA program

J. SI subunit of measure for the radiation quantity, "absorbed dose"

K. Method for comparing the amount of radiation received from a radiologic procedure with natural background radiation received over a specified period, such as days, weeks, months, or years

L. Produces positively and negatively charged particles (ions) when passing through normal matter

M. Type of approach in patient care that has gained an increasing awareness in recent years

N. Year in which x-ray was discovered

O. Requires monitoring of patient dose in CT and in interventional procedures

P. Acronym for *as low as reasonably achievable*

Q. Responsibility of facilities and radiographers that provide imaging services

R. A consequence of ionization in human cells

S. Based on evidence that living tissue of animals and humans can be damaged by exposure to ionizing radiation

T. Fear of being exposed to radiation

21. ___L___ Ionizing radiation

22. ___S___ Justification for reduction of unnecessary radiation exposure.

23. ___M___ Team approach

24. ___Q___ To provide high-quality imaging services

25. ___V___ Nonoccupational doses

U. Have the responsibility to select technical exposure factors that significantly reduce radiation exposure to patients and themselves

V. Radiation exposure received by persons not employed in the medical imaging profession (e.g., patients, the general public)

W. Conducted to provide data on systems as they exist in the United States on the date of the latest survey

X. One of the three cardinal principles of radiation protection

Y. Synonymous with the acronym ALARA

Exercise 2: Multiple Choice

Select the answer that *best* completes the following questions or statements.

1. Which of the following *increases* radiation exposure to the patient and potentially to the radiographer?
   A. Production of optimal quality images with the first exposure
   B. Use of appropriate radiation protection procedures
   C. Repeated radiographic exposures as a result of technical error or carelessness
   D. Limited radiographic examination, as ordered by the radiologist

2. To implement an effective radiation safety program in a facility that provides imaging services, the employer must provide all of the following *except:*
   A. An appropriate environment in which to execute an ALARA program and the necessary resources to support the program
   B. X-ray equipment that can produce only very low kilovoltage and very high milliamperage
   C. A written policy statement describing this ALARA program and identifying the commitment of management to keeping all radiation exposure ALARA that is available to all employees in the workplace
   D. Periodic exposure audits to determine how radiation in the workplace may be lowered

3. Radiation has been present on Earth since:
   A. Its beginning
   B. The fourteenth century
   C. The eighteenth century
   D. The twentieth century

4. Occupational and nonoccupational doses will remain well below maximum allowable levels when:
   A. Radiographers and radiologists keep exposure as low as reasonably achievable.
   B. Referring physicians stop ordering imaging procedures.
   C. Orders for imaging procedures are determined only by medical insurance companies.
   D. Patients assume sole responsibility for ordering their imaging procedures.

5. How can humans safely control the use of radiant energy?
   1. By using the knowledge of radiation-induced hazards that has been gained over many years
   2. By employing effective methods to limit or eliminate radiation-induced hazards
   3. By completely eliminating the use of radiation in the healing arts
   A. 1 and 2 only
   B. 1 and 3 only
   C. 2 and 3 only
   D. 1, 2, and 3

6. In medicine, when radiation safety principles are correctly applied during imaging procedures, the energy deposited in living tissue by the radiation can be limited. This results in:
   A. Completely eliminating the possibility for reducing the potential for adverse effects
   B. No change in the possibility for reducing the potential for adverse effects
   C. Increasing the potential for adverse biologic effects
   D. Reducing the potential for adverse biologic effects

7. To reduce radiation exposure to the patient:
   1. Reduce the amount of the x-ray "beam on" time
   2. Use as much distance as warranted between the x-ray tube and the patient for the examination
   3. Always shield the patient with appropriate gonadal and/or specific area shielding devices
   A. 1 and 2 only
   B. 1 and 3 only
   C. 2 and 3 only
   D. 1, 2, and 3

8. X-rays:
   1. Can have varying degrees of penetration in normal biologic tissue
   2. Can be focused by a lens
   3. Are invisible
   A. 1 and 2 only
   B. 1 and 3 only
   C. 2 and 3 only
   D. 1, 2, and 3

9. Cardinal principles of radiation protection include:
    1. Time
    2. Distance
    3. Shielding
    A. 1 and 2 only
    B. 1 and 3 only
    C. 2 and 3 only
    D. 1, 2, and 3

10. For CT the Joint Commission requires:
    1. Annual education of staff in dose reduction techniques
    2. Minimum qualifications for medical physicists
    3. Documentation of CT radiation dose
    4. Management of CT protocols to minimize radiation dose
    A. 1, 2, and 3 only
    B. 1, 3, and 4 only
    C. 2, 3, and 4 only
    D. 1, 2, 3, and 4

11. Effective radiation protection measures take into consideration:
    1. Both human and environmental physical determinants
    2. Technical elements
    3. Procedural factors
    A. 1 and 2 only
    B. 1 and 3 only
    C. 2 and 3 only
    D. 1, 2, and 3

12. When illness or injury occurs or when a specific imaging procedure for health screening purposes is prudent, a patient may:
    A. Be forced by the referring physician to assume a large risk of exposure to ionizing radiation to obtain unnecessary diagnostic medical information
    B. Be forced by the referring physician to assume the relatively large risk of exposure to ionizing radiation to obtain essential diagnostic information
    C. Elect to assume the relatively large risk of exposure to ionizing radiation to obtain essential diagnostic medical information
    D. Elect to assume a relatively small risk of exposure to ionizing radiation to obtain essential diagnostic medical information

13. Any radiation exposure that *does not* benefit a person in terms of diagnostic information obtained from diagnostic images for the clinical management of medical needs is termed:
    A. Artificial radiation
    B. Enhanced natural background radiation
    C. Man-made radiation
    D. Unnecessary radiation

14. The ALARA philosophy should:
    1. Be a main part of every health care facility's personnel radiation control program
    2. Be maintained because at this time there are no firm dose limits established for the amount of radiation that patients may receive for individual imaging procedures
    3. Be maintained and show all reasonable actions that will reduce dose to patients and personnel below required limits have been considered
    A. 1 and 2 only
    B. 1 and 3 only
    C. 2 and 3 only
    D. 1, 2, and 3

15. When an imaging procedure is justified in terms of medical necessity, diagnostic efficacy is achieved when optimal-quality images, revealing the presence or absence of disease, are obtained with:
    A. Maximal radiation exposure to the patient
    B. Minimal radiation exposure to the patient
    C. Scattered radiation exposure to the patient
    D. Secondary radiation exposure to the patient

16. For the welfare of patients and the workers, facilities providing imaging services must have:
    A. An effective radiation safety program
    B. An inspection of the imaging department every day by nationally recognized authorities
    C. An inspection of the imaging department every day by state-recognized authorities
    D. A strong legal team to suppress potential lawsuits that result from poor radiologic practice

17. When radiation is safely and prudently used in the imaging of patients, the benefit of the exposure can be _____ and the potential risk of biologic damage is _____
    A. Minimized, maximized
    B. Maximized, minimized
    C. Minimized, minimized
    D. Maximized, maximized

18. Which of the following cardinal principles of radiation protection can be applied to both the patient and the radiographer?
    1. Time
    2. Distance
    3. Shielding
    A. 1 and 2 only
    B. 1 and 3 only
    C. 2 and 3 only
    D. 1, 2, and 3

4

19. Which of the following recommend the use of background equivalent radiation time for improving patient understanding and reducing fear and anxiety associated with having an x-ray procedure?
   A. Environmental Protection Agency
   B. Occupational Safety and Health Administration
   C. National Council on Radiation Protection and Measurements
   D. Nuclear Regulatory Commission

20. BERT is a:
   A. Method of comparison
   B. Method of optimizing radiation protection
   C. Radiation quantity
   D. Radiation unit

21. Which of the following terms is an attempt to provide a quantity that is a measure of general harm in humans?
   A. Absorbed dose
   B. Effective dose
   C. Exposure
   D. Diagnostic efficacy

22. Typically, people are more likely to accept a risk if they perceive that:
   A. They have no other options.
   B. They have positive assurance that they will have a good outcome in terms of prognosis.
   C. The potential benefit to be obtained is greater than the risk involved.
   D. The radiologic procedure will absolutely not cause any pain or discomfort.

23. The most effective tool for diagnosing breast cancer continues to be:
   A. Posteroanterior (PA) and lateral chest x-ray examinations
   B. Clinical breast self-examination
   C. Clinical breast examination by a physician
   D. High-quality mammography

24. The millisievert (mSv), a subunit of the sievert (Sv), is equal to:
   A. 1/10,000 of a Sv
   B. 1/1000 of a Sv
   C. 1/100 of a Sv
   D. 1/10 of a Sv

25. Repetition of a radiographic exposure because of poor patient positioning results in:
   A. No significant change in total radiation exposure to the patient or the radiographer
   B. A slight decrease in total radiation exposure to the patient and the radiographer
   C. An increase in total radiation exposure to the patient and the radiographer
   D. A significant decrease in total radiation exposure to the patient and the radiographer

Exercise 3: True or False

Circle *T* if the statement is true; circle *F* if the statement is false.

1. T F X-rays are a form of nonionizing radiation.

2. T F The millisievert (mSv) is the SI subunit of EfD.

3. T F The ability of x-rays to cause injury in normal biologic tissue just became apparent recently.

4. T F A threshold exists for radiation-induced malignant disease.

5. T F BERT is based on an annual U.S. population exposure of approximately 1 mSv per year.

6. T F Diagnostic efficacy provides the basis for determining whether an imaging procedure or practice is justified.

7. T F The basic principles of time, distance, and shielding can be applied for the safety of both the patient and the radiographer.

8. T F Man-made radiation is more dangerous than an equal amount of natural radiation.

9. T F Humans are not continuously exposed to sources of ionizing radiation.

10. T F BERT is a method of explaining radiation to the public.

11. T F Radiologic technologists and radiologists are educated in the safe operation of radiation-producing imaging equipment.

12. T F After ordering an x-ray examination or procedure, the referring physician must accept basic responsibility for protecting the patient from nonuseful radiation exposure.

13. T F   It is the responsibility of the referring physician to provide the necessary resources and appropriate environment in which to execute an ALARA program in a health care facility.

14. T F   A health care facility must have a written policy statement describing the Radiation Safety Program. The statement must also identify the commitment of management to keep all radiation exposure ALARA and must be available to all employees in the workplace.

15. T F   In general terms, risk can be defined as the probability of injury, ailment, or death resulting from an activity.

16. T F   BERT implies risk from radiation exposure.

17. T F   The Joint Commission specifies that all imaging equipment that uses ionizing radiation be regularly tested by qualified personnel and properly maintained.

18. T F   NEXT stands for Nationwide Evaluation of X-ray Trends.

19. T F   Production of high-energy x-ray photons is a consequence of ionization in human cells.

20. T F   Radiation produced from an x-ray tube is an example of controllable radiant energy.

21. T F   Various methods of radiation protection may be applied to ensure safety for persons employed in radiation industries, including medicine, and for the population at large.

22. T F   If a radiographer makes an error in selecting technical radiographic exposure factors for a specific projection of an anatomic body part, the projection can be repeated without an increase in radiation dose for the patient and a potential dose increase for the radiographer.

23. T F   Most patients are unaware that most of their background radiation comes from artificial radioactivity in their own body.

24. T F   Diagnostic efficacy is not an important part of radiation protection in the healing arts.

25. T F   Radiology departments, or individual radiologic technologists, can "pledge" to image gently.

Exercise 4: Fill in the Blank

Using the following Word Bank, fill in the blanks with the word or words that best complete the statements.

ALARA (may be used three times)	energy	more
	exposure	occupational
audit	far outweigh	protective (may be used two times)
beneficial	first	
benefits	follow-up	smallest
BERT	gonadal	specific area
biologic effects	innate	subunit
chance	justified	time
destructive	lowest	unstable
education	maximized	unsafe

1. BERT emphasizes that radiation is a(n) _____ part of our environment.

2. Radiation exposure should always be kept at the _____ possible level for the general public.

3. _____ is the amount of ionization produced in air when ionizing radiation is present.

4. When ionizing radiation is used to obtain a mammogram for the welfare of a patient, the directly realized _____ of the exposure to this radiant energy ____ _____ any slight _____ of inducing a radiogenic malignancy or any genetic defect.

5. In medicine, when radiation safety principles are correctly applied during imaging procedures, the _____ deposited in living tissue by the radiation can be limited, thereby reducing the potential for adverse _____ _____.

6. Diagnostic efficacy is _____ when essential images are produced with the least radiation exposure to the patient.

7. The rationale for _____ comes from evidence compiled by scientists over the past century.

8. Diagnostic efficacy provides the basis for determining whether an imaging procedure or practice is _____.

9. To use _____ as a basic principle for radiation, a radiographer can reduce the duration of unnecessary exposure.

10. Patients not only should be made aware of what a specific procedure involves and what type of cooperation is required but also must be informed of what needs to be done, if anything, as a _____ to their examination.

11. There is no existing data regarding any _____ effects from the x-rays used in examinations.

12. For many regulatory agencies the _____ principle provides a method for comparing the amount of radiation used in various health care facilities in a particular area for specific imaging procedures.

13. The _____ concept should serve as a guide for the selection of technical exposure factors.

14. _____ does not imply radiation risk; it is simply a means for comparison.

15. The goal of reducing retake rates is to obtain optimal radiographic images with the _____ exposure.

16. Radiologic technologists and radiologists use _____ devices whenever possible.

17. Management in a health care facility should perform a periodic exposure _____ to determine how radiation exposure in the workplace may be lowered.

18. Children are significantly _____ sensitive to ionizing radiation than are adults.

19. The millisievert (mSv) is a _____ of the sievert (Sv).

20. X-rays are a form of _____ radiation; therefore their use in medicine for the detection of disease and injury requires _____ measures.

21. Imaging facilities must have an effective radiation safety program that provides patient protection and patient _____.

22. Ionizing radiation, such as x-rays, has both a _____ and a _____ potential.

23. Radiographers should select the _____ radiation exposure that produces useful radiographic images.

24. Creation of _____ atoms is a consequence of ionization in healthy tissue.

25. Radiation workers are required to perform their _____ practices in a manner consistent with the ALARA principle.

Exercise 5: Labeling
Label the following illustration and table.

A. X-ray tube.

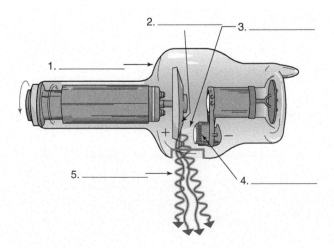

B. Typical adult patient effective dose (EfD) and background equivalent radiation time (BERT) values.

Radiologic Procedure	EfD mSv	BERT (Amount of Time to Receive the Same EfD from Nature)
1. Dental, intraoral	_____	1 wk
2. Chest radiograph	_____	10 days
3. Lumbar spine	_____	1 yr
4. Abdomen	_____	4 mo
5. CT chest	_____	3.6 yr
6. CT abdomen/pelvis	_____	4.5 yr

Sources: Adapted from Wall BF: *Patient dosimetry techniques in diagnostic radiology,* York, UK, 1988, Institute of Physics and Engineering in Medicine, pp 53, 117; Cameron JR: *Med Phys World,* 15:20, 1999; Stabin MG: *Radiation protection and dosimetry: an introduction to health physics,* New York, 2008, Springer.
CT, Computed tomography; *mSv,* millisievert.

Exercise 6: Short Answer

Answer the following questions by providing a short answer.

1. How can humans safely control the use of radiant energy?

_____

_____

2. How can radiologic technologists reduce radiation exposure to patients and to themselves?

_____

_____

3. As ionizing radiation passes through matter, what is the event that may cause injury in normal biologic tissue?

_____

_____

4. What are the three cardinal principles of radiation protection?

_____

_____

5. How can imaging personnel apply the three cardinal principles of radiation protection to minimize occupational exposure?

_____

_____

6. What principle can be used as a method for comparing the amount of radiation used in various health care facilities in a particular area for specific imaging procedures?

_____

_____

7. What is the goal of modern radiation protection programs?

_____

_____

8. Regarding the ALARA program in a hospital setting, what are three responsibilities for the program that are entrusted to the radiation safety officer by the administration?

_____

_____

9. How is risk weighed against benefit in medical radiography?

_____

_____

10. List four good practices that apply to radiologic technologists and radiologists.

_____

_____

11. List six consequences of ionization in human cells.

_____

_____

12. If a patient is having a chest x-ray examination and the patient asks the radiographer, "How much radiation will I receive from this x-ray?" how should the radiographer respond?

_____

_____

13. On what are reference values for patient dose based?

_____

_____

14. For all medical imaging procedures, what concept or principle should the selection of exposure factors always follow?

_____

_____

15. List three advantages of using the BERT method to compare the amount of radiation received with the natural background radiation received over a given period.

_____

_____

16. What are the radiation workers' responsibilities to maintain an effective radiation safety program?

_____

_____

17. What are the two objectives of the Image Wisely campaign?

_____

_____

18. What are adverse biologic effects?

_____

_____

19. How fast do x-rays travel in a straight line until they interact with atoms?

_____

_____

20. What is the responsibility of the technologist with regard to calculation of radiation dose for a specific patient?

_____

_____

Exercise 7: General Discussion or Opinion Questions

The following questions are intended to allow students to express their knowledge and understanding of subject matter or to present a personal opinion on a specific topic. The questions may be used to stimulate class discussion. Because answers to these questions may vary, determination of an answer's acceptability is left to the discretion of the course instructor.

1. Discuss the value of team concept as it relates to medical imaging.

2. How can imaging professionals help ensure that both occupational and nonoccupational radiation doses remain well below maximum allowable levels?

3. How can the cardinal rules of radiation protection be applied in the clinical setting?

4. How can a radiographer maintain radiation exposure ALARA on a daily basis in a clinical setting?

5. In addition to CT and interventional procedures, how will required monitoring of patient dose for all modalities in radiology be beneficial?

6. Describe the value of patient education with regard to radiation procedures and radiation safety.

7. Discuss the importance of diagnostic efficacy as it relates to medical x-ray procedures and radiation safety for the patient.

8. Discuss the responsibility of the employer in a health care facility for maintaining the ALARA concept in the workplace.

9. Applying the BERT method, explain how a radiographer could respond to a patient who asks how much radiation he or she will receive from a routine x-ray series of the lumbar spine.

10. Explain how reference values can be used to benefit an individual health care facility.

The student should take this test after reading Chapter 1, finishing all accompanying textbook and workbook exercises, and completing any additional activities required by the course instructor. The student should complete the post-test with a score of 90% or higher before advancing to the next chapter. (Each of the following 20 questions are worth 5 points.)
Score = _____ %

1. Define the term *radiation protection.*

   _____

   _____

2. What term (and acronym) is used to express the principle of keeping radiation exposure to a level that minimizes the potential for adverse biologic damage to humans?

   _____

3. Who should justify the need for every radiation procedure and accept basic responsibility for protecting the patient from nonuseful radiation exposure?

   _____

4. The directly realized benefits of exposing patients to ionizing radiation should far outweigh any slight _____ of inducing a radiogenic malignancy or genetic defects.

5. What must imaging facilities have that provides for patient protection and patient education?

   _____

   _____

6. What is the need for safeguarding against unnecessary radiation exposure based on?

   _____

   _____

7. One millisievert (mSv) is equal to:
   A. 1/10 of a Sv
   B. 1/100 of a Sv
   C. 1/1000 of a Sv
   D. 1/10,000 of a Sv

8. What is the SI subunit of measure for absorbed dose?

   _____

   _____

9. The degree to which the diagnostic study accurately reveals the presence or absence of disease in a patient, while adhering to radiation safety guidelines, defines:
   A. ALARA
   B. BERT
   C. Diagnostic efficacy
   D. Optimization

10. Any radiation exposure that does not benefit a person in terms of diagnostic information obtained from diagnostic images for the clinical management of medical needs is called:
   A. Enhanced natural background radiation
   B. Environmental radiation
   C. Manmade radiation
   D. Unnecessary radiation

11. What is the goal of modern radiation protection programs?

   _____

   _____

12. What is the most effective tool for diagnosing breast cancer early?

   _____

   _____

13. What is the name of the campaign that delivers the message that CT saves children's lives but that patient dose should be lowered by "child sizing" the kV and mA x-ray machine settings, by scanning only the indicated anatomic area, and by removing multiphase scans from the pediatric protocol?

   _____

14. What method can a radiographer use to compare the amount of radiation received during a routine radiographic procedure with natural background radiation received over a specific period?

   _____

15. Optimization for radiation protection is synonymous with the term:
   A. ALARA
   B. BERT
   C. FDA
   D. NEXT

16. The cardinal principles of radiation protection are:
      1. Time
      2. Distance
      3. Shielding
   A. 1 only
   B. 2 only
   C. 3 only
   D. 1, 2, and 3

17. In a hospital setting, who does the administration charge to be directly responsible for the execution, enforcement, and maintenance of the ALARA program?

   _____

   _____

18. Radiographers should select the _____ radiation exposure that will produce useful images and avoid errors that result in _____ radiographic exposures.

19. BERT does not imply radiation risk; it is simply a means for _____.

20. True or False: Man-made radiation is more dangerous than an equal amount of natural radiation.

   _____

   _____

2 Radiation: Types, Sources, and Doses Received

There are different types and sources of radiation. Some types of radiation produce damage in biologic tissue, whereas others do not. Some sources of radiation are considered natural sources because they are always present in the environment. However, other sources are created by humans for specific purposes and therefore are classified as manmade. The radiation dose to the global population from both sources contributes a percentage of the total amount of radiation that humans receive during their lifetime. Chapter 2 presents an overview of the various types and sources of radiation as well as the doses that are typically received from both natural and manmade sources. Specific topics covered in this chapter include discussion of not only the various types and sources of radiation but also the electromagnetic spectrum, ionizing and nonionizing radiation, particulate radiation, an introduction to the concept of radiation dose, and biologic damage potential.

CHAPTER HIGHLIGHTS

- Radiation is kinetic energy and exists in many forms.
- For radiation protection purposes, the electromagnetic spectrum can be divided into two categories: ionizing and nonionizing radiation.
- X-rays, gamma rays, and ultraviolet radiation with energy greater than 10 eV are classified as ionizing radiations.
- Low-energy ultraviolet radiation, visible light, infrared rays, microwaves, and radio waves are classified as nonionizing radiations.
- X-rays are classified as electromagnetic radiation.
- The process of ionization is the foundation of the interaction of x-rays with human tissue. It makes the x-rays valuable for creating images but has the undesirable result of potentially producing some damage in biologic material.
- Alpha particles, beta particles, neutrons, and protons are particulate radiations. They vary in their ability to penetrate matter.
- Radiation absorbed dose is usually measured in units of milligray (mGy).
- Equivalent dose (EqD) takes into account the type of radiation that was absorbed. It provides an overall dose value that includes the different degrees of tissue interaction that could be caused by the different types of radiation. The millisievert (mSv) is the most common unit of measure of equivalent dose.
- Equivalent dose enables the calculation of the effective dose.
- The effective dose (EfD) is intended to be the best estimate of overall harm that might be produced by a

given dose of radiation in human tissue. It takes into account both the type of radiation and the part of the body irradiated. The millisievert is also the unit of measure for the effective dose.

- Ionizing radiation produces electrically charged particles that can cause biologic damage on molecular, cellular, and organic levels in humans.
- Sources of ionizing radiation may be natural or manmade.
  - □ Natural sources include radioactive materials in the crust of the earth, cosmic rays from the sun and beyond the solar system, internal radiation from radionuclides deposited in humans through natural processes, and terrestrial radiation in the environment.
  - □ Manmade sources include consumer products containing radioactive material, air travel, nuclear fuel, atmospheric fallout from nuclear weapons testing, nuclear power plant accidents whatever their origin, and medical radiation from diagnostic x-ray machines and radiopharmaceuticals in nuclear medicine procedures.
  - □ Although there has not been much change in the amount of natural background radiation to the U.S. population since 1987, there have been significant increases in the amount of radiation exposure resulting from medical imaging procedures such as computed tomography (CT) scanning, cardiac nuclear medicine examinations, and interventional procedures.
  - □ The most recently available data indicate that 37% of natural background radiation exposure comes primarily from the gaseous radionuclide radon and, to a much lesser degree, from the radionuclide thoron.
  - □ The Environmental Protection Agency considers radon to be the second leading cause of lung cancer in the United States.
  - □ The recommended action limit for radon in homes is 4 picocuries per liter (pCi/L) of air.
  - □ Natural background radiation in the United States results in an estimated average annual individual EqD of 3.0 mSv.
  - □ Manmade radiation exposure contributes about 3.3 mSv to the average annual radiation exposure of the U.S. population.
  - □ The total average annual EfD from natural background and manmade radiations combined is about 6.3 mSv.
  - □ Thyroid cancer continues to be the main adverse health effect of the 1986 Chernobyl nuclear power plant accident.
  - □ The amount of ionizing radiation actually received by a patient from diagnostic x-ray procedures may be indicated in terms such as entrance skin exposure (ESE), bone marrow dose, and gonadal dose. In pregnant women, fetal dose can also be estimated.

Exercise 1: Matching

Match the following terms with their definitions or associated phrases.

1. ___K___ Fukushima Daiichi

2. ___X___ Fallout

3. ___F___ Electromagnetic wave

4. ___L___ Ionization-type smoke detector alarm

5. ___A___ mGy_t

6. ___B___ Energy

7. ___H___ EqD

8. ___Y___ Radionuclides

9. ___G___ Organic damage

10. ___P___ Frequency

11. ___I___ EfD

12. ___E___ Genetic damage

13. ___T___ Enhanced natural sources

14. ___C___ Ionization

15. ___W___ Protons

16. ___D___ Wavelength

17. ___O___ Cellular damage

18. ___R___ Terrestrial radiation

19. ___N___ Radiation

20. ___U___ Beta particle

21. ___J___ Helical

22. ___S___ Alpha particle

23. ___M___ Electromagnetic spectrum

24. ___Q___ Cosmic rays

25. ___V___ Atomic number

A. SI subunit that can be used for measuring radiation exposure at skin entrance

B. Specified in electron volts (eV)

C. Process that is the foundation of interactions of x-rays with human tissue

D. Specified in meters

E. Biologic effects of ionizing radiation or other agents on generations yet unborn

F. Electric and magnetic fields that fluctuate rapidly as they travel through space, including radio waves, microwaves, visible light, and x-rays

G. Genetic or somatic changes in a living organism (e.g., mutation, cataracts, and leukemia) caused by excessive cellular damage from exposure to ionizing radiation

H. Radiation quantity that takes into account the type of ionizing radiation that was absorbed

I. Radiation quantity intended to be the best estimate of overall harm that might be produced by a given dose of radiation in human tissue

J. Another name for multislice spiral computed tomography

K. Nuclear power plant severely damaged as a consequence of a 9.0-magnitude earthquake that triggered a tsunami in 2011

L. Consumer product containing radioactive material

M. The full range of frequencies and wavelengths of electromagnetic waves

N. Kinetic energy that passes from one location to another

O. Injury on the cellular level caused by sufficient exposure to ionizing radiation at the molecular level

P. Given in units of hertz (Hz) (i.e., cycles per second)

Q. Rays of extraterrestrial origin that result from nuclear interactions that have taken place in the sun and other stars

R. Long-lived radioactive elements present in variable quantities in the crust of the earth and emitting densely ionizing radiations

S. Containing two protons and two neutrons

T. Ionizing radiation that has always been part of the environment but has grown larger because of accidental or deliberate human actions, such as mining of radioactive materials

U. Identical to a high-speed electron, except it is emitted from the nuclei of radioactive atoms instead of originating in atomic shells outside of the nucleus

V. The number of protons contained within the nucleus of an atom

W. Positively charged components of an atom

X. Radiation produced as a consequence of nuclear weapons testing and chemical explosions in nuclear power plants

Y. Internal radiation from radioactive atoms that make up a small percentage of the human body's tissue

Exercise 2: Multiple Choice

Select the answer that *best* completes the following questions or statements.

1. Of the following radiations, which are classified as ionizing radiation?
   1. Infrared rays, low-energy ultraviolet radiation, and microwaves
   2. Low-energy ultraviolet radiation, radio waves, and visible light
   3. Ultraviolet radiation with energy greater than 10 eV, gamma rays, and x-rays
   A. 1 only
   B. 2 only
   C. 3 only
   D. 1, 2, and 3

2. The amount of energy received by an individual is termed:
   A. Electromagnetic energy
   B. Linear acceleration
   C. Radioactive decay
   D. Radiation dose

3. The most recently available data indicate that the gaseous radionuclide radon and, to a much lesser degree, the radionuclide thoron account for what percentage of natural background radiation exposure?
   A. 15%
   B. 25%
   C. 37%
   D. 55%

4. Of the following radiations, which are classified as particulate radiations?
   1. X-rays and gamma rays
   2. Alpha particles and beta particles
   3. Gamma rays and ultraviolet radiation with energy greater than 10 eV
   A. 1 only
   B. 2 only
   C. 3 only
   D. 1, 2, and 3

5. Beta particles are:
   A. 8 times lighter than alpha particles
   B. 80 times lighter than alpha particles
   C. 800 times lighter than alpha particles
   D. 8000 times lighter than alpha particles

6. Which of the following places human beings in closer contact with extraterrestrial radiation?
   A. Posteroanterior and lateral digital radiographic images of the chest
   B. Deep-sea diving
   C. A flight on a commercial airplane
   D. Visit to a nuclear power plant

7. What do airport surveillance systems, ionization-type smoke detector alarms, and nuclear power plants have in common?
   A. They are all sources of natural background radiation.
   B. They each contribute 0.05 mSv per year to the equivalent dose received by the global population.
   C. They are not sources of ionizing radiation.
   D. They are all sources of manmade radiation.

8. From which of the following sources do human beings receive the *largest* dose of ionizing radiation?
   A. Radioactive fallout from atomic weapons testing
   B. Medical radiation procedures
   C. Cosmic rays
   D. The area surrounding a nuclear reactor

9. Thoron is a radioactive decay product of an isotope of:
   A. Carbon
   B. Iodine
   C. Radon
   D. Strontium

10. Of the following groups of people, which group is most likely to experience adverse health effects as a consequence of *substantial* exposure to ionizing radiation?
    A. Employees on duty at TMI-2 at the time of the 1979 nuclear power plant accident
    B. Members of the general population living within 50 miles of the TMI-2 nuclear reactor at the time of the 1979 accident
    C. Members of the general population living near Kiev in the former Soviet Union at the time of the 1986 accident at the Chernobyl nuclear power plant
    D. News reporters visiting the former Soviet Union 10 years after the 1986 Chernobyl accident

11. Which of the following is a radiation quantity that provides an overall dose value that includes the different degrees of tissue interaction that could be caused by the different types of radiation?
    A. Absorbed dose
    B. Effective dose
    C. Equivalent dose
    D. Exposure

Chapter 2 Radiation: Types, Sources, and Doses Received

12. A 3-year pilot research project was launched in the Republic of Belarus in 1996, in the aftermath of the Chernobyl nuclear accident, to empower local citizens in making their own decisions regarding reconstruction of their overall quality of life; this project was known as the:
    A. ALARA program
    B. Belarus Health Impact Study
    C. Chernobyl Rehabilitation Taskforce
    D. ETHOS Project

13. The average U.S. inhabitant received an EqD of approximately _____ per year from extraterrestrial radiation.
    A. 0.3 mSv
    B. 0.6 mSv
    C. 0.9 mSv
    D. 1.0 mSv

14. The amount of radiation a patient receives may be indicated in terms of:
    1. Entrance skin exposure
    2. Bone marrow dose
    3. Gonadal dose
    A. 1 and 2 only
    B. 1 and 3 only
    C. 2 and 3 only
    D. 1, 2, and 3

15. The most highly exposed Chernobyl liquidators, who worked at the Chernobyl nuclear power complex after the disaster, demonstrated a statistically significant rise in the number of:
    A. Leukemia cases
    B. Liver cancer cases
    C. Pancreatic cancer cases
    D. Prostate cancer cases

16. Ultraviolet radiation less than 10 eV, visible light, infrared rays, microwaves, and radio waves are considered to be nonionizing because they:
    A. Have sufficient kinetic energy to eject electrons from atoms
    B. Do not have sufficient kinetic energy to eject electrons from atoms
    C. Have sufficient potential energy to eject electrons from atoms
    D. Do not have sufficient potential energy to eject electrons from atoms

17. Which of the following is a naturally occurring process by which instability of the nucleus is relieved through various types of nuclear spontaneous emissions?
    A. Electromagnetic radiation
    B. Electromagnetic ionization
    C. Radioactive decay
    D. Radioactive fallout

18. The frequency of exposure to manmade radiation in medical applications continues to increase rapidly among all age groups in the United States because of:
    1. Health insurance requirements
    2. Medicolegal considerations
    3. Physicians relying more often on unneeded expensive, sophisticated technology to assist them in making diagnoses for patient care to protect themselves from often frivolous lawsuits, instead of ordering much less expensive and much lower radiation dose procedures
    A. 1 and 2 only
    B. 1 and 3 only
    C. 2 and 3 only
    D. 1, 2, and 3

19. Radioactive elements in the crust of the earth and in the human body may be classified as:
    A. Enhanced natural sources of ionizing radiation
    B. Enhanced manmade sources of ionizing radiation
    C. Natural sources of ionizing radiation
    D. Unnatural sources of ionizing radiation

20. Medical radiation procedures account for:
    A. The largest manmade dose of ionizing radiation received by humans
    B. The second largest manmade dose of ionizing radiation received by humans
    C. The smallest manmade dose of ionizing radiation received by humans
    D. Negligible manmade doses of ionizing radiation received by humans

21. Which of the following commonly used building materials contain(s) radon?
    1. Bricks
    2. Concrete
    3. Gypsum wallboard
    A. 1 and 2 only
    B. 1 and 3 only
    C. 2 and 3 only
    D. 1, 2, and 3

22. The authority that directs and coordinates health programs within the United Nations System is the:
    A. International Atomic Energy Agency
    B. National Council on Radiation Protection
    C. World Health Organization
    D. United States Nuclear Regulatory Commission

23. Beta particles are identical to _____ except for their origin.
    A. Alpha particles
    B. Gamma rays
    C. High-speed electrons
    D. X-rays

24. Which of the following identifies an element and determines its placement in the periodic table of elements?
    A. Atomic number
    B. Atomic weight
    C. Combining power
    D. Valence

25. White blood cells that defend the body against foreign invaders by producing antibodies to combat disease are:
    A. Erythrocytes
    B. Granulocytes
    C. Lymphocytes
    D. Osteocytes

Exercise 3: True or False

Circle *T* if the statement is true; circle *F* if the statement is false.

1. T F The number of protons in the nucleus of an atom constitutes the atomic number, or Z.

2. T F The total average annual EfD from natural background and manmade radiations combined is 3.6 mSv.

3. T F To reduce the possibility of genetic damage in future generations, the increase in frequency of radiation exposure in medicine must be counterbalanced by controlling the amount of patient exposure in individual imaging procedures.

4. T F Because humans are unable to control natural background radiation, exposure from artificial sources that can be controlled must be limited to protect the general population from further biologic damage.

5. T F Sunspots indicate regions of decreased electromagnetic field activity and are occasionally responsible for ejecting particulate radiation into space.

6. T F Radio waves, microwaves, visible light, and x-rays are forms of electromagnetic waves.

7. T F Particulate radiations do not vary in their ability to penetrate matter.

8. T F EfD enables the calculation of the EqD.

9. T F The actual radiation exposure experienced by commercial flight crews (pilots, flight attendants, etc.) sometimes exceeds that of workers at nuclear plants.

10. T F Most radiation-induced cancers have a latent period of 15 years or more.

11. T F Atmospheric nuclear testing has escalated since 1980.

12. T F Nuclear power plants that produce nuclear fuel for generation of power contribute significantly to the annual EqD of the U.S. population during their normal operating cycles.

13. T F Plans were made to cover the remains of Chernobyl reactor unit 4 and the concrete sarcophagus that entombs it with a weatherproof, massive aluminum vault.

14. T F Sources of ionizing radiation may be natural or manmade.

15. T F If emitted from a radioisotope deposited in the body (e.g., in the lungs), alpha particles cannot be absorbed in epithelial tissue and therefore are not damaging to that tissue.

16. T F Because it is extremely difficult to measure the amount of radiation people received in the area near the Fukushima Daiichi Nuclear Plant, the long-term effects, such as an increased incidence of cancer in the exposed population, cannot be accurately determined.

17. T F Because of the large variety of radiologic equipment and differences in imaging procedures and in individual radiologist and radiographer technical skills, the patient dose for each examination varies according to the facility providing imaging services.

18. T F Wavelength is the distance between successive crests or troughs in a wave.

19. T F An electron has approximately the same mass as a proton.

20. T F Changes in white blood cell count are a classic example of molecular damage caused by significant exposure to ionizing radiation.

21. T F Wave-particle duality means that electromagnetic radiation travels through space in the form of a wave but can interact with matter as a particle of energy called a photon.

17

22. T   F   Nonsmokers exposed to high radon levels face a higher risk of lung cancer than do smokers.

23. T   F   The solar contribution to the cosmic ray background decreases during periods of high sunspot activity.

24. T   F   Neutrons are electrically neutral components of an atom.

25. T   F   Radon initially does not cling to or interact with the atoms of other particles.

Exercise 4: Fill in the Blank

Using the following Word Bank, fill in the blanks with the word or words that best complete the statements.

0.08 mGy	ETHOS Project	radionuclides (may be used two times)
4	fetal dose	
40	greatest	radiopharmaceuticals
alpha particles	higher	radium
atmosphere	lowest	radon
constant	magnetic field	solar flare
cosmic	millisievert (mSv)	terrestrial
dose rates	molten	thyroid
electromagnetic spectrum	noble	unplanned
equivalent dose	radiation dose	x-ray machines

1. The actual _____ _____ to the global population from atmospheric fallout from nuclear weapons testing is not received all at once. It is instead delivered over a period of years at changing _____ _____.

2. Unfortunate accidents involving nuclear reactors can occur. This can lead to substantial, _____ radiation exposure for humans and the environment.

3. The aim of the _____ _____ was to rebuild acceptable living conditions for local citizens in contaminated territories in the Ukraine region of Russia by actively involving them in the reconstruction process.

4. In pregnant woman, _____ _____ may be estimated.

5. The full range of frequencies and wavelengths of electromagnetic waves is known as the _____ _____.

6. The quantity of _____ radiation present in any area depends on the composition of the soil or rocks in that geographic region.

7. _____ radiations consist predominantly of high-energy protons.

8. The tissues of the human body contain many naturally existing _____ that have been ingested in minute quantities from various foods or inhaled as particles in the air.

9. If a person spends 10 hours flying aboard a commercial aircraft during a period of normal sunspot activity, that individual will receive a radiation _____ _____ that is about equal to the dose received from one chest x-ray examination.

10. Medical radiation exposure results from the use of diagnostic _____ _____ and _____ in medicine.

11. The amount of natural background radiation remains fairly _____ from year to year.

12. A tremendous explosion on the surface of the sun is called a _____ _____.

13. The average dose received by the exposed population living within a 50-mile radius of the TMI nuclear power station was determined to be _____.

14. The most common unit of measure for equivalent dose is the _____.

15. The Environmental Protection Agency (EPA) considers _____ to be the second leading cause of cancer in the United States.

16. _____ in the soil and air add to the human radiation dose burden.

17. The amount of cosmic rays varies with altitude relative to the earth's surface. The _____ intensity occurs at high altitudes, where there is less attenuation as a result of the low atmospheric density, whereas the _____ intensity occurs at sea level.

18. Because _____ _____ lose energy quickly as they travel a short distance, they are considered virtually harmless as an external source of radiation.

19. The earth's _____ and _____ _____ help shield it from cosmic rays.

20. _____ cancer continues to be the main adverse health effect of the 1986 accident at the Chernobyl nuclear power plant.

21. The EPA recommends that action be taken to reduce levels of radon in homes in the United States to a concentration less than _____ picocuries per liter (pCi/L) of air.

22. Radon is the first decay product of _____, a metallic chemical element.

23. During the accident at the TMI-2 nuclear power plant in March 1979, the U.S. Department of Energy estimated that about _____% of the material in the TMI-2 nuclear reactor core reached a _____ state.

24. In cooler months, when homes and buildings are tightly closed, radon levels are usually _____.

25. Radon is considered to be a _____ gas.

Exercise 5: Labeling
Label the following illustration and tables.

A. Percentage contribution of each natural and manmade radiation source to the total collective effective dose for the population of the United States, 2006.

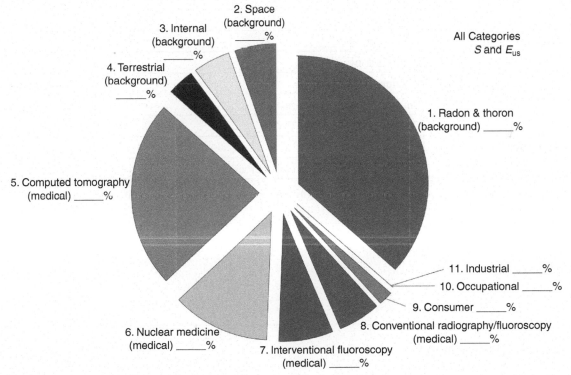

From National Council on Radiation Protection and Measurements (NCRP): *Ionizing radiation exposure of the population of the United States,* Report No. 160, Bethesda, Md, 2009, NCRP.

Chapter **2** **Radiation: Types, Sources, and Doses Received**

B. Radiation equivalent dose and subsequent biologic effects of acute whole-body exposure.*

Radiation Equivalent Dose (EqD)	Subsequent Biologic Effect
1. _____ Sv	Blood changes (e.g., measurable hematologic depression, substantial decreases within a few days in the number of lymphocytes or white blood cells that are the body's primary defense against disease)
2. _____ Sv	Nausea, diarrhea
3. _____ Sv	Erythema (diffuse redness over an area of skin after irradiation)
4. _____ Sv	If dose is to gonads, temporary sterility
5. _____ Sv	50% chance of death; lethal dose (LD) for 50% of population over 30 days (LD 50/30)
6. _____ Sv	Death

Adapted from *Radiologic health,* unit 4, slide 17, Denver, Multi-Media Publishing (slide program).
*Radiation exposures are delivered to the entire body over a period of less than a few hours.

C. Average annual radiation equivalent dose (EqD) for estimated levels of radiation exposure for humans.

Category	Type of Radiation	mSv
Natural	Radon	_____
	Cosmic	_____
	Terrestrial and internally deposited radionuclides	_____
	Total	_____
Medical imaging	CT scanning	_____
	Radiography	_____
	Nuclear medicine	_____
	Interventional procedures	_____
	Total	_____
Other manmade		_____
	Total annual EqD from all sources	_____

Adapted from Bushong SC: *Radiologic science for technologists: physics, biology, and protection,* ed 10, St. Louis, 2013, Mosby.

Exercise 6: Short Answer

Answer the following questions by providing a short answer.

1. What is energy?

_____

_____

2. What is an electron volt (eV)?

_____

_____

3. How does ionizing radiation damage biologic tissue?

_____

_____

4. What is an important determinant of the extent of biologic harm that may occur in humans?

_____

_____

5. Describe what can happen to a living organism if excessive cellular damage occurs as a consequence of radiation exposure.

_____

_____

6. What is the origin of cosmic rays? From what do they result?

_____

_____

7. Name four radionuclides found in small quantities in the human body.

_____

_____

8. Why is it impossible to estimate accurately the total annual equivalent dose from fallout?

_____

_____

9. Why is it necessary to control artificial sources of radiation?

_____

_____

10. For radiation protection purposes what are the two categories of the electromagnetic spectrum?

_____

_____

11. Why are radiations such as visible light and radio waves considered to be nonionizing?

_____

_____

12. What are mesons?

_____

_____

13. What subunit of a sievert (Sv) is equal to 1/1000 of a Sv?

_____

14. List seven sources of manmade, or artificial, ionizing radiation.

_____

_____

_____

21

15. What disease continues to be the main adverse health effect of the 1986 accident at the Chernobyl nuclear power plant?

_____

_____

16. What was the average dose received by the exposed population living within a 50-mile radius of the Three Mile Island nuclear power station at the time of the accident that occurred in 1979?

_____

_____

17. List three ways to indicate the amount of radiation received by a patient.

_____

_____

18. What radiation quantity enables the calculation of the effective dose?

_____

_____

19. In the electromagnetic spectrum with what are higher frequencies associated?

_____

_____

20. In terms of ability to penetrate biologic matter, how do alpha particles compare with beta particles? Why are alpha particles considered virtually harmless as an external source of radiation?

_____

_____

Exercise 7: General Discussion or Opinion Questions

The following questions are intended to allow students to express their knowledge and understanding of subject matter or to present a personal opinion on a specific topic. The questions may be used to stimulate class discussion. Because answers to these questions may vary, determination of an answer's acceptability is left to the discretion of the course instructor.

1. Since the 1979 TMI-2 nuclear power plant accident, what detectable effects have been observed in the population living in the community near the plant? What is the current status of TMI-2, and what will eventually happen to this power plant?

2. What mental and adverse physical health effects have been attributed to the 1986 disaster at the Chernobyl nuclear power plant from the time of the accident to the present time? Discuss the consequences of this accident for plant workers, the exposed population, and the remaining global population since the time of the accident. Describe what is expected to replace the sarcophagus that covers the remains of the reactor 4 unit.

3. Discuss the significance of the ETHOS Project, and explain the value of this program to the community in the Republic of Belarus.

4. Explain why medical radiation has increased since the 1980s, and discuss the impact this increase in exposure can have on the population of the United States.

5. Using the information in Table 2.1 in the text, compare the use, frequency, wavelength, and energy of the radiations that make up the electromagnetic spectrum.

6. Discuss the Fukushima Daiichi nuclear plant crisis of 2011 and the possibility of long-term effects of radiation on the exposed population.

7. Explain how the usage of ionizing radiation in medicine has changed from the early 1980s to the present time.

8. Discuss the biologic damage potential of ionizing radiation as it penetrates tissues in the human body.

9. Describe the various sources of natural background radiation and their impact on humans and the environment.

10. Describe the health impact of radon exposure for humans.

POST-TEST

The student should take this test after reading Chapter 2, finishing all accompanying textbook and workbook exercises, and completing any additional activities required by the course instructor. The student should complete the post-test with a score of 90% or higher before advancing to the next chapter. (Each of the following 20 questions are worth 5 points.)
Score = _____ %

1. Define the term *radiation*.

   _____

   _____

2. List three electromagnetic radiations that are classified as ionizing radiations.

   _____

3. What process is the foundation of the interactions of x-rays with human tissue?

   _____

4. True or False: As an external source of radiation, alpha particles are more penetrating than are beta particles.

   _____

5. What radiation quantity is used to express both occupational and nonoccupational dose limits, and what metric subunit is used?

   _____

6. What does ionizing radiation produce that can cause biologic damage on the molecular, cellular, and organic levels in humans?

   _____

7. Smokers exposed to high radon levels face a higher risk of _____ _____ than do nonsmokers.

8. What is the SI subunit of measure for EqD?

   _____

9. Which of the following radiation quantities takes into account both the type of radiation and the part of the body irradiated and is intended to be the best estimate of overall harm that might be produced by a given dose of radiation in human tissue?
   A. Absorbed dose
   B. Effective dose
   C. Equivalent dose
   D. Exposure

10. *Z number* refers to the number of:
    A. Electrons in the outer shell of an atom
    B. Electrons in the nucleus of an atom
    C. Neutrons in the nucleus of an atom
    D. Protons in the nucleus of an atom

11. Bone marrow dose, gonadal dose, and ESE (which includes skin and glandular dose) may be used to indicate:

    _____

12. What is the term used for the full range of frequencies and wavelengths of electromagnetic waves?

    _____

13. The radioactive elements in the crust of the earth and in the human body are considered what type of sources of ionizing radiation?

    _____

14. Changes in blood count are a classic example of _____ damage that results from nonnegligible exposure to ionizing radiation.

15. The EPA considers the second leading cause of lung cancer in the United States to be:
    A. Diagnostic x-rays
    B. Normal exposure to natural background radiation
    C. Radon
    D. Cosmic rays

16. Which of the following is a consumer product that contains radioactive material?
    1. Airport surveillance systems
    2. Electron microscopes
    3. Ionization-type smoke detector alarms
    A. 1 and 2 only
    B. 1 and 3 only
    C. 2 and 3 only
    D. 1, 2, and 3

17. Are alpha particles more harmful as an external source of radiation or as an internal source of radiation?

    _____

18. Why are the long-term effects, such as an increased incidence of cancer in the exposed population near the Fukushima Daiichi nuclear power plant at the time of the accident caused by natural disaster and resulting tsunami, not able to be accurately determined?

    _____

19. What disease continues to be the main adverse health effect of the 1986 accident at the Chernobyl nuclear power plant?

    _____

20. What is the term for radiation damage to generations yet unborn?

    _____

3 | Interaction of X-Radiation with Matter

Chapter 3 reviews fundamental physics concepts that relate to radiation absorption and scatter. The processes of interaction between radiation and matter are emphasized because a basic understanding of the subject is necessary for radiographers to optimally select technical exposure factors, such as the peak kilovoltage (kVp) and the milli-ampere-seconds (mAs). Selection of the appropriate techniques can minimize the radiation dose to the patient while producing optimal-quality images.

CHAPTER HIGHLIGHTS

- Peak kilovoltage (kVp) controls the quality, or penetrating power, of the photons in the x-ray beam and to some degree also affects the quantity, or number of photons, in the beam.
- Because radiographers select the technical exposure factors, they are responsible for the radiation dose the patient received during an imaging procedure
- The amount of energy absorbed by the patient per unit mass is called the absorbed dose.
- Biologic damage in the patient may result from absorption of x-ray energy. However, some small amount of radiation dose is necessary to produce a diagnostic image.
- Variations in x-ray absorption properties of various body structures make radiographic imaging of human anatomy possible.
- Radiographers receive less radiation exposure when the patient's dose is minimal because less radiation is scattered from the patient during an imaging procedure.
- The anode of an x-ray tube is usually made of tungsten or an alloy of tungsten and rhenium.
- The units kVp and kilovolt (kV) refer to the voltage on the x-ray tube, whereas kiloelectron volt (keV) refers to the energy of specific x-rays.

- Attenuation results when, through the processes of absorption and scatter, the intensity of the primary photons in an x-ray beam decreases as it passes through matter.
- Scattered radiation can result in diminished contrast of the image by adding additional, undesirable exposure to the image receptor (radiographic fog). In fluoroscopy, Compton-scattered photons may expose personnel who are present in the room to scattered radiation.
- Two interactions of x-radiation are central in diagnostic radiology: photoelectric absorption and Compton scattering. The photoelectric absorption is the basis of useful radiographic imaging, whereas Compton scattering is its bane.
- For each radiographic procedure, an optimal peak kilovoltage (kVp) and milliampere-seconds (mAs) combination exists that minimizes the dose to the patient and produces an acceptable image.
  □ Within the energy range of diagnostic radiology (23 to 150 kVp), which also includes mammography, when kVp is decreased, the number of photoelectric interactions increases and the number of Compton interactions decreases; however, the patient absorbs more energy, and therefore the dose to the patient increases.
  □ When kVp is increased, the patient receives a lower dose, but image quality may be compromised.
  □ kVp selection is usually based on the type of procedure and body part imaged.
- Radiographers must balance other variables, such as type of image receptor used, patient thickness, and degree of muscle tissue, to arrive at technical exposure factors that will provide an acceptable image yet stay within the standards of radiation protection.
- Coherent scattering is most likely to occur at less than 10 keV; pair production and photodisintegration occur far above the range of diagnostic radiology.

Exercise 1: Matching

Match the following terms with their definitions or associated phrases.

1. _____ Absorption

2. _____ Permanent inherent filtration
3. _____ Photoelectric absorption

4. _____ Fluorescent yield

5. _____ mAs
6. _____ kVp
7. _____ Deuteron

8. _____ Compton scattering
9. _____ Effective atomic number (Z_{eff})

10. _____ Aluminum
11. _____ Positron

12. _____ Radiographic fog

13. _____ Attenuation

14. _____ Exposure of the image receptor
15. _____ Photoelectron

16. _____ Tungsten and rhenium

17. _____ Pair production

18. _____ 13.8
19. _____ Annihilation radiation

20. _____ $E = mc^2$

21. _____ 7.4

22. _____ Absorbed dose
23. _____ X-ray photons

24. _____ Negative contrast media

25. _____ Image formation photons

A. Reduction in the number of primary photons in the x-ray beam through absorption and scatter as the beam passes through the patient in its path

B. Effective atomic number of compact bone

C. Interaction of an x-ray photon with a loosely bound outer-shell electron of an atom

D. The product of electron tube current and the amount of time in seconds that the x-ray tube is activated

E. Effective atomic number of soft tissue

F. Metal alloys of which the anode of an x-ray tube can be made

G. Transference of electromagnetic energy from the x-rays to the atoms of the patient's biologic material

H. By-product of photoelectric interaction

I. Undesirable, additional exposure on a completed radiographic image that can be caused by scattered radiation

J. Proton-neutron combination

K. Interaction between an x-ray photon and an inner-shell electron of an atom

L. Metal that hardens the x-ray beam by removing low-energy components that would serve to only increase patient dose

M. Determines the highest energy level of photons in the x-ray beam, equal to the highest voltage established across the x-ray tube

N. Positively charged electron

O. Combination of the x-ray tube glass wall and the added aluminum placed within the collimator

P. Refers to the number of x-rays emitted per inner-shell vacancy

Q. A composite Z value by weight for a material that is composed of multiple chemical elements

R. The darkness of a region of a radiographic image

S. Interaction in which the energy of the incoming photon is transformed into two new particles, a negatron and a positron

T. Radiation in the form of two oppositely moving 0.511-MeV photons generated as the result of mutual annihilation of matter and antimatter

U. Mathematic expression of Albert Einstein's famous concept of mass-energy equivalence

V. The amount of energy absorbed by the patient per unit mass

W. X-ray photons that emerge from human tissue and strike the radiographic image receptor after passing through the patient being radiographed

X. Agents that result in areas of increased brightness on a radiographic image

Y. Particles associated with electromagnetic radiation that have neither mass nor charge and travel at the speed of light

Exercise 2: Multiple Choice

Select the answer that *best* completes the following questions or statements.

1. When a technical exposure factor of 100 kVp is selected, which of the following occurs?
   A. The electrons will be accelerated from the anode to the cathode with an average effective energy of 33 keV.
   B. The electrons will be accelerated from the cathode to the anode with an average effective energy of 33 keV.
   C. The beam will contain all photons having an effective energy of 100 keV.
   D. The beam will contain photons having energies of 100 keV or less, with an average effective energy of approximately 33 keV.

2. The passage of primary x-ray photons through a patient *without* interaction in body tissue is called:
   A. Absorption
   B. Attenuation
   C. Indirect transmission
   D. Direct transmission

3. In which of the following x-ray interactions with matter is the energy of the incident photon *completely* absorbed?
   A. Compton
   B. Photoelectric
   C. Incoherent
   D. Rayleigh

4. What is the result of coherent scattering?
   A. Usually just a small angle change in the direction of the incident photon
   B. Transfer of all energy of the incident x-ray photon to the atoms of the irradiated object
   C. Production of a negatron and a positron
   D. Transfer of only some of the energy of the incident x-ray photon to the atoms of the irradiated object

5. A technical exposure factor of 100 kVp means that the electrons bombarding the target of the x-ray tube have a *maximum* energy of:
   A. 1000 electron volts (eV), or 1 keV
   B. 10,000 eV, or 10 keV
   C. 100,000 eV, or 100 keV
   D. 1,000,000 eV, or 1000 keV

6. A Compton scattered electron:
   A. Annihilates another electron
   B. Is absorbed within a few microns of the site of the original Compton interaction
   C. Causes pair production
   D. Engages in the process of photodisintegration

7. Most scattered radiation produced during radiographic procedures is the *direct* result of which of the following?
   A. Photoelectric absorption
   B. Nuclear decay
   C. Image-formation electrons
   D. Compton interactions

8. A reduction in the number of primary photons in the x-ray beam through absorption and scatter as the beam passes through the patient in its path defines:
   A. Annihilation
   B. Attenuation
   C. Photodisintegration
   D. Radiographic fog

9. *Before* interacting with matter, an incoming x-ray photon may be referred to as which of the following?
   A. Attenuated photon
   B. Primary photon
   C. Ionized photon
   D. Scattered photon

10. Within the energy range of diagnostic radiology (23 to 150 kVp), which includes mammography, when kVp is *decreased,* the patient dose:
    A. Decreases
    B. Increases
    C. Remains the same
    D. Doubles

11. Which of the following statements *best* describes mass density?
    A. It is the number of electrons per gram of tissue.
    B. It is the same as radiographic density.
    C. It relates the way the effective atomic number of biologic tissues influences absorption.
    D. It is measured in grams per cubic centimeter.

12. Of the following interactions between x-radiation and matter, which only occur above the range of diagnostic radiology?
    1. Photoelectric absorption
    2. Pair production
    3. Photodisintegration
    A. 1 and 2 only
    B. 1 and 3 only
    C. 2 and 3 only
    D. 1, 2, and 3

13. For a diagnostic radiologic examination, the selection of technical exposure factors using an *optimal* kVp and mAs combination:
    A. Produces an x-ray image of acceptable quality but increases patient dose
    B. Produces an x-ray image of acceptable quality while minimizing patient dose
    C. Produces an x-ray image of acceptable quality without affecting patient dose
    D. Affects neither the quality of the completed radiographic image nor patient dose

14. The quality, or penetrating power, of an x-ray beam is controlled by:
    A. The absorption characteristics of the patient being radiographed
    B. Fluorescent yield
    C. mAs
    D. kVp

15. Small-angle scatter:
    A. Degrades the appearance of a completed radiographic image by blurring the sharp outlines of dense structures
    B. Enhances the appearance of a completed radiographic image by clearly delineating the sharp outlines of dense structures
    C. Affects the appearance of a completed radiographic image only when contrast medium is used for visualization of a tissue or structure
    D. Occurs only in therapeutic radiologic ranges

16. Within the energy range of diagnostic radiology, as absorption of electromagnetic energy in biologic tissue increases, the potential for biologic damage:
    A. Decreases slightly
    B. Decreases significantly
    C. Increases
    D. Remains the same

17. Which of the following terms are synonymous?
    1. Coherent scattering
    2. Classical scattering
    3. Unmodified scattering
    A. 1 and 2 only
    B. 1 and 3 only
    C. 2 and 3 only
    D. 1, 2, and 3

18. Noninteracting and small-angle scattered photons comprise:
    A. Absorbed photons
    B. Attenuated photons
    C. Exit, or image formation, radiation
    D. Compton scatter

19. *Direct transmission* means that x-ray photons:
    A. Are absorbed in biologic tissue on interaction
    B. Are completely scattered within biologic tissue on interaction
    C. Pass through biologic tissue without interaction
    D. Pass through biologic tissue with some interaction

20. Which of the following has the same mass and magnitude of charge as a negatron?
    A. Deuteron
    B. Neutron
    C. Positron
    D. Proton

21. Which of the following interactions between x-radiation and matter *does not* occur within the range of diagnostic radiology?
    A. Coherent scattering
    B. Compton scattering
    C. Photoelectric absorption
    D. Pair production

22. kVp controls:
    A. Absorption characteristics of the body part being radiographed
    B. Fluorescent yield
    C. Random interaction of x-ray photons with the image receptor
    D. Quality, or penetrating power, of the x-ray photons in the beam

23. *Primary radiation* is synonymous with:
    A. Direct radiation
    B. Compton scatter
    C. Elastic scatter
    D. Rayleigh radiation

24. Which of the following are radiographic image receptors?
    1. Radiographic grid
    2. Digital radiography receptor
    3. Phosphor plate
    4. Radiographic film
    A. 1 and 2 only
    B. 1 and 4 only
    C. 2, 3, and 4 only
    D. 1, 2, 3, and 4

25. The process most responsible for the contrast between bone and soft tissue in a diagnostic radiographic image is:
    A. Coherent scattering
    B. Compton scattering
    C. Photoelectric absorption
    D. Photodisintegration

Exercise 3: True or False

Circle *T* if the statement listed below is true; circle *F* if the statement is false.

1. T F The radiographer also benefits when patient dose is minimal because less radiation is scattered from the patient.

2. T F The optimal x-ray image is formed when only indirect transmission photons reach the image receptor.

3. T F Coherent scattering does not contribute noticeably to radiographic fog in mammography because, during this imaging procedure, breast tissue is gently but firmly compressed.

4. T F During the process of Compton scattering, an x-ray photon interacts with an inner-shell electron of an atom of the irradiated object.

5. T F A photoelectron usually is absorbed within a few micrometers of the medium through which it travels, thereby increasing patient dose and contributing to biologic damage in tissue.

6. T F Absorption properties of different body structures must be identical to make diagnostically useful images possible.

7. T F The intensity of radiation scatter in various directions is a major factor in the planning of protection for medical imaging personnel during a radiologic examination.

8. T F The effective atomic number (Z_{eff}) of air is 13.8.

9. T F In the radiographic kilovoltage range, compact bone with a high calcium content by weight undergoes much more photoelectric absorption than does an equal mass of soft tissue and air.

10. T F The use of positive contrast media leads to a decrease in absorbed dose in the body structures that contain them.

11. T F Compton scattering results in all-directional scatter.

12. T F A Compton scattered electron is also known as an *Auger electron*.

13. T F Annihilation radiation is used in an imaging modality employed in nuclear medicine called positron emission tomography (PET).

14. T F For each radiographic procedure, an optimal kVp and mAs combination exists that minimizes the dose to the patient and produces an acceptable radiographic image.

15. T F A photoelectron may interact with other atoms, but it cannot cause excitation or ionization of those atoms.

16. T F *Attenuation* is any process that increases the intensity of the primary photon beam directed toward a destination such as the radiographic image receptor.

17. T F During the process of photoelectric absorption, the atom also emits primary radiation when the outer-shell electron fills the inner-shell vacancy.

18. T F The minimum energy required to produce an electron-positron pair is 0.022 mega-electron volts (MeV).

19. T F The target in the x-ray tube is also known as the *cathode.*

20. T F If an electron is drawn across an electrical potential difference of 1 volt (V), it has acquired an energy of 1 eV.

21. T F The term *exit photons* is synonymous with the term *image formation photons.*

22. T F The by-products of photoelectric absorption include photoelectrons and characteristic x-ray photons.

23. T F The atomic number of tungsten is 94.

24. T F Biologic damage in the patient may result from the absorption of x-ray energy.

25. T F Selection of kVp usually is based on the type of procedure and body part to be radiographed.

Exercise 4: Fill in the Blank

Using the following Word Bank, fill in the blanks with the word or words that best complete the statements.

absorption (may be used two times)	electrical voltage	milliampere-seconds (mAs)
Auger	electrons (may be used two times)	one-third
backscatter	energy (may be used two times)	pathologic
coherent (classical, elastic, or unmodified) (may be used two times)	fluorescent	photoelectric (may be used two times)
Compton (may be used two times)	glass window	photons
	image	positively
darker	increase	random
decreases	intensity	recoil
degrade	kinetic	sidescatter
	manmade	small-angle

1. X-rays are carriers of _____ electromagnetic energy.

2. As _____ interact with the atoms of the tube target, x-ray _____ are produced. They emerge from the target with a broad range, or spectrum, of energies and leave the x-ray tube through a glass window.

3. The energy of the electrons inside the x-ray tube is generally specified in terms of the _____ _____ applied across the tube.

4. In clinical situations, scattered photons reach the image receptor and _____ image quality.

5. In a diagnostic x-ray beam, the ultimate destination of photons is the _____ receptor.

6. In the process of _____ scattering, because the wavelengths of both incident and scattered waves are the same, no net energy has been absorbed by the atom.

7. Compton scatter may be directed forward as _____ _____, backward as _____, and laterally as _____.

8. _____ scattering and _____ absorption in tissue are equally probable at about 35 keV.

9. When an inner-shell electron is removed from an atom in a photoelectric interaction, thus causing an inner-shell vacancy, the energy liberated when this vacancy is filled can be transferred to another electron of the atom, thereby ejecting the electron, instead of emerging from the atom as characteristic radiation. Such an emitted electron is called an _____ electron.

10. Biologic damage may result from the _____ of x-ray energy.

11. A diagnostic x-ray beam is produced when a stream of very energetic _____ bombards a _____ charged target in a highly evacuated glass tube.

12. Although all photons in a diagnostic x-ray beam do not have the same _____, the most energetic photons in the beam can have no more _____ than the electrons that bombard the target.

13. For a typical diagnostic x-ray unit, the mean photon energy in the x-ray beam is about _____ the energy of the most energetic photon.

14. The _____ of radiation scatter in various directions is a major factor in the planning of protection for medical imaging personnel during a radiologic examination.

15. _____ is the product of electron tube current and the amount of time in seconds that the x-ray tube is activated.

16. The less a given structure attenuates radiation, the _____ its radiographic image will be, and vice versa.

17. Use of a positive contrast medium leads to an _____ in absorbed dose in the body structures that contain it.

18. The _____ _____ of the x-ray tube permits passage of all but the lowest-energy components of the x-ray spectrum.

19. Characteristic photons are also termed _____ radiation.

20. _____ scattering is most likely to occur at low energy, typically less than 10 keV.

21. The interaction of x-ray photons with biologic matter is _____.

22. _____ conditions such as degenerative arthritis contribute to differences in x-ray absorption in biologic tissue.

23. Variations in the x-ray _____ properties of various body structures make radiographic imaging of human anatomy possible.

24. A Compton scattered electron is also known as a secondary, or _____, electron.

25. An incoming x-ray photon has _____ energy.

Exercise 5: Labeling
Label the following illustrations.

A. Primary, exit, and attenuated photons.

B. Process of photoelectric absorption.

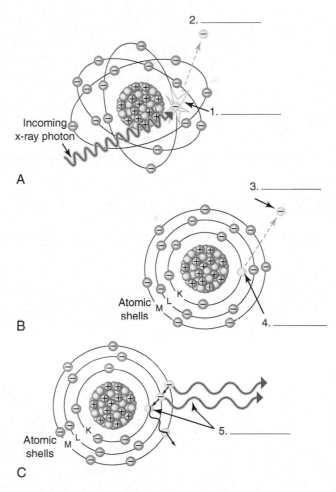

Primary
1 2 3 4

1. _____

2. _____

3. _____

4. _____

5. _____

6. _____

No interaction

Primary − Exit = Attenuation

2. _____

1. _____

Incoming x-ray photon

A

3. _____

Atomic shells

4. _____

K
L
M

B

Atomic shells

5. _____

K
L
M

C

C. Process of Compton scattering.

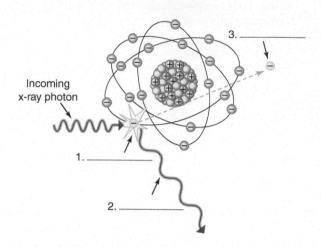

Incoming x-ray photon

1. _____

2. _____

3. _____

Exercise 6: Short Answer
Answer the following questions by providing a short answer.

1. Name five types of interactions that can occur between x-radiation and matter.

_____

_____

2. How is a radiographer responsible for the radiation dose the patient receives during a diagnostic x-ray procedure?

_____

_____

3. What is responsible for producing diagnostically useful images in which different anatomic structures can be perceived and distinguished?

_____

_____

4. What is the best way for the radiographer to decrease the amount of radiographic fog that is produced by small-angle scatter?

_____

_____

5. How is the energy of the electrons inside a diagnostic x-ray tube usually specified?

_____

_____

6. What is the minimum energy required to produce an electron-positron pair?

_____

7. Of what does positive contrast media consist?

_____

_____

8. Name three unstable nuclei used in PET scanning.

_____

_____

9. What type of energy does a photoelectron have?

_____

_____

10. What can happen to the radiographic image when scattered radiation emerges from the patient and strikes this image receptor?

_____

_____

11. During a fluoroscopic procedure, how can radiographers protect themselves from scattered radiation?

_____

_____

12. During the process of coherent scattering, why is any net energy not absorbed by the atom with which the incident x-ray photon interacts?

_____

_____

13. How is mass density measured?

_____

_____

14. Within the energy range of diagnostic radiology, what impact does the difference of photoelectric absorption in body tissue have on radiographic contrast in the recorded image?

_____

_____

15. In what image modality is annihilation radiation used?

_____

_____

Exercise 7: General Discussion or Opinion Questions

The following questions are intended to allow students to express their knowledge and understanding of the subject matter or to present a personal opinion. The questions may be used to stimulate class discussion. Because answers to these questions may vary, determination of an answer's acceptability is left to the discretion of the course instructor.

1. Discuss the importance of photoelectric absorption in radiography, and explain the impact of this x-ray interaction on patient dose.

2. Describe how a radiographer can limit the production of scattered radiation in a general radiography x-ray room and in a fluoroscopic room during a procedure.

3. Discuss the use of positive contrast media in radiography. How does the use of such media affect patient dose?

4. Discuss the probability of photon interaction with matter.

5. How can radiographers select technical exposure factors for routine x-ray procedures to minimize the radiation dose to the patient and to themselves, while producing an optimal-quality image?

POST-TEST

The student should take this test after reading Chapter 3, finishing all accompanying textbook and workbook exercises, and completing any additional activities required by the course instructor. The student should complete the post-test with a score of 90% or higher before advancing to the next chapter. (Each of the following 20 questions are worth 5 points.)
Score = _____ %

1. Use of a barium- or iodine-based contrast medium significantly enhances the occurrence of _____ absorption in biologic tissue and results in an increase in the radiation dose to the patient.

2. Define the term *attenuation*.

   _____

   _____

3. For each radiographic procedure, an optimal kVp and mAs combination exists that _____ the dose to the patient while producing an optimal-quality image.

4. In fluoroscopy, Compton scattered photons can expose imaging _____ who are present in the room.

5. During the process of Compton scattering, the energy of the incident x-ray photon is _____ absorbed.

6. What controls the quality, or penetrating power, of an x-ray beam?

   _____

7. The interactions of x-ray photons with biologic matter are _____; it is impossible to predict with certainty what will happen to a single photon when it enters human tissue.

8. Pair production and _____ do not occur within the range of diagnostic radiology.

9. Which interaction of x-radiation with matter is most responsible for the contrast between bone and soft tissue that is seen on an optimal-quality image?

   _____

10. Scattered radiation can result in:
    1. A higher-quality diagnostic image
    2. Exposure to personnel who are present in a fluoroscopic room during a procedure
    3. Radiographic fog on an image
    A. 1 and 2 only
    B. 1 and 3 only
    C. 2 and 3 only
    D. 1, 2, and 3

11. A positron is considered a:
    A. Form of antimatter
    B. Modified proton
    C. Form of small-angle scatter
    D. By-product of the photoelectric interaction

12. The symbol Z_{eff} indicates:
    A. Atomic number
    B. Effective atomic number
    C. Mass number
    D. The number of vacancies in an atomic shell

13. Of the following x-radiation interactions with matter, which is most likely to occur at less than 10 keV?
    A. Coherent scattering
    B. Compton scattering
    C. Photoelectric absorption
    D. Pair production

14. Which of the following terms are synonymous?
    A. Classical scattering and photoelectric absorption
    B. Compton scattering and photodisintegration
    C. Photoelectric absorption and Compton scattering
    D. Characteristic radiation and fluorescent radiation

15. PET makes use of:
    A. Annihilation radiation
    B. Compton scattered photons
    C. Photoelectrons
    D. Bremsstrahlung

16. What is the effective atomic number of compact bone?

    _____

17. What term is used for the energy absorbed by the patient per unit mass?

    _____

18. To ensure the quality of the radiographic image and the patient's safety, both the radiologist and the radiographer should choose the highest-energy x-ray beam that permits adequate radiographic _____ for all radiography.

19. _____ scattering results in all-directional scatter.

20. To what does the term *fluorescent yield* refer?

    _____

4 Radiation Quantities and Units

Chapter 4 covers the evolution of radiation quantities and units. As the potentially harmful effects of ionizing radiation became known, the medical community sought to reduce these effects throughout the world by developing standards for measuring and limiting radiation exposure. To be able to control patient and personnel exposure in a consistent and uniform manner, diagnostic imaging personnel must become familiar with the radiation quantities and units covered in this chapter.

CHAPTER HIGHLIGHTS

- German physics professor Wilhelm Conrad Roentgen discovered "x-rays" on November 8, 1895, during an experiment investigating the nature of cathode rays and fluorescent materials.
- Many individuals who were exposed to substantial doses of x-rays in the early years after their discovery developed somatic damage from the exposure.
- *Skin erythema dose* was used from 1900 to 1930 as the unit for measuring radiation exposure. Eventually a tolerance dose was established for occupationally exposed individuals that could be regarded as a threshold dose. *Maximum permissible dose (MPD)* replaced *tolerance dose* in the early 1950s. In 1977 *dose equivalent* or *effective dose equivalent* replaced the MPD. In 1991 the International Commission on Radiological Protection (ICRP) replaced *effective dose equivalent* with the term *effective dose,* which is still in use today.
- Effective dose (EfD) is based on the energy deposited in biologic tissue by ionizing radiation. It takes into account both the type of radiation and the variable sensitivity of the tissues exposed to the radiation. EfD is expressed in the SI unit sievert (Sv) or in subunits of the sievert.
- In 1980 the International Commission on Radiation Units and Measurement (ICRU) adopted SI units for use with ionizing radiation. Many developed countries, particularly in Europe, have already made a complete transition to SI units. In the United States, this transition is not as yet fully complete and some conventional units are still in use.
- SI radiation units are preferred for specifying radiation quantities because the traditional system of units does not fit into the metric system that provides "one unified system of units for all physical quantities."
- Coulomb per kilogram (C/kg) is used for specifying x-ray or gamma ray exposure in air only. This exposure unit is equal to an electrical charge of 1 coulomb produced in a kilogram of dry air by ionizing radiation.

- Air kerma is an SI quantity that is used to express radiation concentration transferred to a point, which may be at the surface of a patient's or radiographer's body.
- Dose area product (DAP) is essentially the sum total of air kerma over the exposed area of the patient's surface.
- Absorbed dose (D) is the amount of energy per unit mass absorbed by an irradiated object.
- The gray (Gy) is used for measuring absorbed dose in air (Gy_a) or for measuring absorbed dose in tissue (Gy_t).
- The number of gray times 1000 equals the number of milligray. The number of grays times 100 equals the number of centigray.
- Linear energy transfer is the amount of energy transferred on average by incident radiation to an object per unit length of track, or passage, through the object and is expressed in units of kiloelectron volts per micrometer (keV/μm).
- Equivalent dose (EqD) and effective dose (EfD) are the quantities of choice for measuring biologic effects when all types of radiation must be considered.
- EqD specifies how the potential for biologic damage from different types and doses of radiation will be equivalent if correct weighting factors are included. To calculate equivalent dose: $EqD = D \times W_R$.
- EfD describes the total biologic damage to a human that is caused by equivalent doses received by specific organs. To calculate effective dose: $EfD = D \times W_R \times W_T$.
- In the SI system, sievert, or its subunits, millisievert and millisievert, is used to specify EqD and EfD. These units are used for occupational radiation exposure.
- Collective effective dose (ColEfD) represents an attempt to describe the radiation exposure of a population or group from low doses of different sources of ionizing radiation. Person-sievert is the radiation unit used to calculate this quantity. According to the ICRP it is not a valid method for computing the potential number of deaths from cancer.
- The radiation dosimetry quantity, total effective dose equivalent (TEDE), is designed to take into account all possible sources of radiation exposure and is used for dose monitoring for occupationally exposed personnel (e.g., nuclear medicine technologists and interventional radiologists) who are likely to receive possibly significant radiation exposure during the course of a year. The whole-body TEDE regulatory limit for exposed personnel is 0.05 Sv and for the general public is 0.001 Sv.
- The committed effective dose equivalent (CEDE) in radiation protection is a measure of the probabilistic health effect on an individual resulting from an intake of radioactive material into the body.

36

Exercise 1: Matching

Match the following terms with their definitions or associated phrases.

1. ___J___ Aplastic anemia
2. ___D___ Linear energy transfer (LET)
3. ___C___ SI
4. ___G___ Leukemia
5. ___E___ Air kerma
6. ___L___ Somatic damage
7. ___O___ Gy
8. ___B___ Dose area product (DAP)
9. ___Y___ One R (traditional unit)
10. ___M___ Person-sievert
11. ___S___ W_R
12. ___N___ Occupational exposure
13. ___H___ EfD
14. ___T___ Crookes tube
15. ___W___ Gamma radiation
16. ___A___ Skin erythema dose
17. ___K___ EqD
18. ___P___ TEDE
19. ___F___ Sv
20. ___X___ D
21. ___I___ Bragg-Gray theory
22. ___U___ Barium platinocyanide
23. ___Q___ Exposure
24. ___R___ Tissue kerma
25. ___V___ Entrance skin surface

A. Unit used from 1900 to 1930 to measure radiation exposure
B. A measure of the amount of radiant energy that has been thrust into a portion of the patient's body surface
C. Allows units to be used interchangeably among all branches of science throughout the world
D. The amount of energy transferred on average by incident radiation to an object per unit length of track, or passage, through the object
E. Kinetic energy released in a unit mass (kilogram) of air
F. SI unit of EqD
G. Blood disorder resulting in abnormal overproduction of white blood cells after exposure to ionizing radiation
H. The product of $D \times W_R \times W_T$
I. Relates the ionization produced in a small cavity within an irradiated medium or object to the energy absorbed in that medium as a result of its radiation exposure
J. Blood disorder resulting from bone marrow failure after exposure to ionizing radiation
K. Product of $D \times W_R$
L. Biologic damage to the body caused by exposure to ionizing radiation
M. SI unit for the radiation quantity ColEfD
N. Radiation exposure received by radiation workers in the course of exercising their professional responsibilities
O. SI unit used to express D
P. Radiation dosimetry quantity that was defined by the Nuclear Regulatory Commission (NRC) to monitor and control human exposure to ionizing radiation. It is a particularly useful dose monitor for occupationally exposed personnel such as nuclear medicine technologists and interventional radiologists, who are likely to receive possibly significant radiation exposure during the course of a year
Q. What occurs when ionizing radiation strikes an object such as the human body
R. The total kinetic energy released in a unit mass of tissue
S. A dimensionless factor (a multiplier) that was chosen for radiation protection purposes to account for differences in biologic impact among various types of ionizing radiation
T. A partially evacuated pear-shaped glass tube
U. Fluorescent material that coated the paper used when x-rays were discovered
V. The surface of the patient that is toward the x-ray tube. This is where the radiation dose to the patient is the highest
W. Short-wavelength, higher-energy electromagnetic waves emitted by the nuclei of radioactive substances
X. The amount of energy per unit mass absorbed by an irradiated object
Y. The photon (either x-ray or gamma ray) exposure that under standard conditions of pressure and temperature produces a total positive or negative ion charge of 2.58×10^{-4} C/kg of dry air

37

Exercise 2: Multiple Choice

Select the answer that *best* completes the following questions or statements.

1. Which of the following factors must be multiplied to determine the EfD from an x-radiation exposure of an organ or body part?
   A. $EqD \times W_R \times D$
   B. $W_T \times W_R \times ColEfD$
   C. $D \times W_R \times W_T$
   D. $D \times C/kg$

2. Which of the following is the SI unit of radiation exposure that is very useful for x-ray equipment calibration?
   A. C/kg
   B. DAP
   C. R
   D. Sv

3. German physics professor Wilhelm Conrad Roentgen discovered "x-rays" on November 8, 1895:
   A. While he was drilling for oil
   B. While he was mining for uranium
   C. During an experiment investigating how to travel through time
   D. During an experiment investigating the nature of cathode rays and fluorescent materials

4. In radiation protection systems no longer in use, a radiation dose to which occupationally exposed persons could be subjected *without* any apparent harmful acute effects, such as erythema of the skin, was known as a(n):
   A. Air kerma
   B. Effective dose
   C. Tolerance dose
   D. Weighted dose

5. Early tissue reactions of radiation include:
   1. Nausea and fatigue
   2. Blood and intestinal disorders
   3. Diffuse redness of the skin and shedding of its outer layer
   A. 1 and 2 only
   B. 1 and 3 only
   C. 2 and 3 only
   D. 1, 2, and 3

6. Which of the following terms describes the amount of energy per unit mass transferred from an x-ray beam to an object in its path such as the human body?
   A. SI
   B. Exposure
   C. Equivalent dose
   D. Absorbed dose

7. The sum total of air kerma over the exposed area of the patient's surface, or in other words, a measure of the amount of radiant energy that has been thrust into a portion of the patient's surface, is known as:
   A. Absorbed dose
   B. Exposure
   C. Dose area product
   D. Total effective dose equivalent

8. Fluoroscopic patient entrance radiation level is now specified in:
   A. keV/mm
   B. $mGy\text{-}cm^2$
   C. mGy_a/min
   D. Person-sievert

9. EfD describes which of the following?
   A. The total biologic damage to a human that is caused by equivalent doses received by specific organs
   B. The electrical charge produced in a kilogram of dry air by ionizing radiation
   C. The dose of ionizing radiation required to cause diffuse redness over an area of skin
   D. The number of electron-ion pairs in a specific volume of air

10. In radiation protection, which of the following is a measure of the probabilistic health effect on an individual resulting from an intake of radioactive material into the body?
    A. TEDE
    B. Gy_t
    C. Gy_a
    D. CEDE

11. Which of the following radiation quantities provides a measure of the overall risk of exposure to humans from ionizing radiation?
    A. D
    B. EfD
    C. EqD
    D. Exposure

12. Which of the following radiation quantities is used to describe exposure of a population or group from low doses of different sources of ionizing radiation?
    A. D
    B. EqD
    C. CEDE
    D. ColEfD

13. A W_R has been established for the following ionizing radiations: x-rays ($W_R = 1$); fast neutrons ($W_R = 20$); and alpha particles ($W_R = 20$). What is the *total* EqD (in sievert) for a person who has received the following exposures: x-rays = 4 Gy_t; fast neutrons = 6 Gy_t; and alpha particles = 3 Gy_t?
    A. 1.84
    B. 18.4
    C. 184
    D. 1840

14. A dimensionless factor, or multiplier, that places risks associated with biologic effects on a common scale is known as the:
    A. D
    B. Background time factor
    C. EqD
    D. W_R

15. Which of the following have similar numeric values?
    1. Quality factor (Q)
    2. W_R
    3. W_T
    A. 1 and 2 only
    B. 1 and 3 only
    C. 2 and 3 only
    D. 1, 2, and 3

16. If a patient undergoing x-ray therapy receives a total dose of 3000 rad, the dose may be recorded as _____ when the SI system is used.
    A. 6000 Gy
    B. 3000 centigray (cGy)
    C. 300 rad
    D. 30 R

17. Which of the following types of radiation has a W_R of 20?
    A. Alpha particles
    B. Gamma radiation
    C. Neutrons, energy, <10 keV
    D. X-radiation

18. Ten sievert equal _____ millisievert.
    A. 10
    B. 100
    C. 1000
    D. 10,000

19. Which of the following is (are) equivalent to 1 gray?
    1. 1 J/kg
    2. 100 cGy
    3. 1000 mGy
    A. 1 only
    B. 2 only
    C. 3 only
    D. 1, 2, and 3

20. Thomas A. Edison invented the:
    A. Cold cathode x-ray tube
    B. Hot cathode x-ray tube
    C. Fluoroscope
    D. Standard ionization chamber

21. In the United States, SI units such as the gray (Gy) and the centigray (cGy) are now used routinely in therapeutic radiology to specify:
    A. Exposure
    B. Effective dose
    C. Equivalent dose
    D. Absorbed dose

22. The ampere is the SI unit of:
    A. Electrical charge
    B. Electrical current
    C. Electrical resistance
    D. X-ray ionization in air

23. In the traditional system of quantities and units, 1 rad is equivalent to an energy transfer of:
    A. 500 erg per gram of irradiated object
    B. 300 erg per gram of irradiated object
    C. 200 erg per gram of irradiated object
    D. 100 erg per gram of irradiated object

24. X-rays, beta particles (high-speed electrons), and gamma rays have been given a numeric adjustment value of 1 because they produce:
    A. No biologic effect in body tissue for equal absorbed doses
    B. Varying degrees of biologic effect in body tissue for equal absorbed doses
    C. High-dose biologic effects in all body tissues for even the smallest dose
    D. Virtually the same biologic effect in body tissue for equal absorbed doses

25. The whole-body TEDE regulatory limit for exposed personnel is _____ and _____ for the general public.
    A. 0.05 sievert, 0.001 sievert
    B. 5 milligray 0.1 milligray
    C. 5 millisievert, 0.5 millisievert
    D. 5 sievert, 1 sievert

Exercise 3: True or False

Circle *T* if the statement is true; circle *F* if the statement is false.

1. T   F   Wilhelm Conrad Roentgen discovered x-rays on November 8, 1895, at the University of Wurzburg in Bavaria, Germany.

2. T   F   When x-rays were discovered, electricity was being passed through a partially evacuated pear-shaped glass tube. Light was seen emanating from a piece of paper coated with calcium tungstate that lay on a bench several feet away.

3. T   F   Cancer deaths among physicians attributed to x-ray exposure were reported as early as 1910.

4. T   F   The British X-ray and Radium Protection Committee was created in 1921 to investigate methods for reducing radiation exposure because the medical community was alarmed by the increasing number of radiation injuries reported.

5. T   F   By the 1950s EfD had replaced the tolerance dose for radiation protection purposes.

6. T   F   In 1991 tissue weighting factors were revised by the NCRP based on data from more recent epidemiologic studies of the Chernobyl survivors.

7. T   F   Fluoroscopic entrance exposure rates are now measured in milligray per minute (mGy_a/min).

8. T   F   The SI unit of absorbed dose, the gray, was named after the English radiobiologist Dorian Gray.

9. T   F   Air kerma actually denotes a calculation of radiation intensity in air.

10. T   F   CEDE is the SI unit used in the calculation of the radiation quantities EqD and EfD.

11. T   F   Air kerma is replacing the traditional quantity, absorbed dose.

12. T   F   In radiation therapy, the cGy is used for recording of the D.

13. T   F   Each type and energy of radiation has a specific W_R.

14. T   F   As the intensity of x-ray exposure of an air volume increases, the number of electron-ion pairs produced decreases.

15. T   F   Absorbed energy is responsible for any biologic damage resulting from exposure of the tissues to radiation.

16. T   F   Skin erythema dose was an accurate way to measure radiation exposure because the same amount of radiation was required to produce an erythema in every patient.

17. T   F   In 1991 the ICRP revised tissue weighting factors based on data from more recent epidemiologic studies of atomic bomb survivors.

18. T   F   EfD provides a measure of the overall risk of exposure to humans from ionizing radiation.

19. T   F   The lower the atomic number of a material, the more x-ray energy it absorbs.

20. T   F   Radiation weighting factors are selected by national and international scientific advisory bodies (NCRP, ICRP) and are based on quality factors and linear energy transfer.

21. T   F   The EqD for measuring biologic effects may be determined and expressed in the SI unit C/kg.

22. T   F   The concept of tolerance dose was originally developed to protect occupationally exposed persons from any apparent acute effects of radiation exposure, such as erythema of the skin.

23. T   F   Anatomic structures in the body possess the same absorption properties.

24. T   F   EfD can be expressed in Sv or mSv.

25. T   F   By the 1970s dosimetry and risk analysis had become quite sophisticated.

Exercise 4: Fill in the Blank

Using the following Word Bank, fill in the blanks with the word or words that best complete the statements.

0.001	energy	organs
0.05	exposure	organ systems
0.1	ionization chamber	pressure
0.2	ionization (charge)	risk (can be used two times)
μGy	ionized	roentgen
absorbed dose	Louis Harold Gray	safety
biologic effect	measure	temperature
cancerous	metric	Wilhelm Conrad Roentgen
coulomb	multiply	workable
Crookes tube	nonhazardous	

1. In late November 1895, _____ _____ _____ produced an x-ray image on a glass plate coated with a light-sensitive emulsion of silver salts, which clearly showed the bones of his wife's hand.

2. A substantial number of the skin lesions on the hands and fingers of early radiation workers such as radiologists and dentists eventually became _____ as a consequence of continued exposure to what was soon found to be ionizing radiation.

3. Modern radiographic and fluoroscopic units have incorporated an ability to determine the entire amount of _____ delivered to the patient by the x-ray beam.

4. In 1937 the traditional unit, roentgen, became internationally adopted as the unit of measurement for _____ to x-radiation and gamma radiation.

5. By the 1970s there was growing recognition that the consequences from radiation exposure to the health of a human as a whole depended on which _____ and _____ _____ had been irradiated.

6. _____ _____ is the amount of energy per unit mass absorbed by an irradiated object.

7. A _____ is the basic unit of electrical charge. It is equal to the amount of electrical charge moving past a point in a conductor in 1 second when an electrical current amounting to 1 ampere is used.

8. X-rays, beta particles (high-speed electrons), and gamma rays produce virtually the same _____ _____ in body tissue for equal absorbed doses.

9. Traditionally, the whole-body TEDE regulatory limit is _____ Sv for occupationally exposed and _____ Sv for the general public.

10. Each tissue weighting factor value denotes the percentage ratio of the summed stochastic (cancer plus genetic) _____ stemming from irradiation of a specific tissue or organ to the all-inclusive _____ when the entire body is irradiated in a uniform fashion.

11. In 1980 the ICRU adopted SI units, a unified system of _____ units, for use with ionizing radiation.

12. Trade and government desk work are considered _____ occupations.

13. Each radiation quantity has its own special unit of _____.

14. To change Sv to mSv, _____ the number of Sv by 1000.

15. In 1921 the British X-ray and Radium Protection Committee was created to investigate methods for reducing radiation exposure from all sources of radiation. The members of the committee were unable to fulfill their responsibility because they could not agree on a _____ unit of radiation exposure.

16. When a volume of air is irradiated with x-rays or gamma rays, the interaction that occurs between the radiation and the neutral atoms in the air causes some electrons to be liberated from those air atoms as they are _____.

17. In 1934 the U.S. Advisory Committee on X-Ray and Radium Protection recommended a tolerance dose equal to _____ roentgen per day. In 1936 the committee reduced this dose to _____ roentgen per day.

18. In 1937 the _____ became internationally adopted as the unit of measurement for exposure to x-radiation and gamma radiation.

19. Neither tolerance dose nor threshold dose is currently used for the purposes of radiation _____.

20. While performing an experiment in his laboratory, the person who discovered x-rays passed electricity through a _____ _____ that this individual had covered with a shield made of black cardboard.

21. _____ _____ _____ was instrumental in developing the most important theory in all of radiation dosimetry.

22. The instrument that can be used to calibrate air kerma is a standard, or free air, _____ _____.

23. The symbol used to indicate microgray is _____.

24. For precise measurement of radiation exposure in radiography, the total amount of _____ an x-ray beam produces in a known mass of air must be obtained.

25. A standard, or free air, ionization chamber contains a specific volume of air at standard atmospheric _____ and _____.

Exercise 5: Labeling

Label the following illustration and tables.

A. Standard, or free air, ionization chamber.

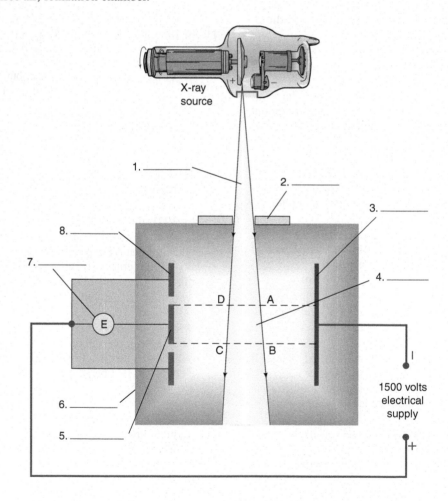

B. Radiation weighting factors for different types and energies of ionizing radiation.

Radiation Type and Energy Range	Radiation Weighting Factor (WR)
X-ray and gamma ray photons, and electrons (every energy)	1. _____
Neutrons, energy <10 keV	2. _____
10 keV-100 keV	3. _____
> 100 keV-2 MeV	4. _____
> 2 MeV-20 MeV	5. _____
> 20 MeV	6. _____
Protons	7. _____
Alpha particles	8. _____

Data adapted from International Commission on Radiological Protection (ICRP): *Recommendations,* ICRP Publication No. 60, New York, 1991, Pergamon Press.

C. Summary of radiation quantities and units.

Type of Radiation	Quantity	SI Unit	Measuring Medium	Radiation Effect Measured
X-radiation or gamma	Exposure	1. C/kg	Air	Ionization of air radiation
All ionizing radiations	2. Absorbed dose	Gray (Gy)	Any object	Amount of energy per unit mass absorbed by object
All ionizing radiations	Equivalent dose (EqD)	3. Sv	Body tissue	Biologic effects
All ionizing radiations	4. EfD	Sievert (Sv)	Body tissue	Biologic effects

Exercise 6: Short Answer

Answer the following questions by providing a short answer.

1. Why did Thomas A. Edison discontinue his x-ray research?

   _____

   _____

2. What unit was used for measuring radiation exposure from 1900 to 1930?

   _____

   _____

3. What is the difference between early tissue reactions and late tissue reactions of ionizing radiation?

   _____

   _____

4. What is a tolerance dose?

   _____

   _____

5. What unit replaced the tolerance dose for radiation protection purposes in the 1950s?

_____

_____

6. In the late 1970s, dose limits were calculated and established to ensure what?

_____

_____

7. What is the Bragg-Gray theory, and what significance does it have?

_____

_____

8. When the human body is exposed to ionizing radiation, for what is absorbed energy responsible?

_____

_____

9. For a precise measurement of radiation exposure in radiography, what must be obtained?

_____

_____

10. Who is responsible for selecting radiation weighting factors, and on what are these factors based?

_____

_____

11. If D is stated in the traditional unit rad, how is the SI equivalent in Gy determined?

_____

_____

12. Consider a patient whose irradiated surface receives an air kerma dose of 0.04 Gy. If the area of the irradiated surface is 100 cm^2, what will the dose area product (DAP) be?

_____

_____

13. What SI unit and traditional unit of measure are used for x-ray equipment calibration? Why can these units be used?

_____

_____

14. If radiation exposure is given in R, how can that value be converted to C/kg?

_____

_____

15. What is the difference between equivalent dose and effective dose?

_____

_____

44

Exercise 7: General Discussion or Opinion Questions

The following questions are intended to allow students to express their knowledge and understanding of the subject matter or to present a personal opinion. The questions may be used to stimulate class discussion. Because answers to these questions may vary, determination of an answer's acceptability is left to the discretion of the course instructor.

1. How were x-rays discovered?

2. How did occupational radiation exposure affect the pioneers of the radiation industry?

3. What problems did medical professionals encounter as they investigated methods for reducing radiation exposure in the early 1900s?

4. What changes in radiation protection criteria led to the use of EfD and EqD for radiation protection purposes?

5. Explain the equivalence of damage caused by radiation from different sources of ionizing radiation.

6. Explain the significance and use of a W_R.

7. Explain the significance and use of a W_T.

8. Summarize the radiation quantities and units currently in use.

9. Discuss the concept of LET and its significance.

10. Discuss the use and benefit of SI units in the field of radiology.

Exercise 8: Calculation Problems

To help the learner understand conversion between the SI system of units and the traditional system, both systems of units are used in Exercise 8. Information for conversions within the SI system is found within Chapter 4 of the textbook. Information for conversions with the traditional system may be found within Appendix A also in the textbook.

Using the information presented here, set up and solve the following problems.

A. The SI unit of the radiation quantity D is the Gy; the traditional unit is the rad. Gy and rad units are easily converted to allow comparison of D values. If D is stated in rad, the equivalent in Gy can be determined by dividing the rad value by 100. If D is stated in Gy, rad can be determined by multiplying the Gy value by 100. Examples of conversion from rad to Gy may be found in Appendix A in the textbook.

1. Convert 8000 rad to Gy.

$$8000 \div 100 = 80 \text{ Gy}$$

2. Convert 8 rad to Gy.

$$8 \div 100 = .08 \, Gy$$

3. Convert 450 rad to Gy.

$$450 \div 100 = 4.5 \, Gy$$

4. Convert 4.5 rad to Gy.

$$.045 \, Gy$$

5. Convert 375 rad to Gy.

$$3.75 \, Gy$$

6. Convert 7 Gy to rad.

$$700 \, rad$$

Chapter 4 Radiation Quantities and Units

7. Convert 25 Gy to rad.

2500 rad

8. Convert 0.4 Gy to rad.

40 rad

9. Convert 0.087 Gy to rad.

8.7 rad

10. Convert 0.96 Gy to rad.

96 rad

B. EqD is used for radiation protection purposes when a person receives exposure from various types of ionizing radiation. The EqD for measuring biologic effects can be determined and expressed in Sv (SI units) or rem (traditional units). The EqD is obtained by multiplying D by W_R. Examples of conversion of rem to Sv may be found in Appendix A of the textbook.

1. A W_R has been established for each of the following ionizing radiations: x-radiation ($W_R = 1$); fast neutrons ($W_R = 20$); and alpha particles ($W_R = 20$). What is the total EqD in Sv for a person who has received the following exposures: x-radiation = 0.6 Gy; fast neutrons = 0.25 Gy; and alpha particles = 0.4 Gy?

.6 Sv
5 Sv   = 13.6 Sv
8 Sv

2. A W_R has been established for each of the following ionizing radiations: x-radiation ($W_R = 1$); fast neutrons ($W_R = 20$); gamma rays ($W_R = 1$); protons ($W_R = 2$); and alpha particles ($W_R = 20$). What is the total EqD in Sv for a person who has received the following exposures: x-radiation = 0.3 Gy; fast neutrons = 0.28 Gy; gamma rays = 0.8 Gy; protons = 0.9 Gy; and alpha particles = 0.4 Gy?

.3 Sv   8 Sv
5.6 Sv   = 16.5 Sv
.8 Sv
1.8 Sv

3. A W_R has been established for each of the following ionizing radiations: x-radiation ($W_R = 1$); fast neutrons ($W_R = 20$); and alpha particles ($W_R = 20$). What is the total EqD in rem for a person who has received the following exposures: x-radiation = 7 rad; fast neutrons = 2 rad; and alpha particles = 5 rad?

7 rem
40 rem   = 147 rem
100 rem

4. A W_R has been established for each of the following ionizing radiations: x-radiation ($W_R = 1$); fast neutrons ($W_R = 20$); gamma rays ($W_R = 1$); protons ($W_R = 2$); and alpha particles ($W_R = 20$). What is the total EqD in rem for a person who has received the following exposures: x-radiation = 3 rad; fast neutrons = 0.35 rad; gamma rays = 6 rad; protons = 2.5 rad; and alpha particles = 8 rad?

3 rem   5 rem
7 rem   100 rem   = 181 rem
6 rem

5. A W_R has been established for each of the following ionizing radiations: x-radiation ($W_R = 1$); fast neutrons, energy = 10 keV ($W_R = 5$); gamma rays ($W_R = 1$); protons ($W_R = 2$); and alpha particles ($W_R = 20$). What is the total EqD in Sv for a person who has received the following exposures: x-radiation = 0.6 Gy; fast neutrons, energy = 10 keV = 0.2 Gy; gamma rays = 4 Gy; protons = 0.8 Gy; and alpha particles = 6 Gy?

.6 Sv   1.6 Sv
1 Sv   120 Sv   = 127.2 Sv
4 Sv

C. The EfD is a quantity used for radiation protection purposes to provide a measure of the overall risk of exposure to ionizing radiation. It incorporates both the effect of the type of radiation used (e.g., x-radiation, gamma, neutron) and the variability in radiosensitivity of the organ or body part irradiated through the use of appropriate weighting factors. These factors determine the overall harm to these biologic components for risk of developing a radiation-induced cancer or, in the case of the reproductive organs, genetic damage. The formula for determining the EfD is as follows: $EfD = D \times W_R \times W_T$. The EfD may be expressed in Sv (SI units) or rem (traditional units). Examples of conversion to rem may be found in Appendix A of the textbook.

1. The W_R for alpha particles is 20, and the W_T for the breast is 0.05. If the breast receives a D of 0.5 Gy from exposure to alpha particles, what is the EfD in Sv?

$$0.5 \times 20 \times .05 = .5 \, Sv$$

2. The W_R for x-radiation is 1, and the W_T for the gonads is 0.2. If the gonads receive a D of 0.4 Gy from exposure to x-radiation, what is the EfD in Sv?

$$.4 \times 1 \times .2 = .08 \, Sv$$

3. The W_R for fast neutrons is 20, and the W_T for the stomach is 0.12. If the stomach receives a D of 6 rad from exposure to fast neutrons, what is the EfD in rem?

$$6 \times 20 \times .12 = 14.4 \, rem$$

4. The W_R for gamma rays is 1, and the W_T for the esophagus is 0.05. If the esophagus receives a D of 25 rad from exposure to gamma rays, what is the EfD in rem?

$$25 \times 1 \times .05 = 1.25 \text{ rem}$$

5. The W_R for x-radiation is 1, and the W_T for red bone marrow is 0.12. If the red bone marrow receives a D of 0.9 Gy from exposure to x-radiation, what is the EfD in Sv?

$$0.9 \times 1 \times .12$$
$$.108 \text{ Sv}$$

D. In addition to EqD and EfD, another dosimetric quantity, the collective effective dose (ColEfD), has been derived and implemented for use in radiation protection to describe internal and external dose measurements. The ColEfD is used to describe radiation exposure of a population or group from low doses of different sources of ionizing radiation. It is determined as the product of the average EfD for an individual belonging to the exposed population or group and the number of persons exposed. Therefore the ColEfD is found by multiplying the average EfD for an individual belonging to the exposed population or group by the number of individuals exposed. The radiation unit for the quantity ColEfD is the person-sievert and is obtained by multiplying the number of persons exposed by the effective dose received.

1. If 400 people receive an average EfD of 0.2 Sv, what is the ColEfD in person-sievert?

80 person sievert

2. If 300 people receive an average EfD of 0.17 Sv, what is the ColEfD in person-sievert?

51 person sievert

3. If 250 people receive an average EfD of 0.24 Sv, what is the ColEfD in person-sievert?

60 person sievert

4. If 1000 people receive an average EfD of 0.10 Sv, what is the ColEfD in person-sievert?

100 person sievert

5. If 100 people receive an average EfD of 0.30 Sv, what is the ColEfD in person-sievert?

30 person sievert

E. Conversion to subunits may also be necessary. In the SI system, to convert Gy to mGy, multiply the number of Gy times 1000 to determine the number of mGy. To convert the number of Sv to mSv, multiply the number of Sv times 1000 to determine the number of mSv.

1. Convert 0.020 Gy to mGy.

20 mGy

2. Convert 0.200 Gy to mGy.

200 mGy

3. Convert 0.030 Sv to mSv.

30 mSv

4. Convert 0.300 Sv to mSv.

300 mSv

POST-TEST

The student should take this test after reading Chapter 4, finishing all accompanying textbook and workbook exercises, and completing any additional activities required by the course instructor. The student should complete the post-test with a score of 90% or higher before advancing to the next chapter. (Each of the following 20 questions are worth 5 points.)
Score = _____ %

1. If 400 people receive an average EfD of 0.2 Sv, what is the ColEfD in person-sievert?

_____

2. Which radiation quantity can be used to compare the average amount of radiation received by the entire body from a specific radiologic examination with the amount received from natural background radiation?

_____

3. What concept helps explain the need for a radiation quality, or modifying, factor?

_____

4. What two SI units can be used for equipment calibration?

_____

_____

5. _____ is a blood disorder resulting in abnormal overproduction of white blood cells after exposure to ionizing radiation.

6. Who is credited with discovering x-rays on November 8, 1895?

_____

7. A W_R has been established for each of the following ionizing radiations: x-radiation ($W_R = 1$); fast neutrons ($W_R = 20$); and alpha particles ($W_R = 20$). What is the total EqD in Sv for a person who has received the following exposures: x-radiation = 5 Gy; fast neutrons = 0.3 Gy; and alpha particles = 0.7 Gy?

_____

_____

8. The W_R for x-radiation is 1, and the W_T for the lungs is 0.12. If the lungs receive a D of 5 Gy from exposure to x-radiation, what is the EfD in Sv?

_____

_____

9. Convert 0.8 Sv to mSv.

_____

10. How is the EqD calculated?

_____

11. The amount of energy per unit mass absorbed by the irradiated object is the definition of:
   A. D
   B. EfD
   C. EqD
   D. X

12. The effective atomic number of bone is:
   A. 7.4
   B. 7.6
   C. 13.8
   D. 20

13. _____ _____ was used as the first measure of exposure for ionizing radiation.

14. What is the basic unit of electrical charge?

_____

15. Which of the following are early tissue reactions of ionizing radiation?
      1. Diffuse redness of the skin
      2. Blood and intestinal disorders
      3. Nausea and vomiting
   A. 1 and 2 only
   B. 1 and 3 only
   C. 2 and 3 only
   D. 1, 2, and 3

16. What radiation dosimetry quantity is used for dose monitoring for occupationally exposed personnel, such as nuclear medicine technologists and interventional radiologists, who are likely to receive possibly significant radiation exposure during the course of a year?

_____

17. In radiation therapy, what SI subunit is used for the recording of D?

_____

18. Many of the skin lesions on the hands and fingers of early radiologists and dentists eventually became _____ as a consequence of continued exposure to ionizing radiation.

19. Define the term *occupational exposure*.

_____

_____

20. On what is EfD based?

_____

_____

References

1. National Council on Radiation Protection and Measurements (NCRP): *Limitation of exposure to ionizing radiation,* Report No. 116, Bethesda, Md, 1993, NCRP.

5 Radiation Monitoring

To ensure that occupational radiation exposure levels are kept well below the annual effective dose (EfD) limit, some means of monitoring personnel exposure must be employed. The radiographer and other occupationally exposed persons should be aware of the various radiation exposure monitoring devices and their functions. Chapter 5 provides an overview of both personnel and area monitoring. In addition, because radiation dosimetry reports still report radiation exposure for workers in traditional units and subunits, the traditional units' numerical values are identified in parentheses after SI units' numerical values.

CHAPTER HIGHLIGHTS

- Personnel monitoring ensures that occupational radiation exposure levels are kept well below the annual effective dose (EfD) limit.
  - Personnel monitoring is required whenever radiation workers are likely to risk receiving 10% or more of the annual occupational EfD limit of 50 mSv (5 rem) in any 1 year as a consequence of their work-related activities.
  - To keep radiation exposure ALARA, most health care facilities issue dosimeter devices when personnel could receive approximately 1% of the annual occupational EfD limit in any month, or approximately 0.5 mSv (50 mrem).
  - The working habits and conditions of diagnostic imaging personnel can be assessed over a designated period through the use of the personnel dosimeter.
  - Even when a protective apron is not normally required, a radiation worker should still wear a personnel monitoring device attached to the clothing on the front of the body at collar level during routine radiographic procedures to detect any potential radiation dose to the thyroid and the head and neck.
  - During high-level radiation procedures, imaging professionals are required to wear both a thyroid shield and a protective lead apron, with the dosimeter worn outside the front of the garment at collar level, so as to provide a reading of the approximate equivalent dose to the thyroid gland and eyes.
  - Commercially available lead aprons typically have either 0.5-mm or 0.25-mm lead equivalent shielding.
  - Pregnant radiation workers may wear a second dosimeter beneath a lead apron to monitor the abdomen during gestation to provide an estimate of the equivalent dose to the embryo-fetus. Many facilities provide pregnant radiographers with a second dosimeter for this purpose.
  - An extremity dosimeter, which is commonly a TLD ring, may be used as a second monitor when performing fluoroscopic procedures that require the hands to be near the primary x-ray beam.
  - In general, personnel dosimeters must be lightweight, portable, durable, and cost efficient.
  - Four types of personnel monitoring devices exist: OSL dosimeters, TLDs (both extremity and for the full body), pocket ionization chambers, and personnel digital ionization dosimeters.
  - Results from personnel monitoring programs must be recorded accurately and maintained for review to meet state and federal regulations. A record of radiation exposure is required by regulatory agencies to be part of the employment record of all radiation workers.
  - Personnel monitoring reports list the deep, eye, and shallow occupational exposure of each covered person on a monthly, quarterly, year-to-date, and lifetime equivalent basis.
  - Whenever the letter *M* appears under the current monitoring period or in the cumulative columns on a radiation monitoring report, it signifies that an equivalent dose below the minimum measurably radiation quantity was recorded during that time.
  - In health care facilities that have a well-structured radiation safety program, personnel monitoring reports are received and reviewed by the radiation safety officer (RSO).
- Area monitoring can be accomplished through the use of radiation survey instruments that fall into several categories.
- When in contact with ionizing radiation, survey instruments respond because of the charged particles that are produced by the radiation interacting with and subsequently ionizing the gas (usually air) in the detector. These instruments measure either the total quantity of electrical charge resulting from the ionization of the gas or the rate at which the electrical charge is produced.
- Three different types of gas-filled radiation detectors serve as field instruments. They include the ionization chamber–type survey meter ("cutie pie"), the proportional counter, and the Geiger-Müller (GM) survey meter.
- Radiation survey instruments for area monitoring must be durable and easy to carry, be able to detect all

55

common types of ionizing radiation, and not be substantially affected by the energy of the radiation or the direction of the incident radiation.

- Ionization chambers can be used to measure the radiation output from both radiographic and fluoroscopic x-ray equipment.

- Medical physicists use ionization chambers connected to electrometers to perform the annual standard measurements required by state, federal, and health care accreditation organizations for radiographic and fluoroscopic devices.

Exercise 1: Matching

Match the following terms with their definitions or associated phrases.

1. _____ Personnel dosimeter

2. _____ Personnel monitoring report

3. _____ Radiation survey instruments

4. _____ OSL

5. _____ Second personnel monitoring device

6. _____ Geiger-Müller meter

7. _____ Control monitor

8. _____ Proportional counter

9. _____ Personnel digital ionization dosimeter

10. _____ Ionization chamber connected to an electrometer

11. _____ Glow curve

12. _____ Check source

13. _____ Doppler shift

14. _____ Extremity dosimeter

15. _____ Exposure monitoring of personnel

16. _____ Radiation safety officer (RSO)

17. _____ Pocket ionization chamber (pocket dosimeter)

18. _____ TLD analyzer

A. A fairly new device that provides radiation workers with an immediate measurement of radiation exposure while including features such as long-term exposure tracking

B. Serves as a basis for comparison with the remaining OSL badges after they have been returned to the monitoring company for processing

C. Device used for personnel monitoring of occupational exposure that contains an Al_2O_3 detector

D. Resembles an ordinary fountain pen but it contains a slender cylindrical (thimble) ionization chamber that measures radiation exposure

E. Cutie pie

F. Contains LiF powder or small chips, which function as a sensing material

G. Measures the amount of ionizing radiation to which a TLD badge has been exposed

H. Worn by a pregnant radiographer to monitor the equivalent dose to the embryo-fetus

I. Used by medical physicists to perform annual standard measurements required by state, federal, and health care accreditation organizations for radiographic and fluoroscopic devices

J. A geometric arrangement of the points in space at which the atoms, molecules, or ions of a crystal occur

K. Provides an indication of the working habits and working conditions of diagnostic imaging personnel

L. Specific gas-filled radiation detectors that detect the presence of radiation and, when properly calibrated, give a reasonably accurate measurement of the exposure and/or exposure rate

M. Lists the deep, eye, and shallow occupational exposures of each covered person on a monthly, year-to-date, and lifetime equivalent basis

N. Device with an audible sound system that alerts the operator to the presence of ionizing radiation

O. Generally used in a laboratory setting to detect alpha and beta radiation and small amounts of other types of low-level radioactive contamination

P. TLD ring that may be used by an imaging professional as a second monitor while performing fluoroscopic procedures that require the hands to be near the primary x-ray beam

Q. Individual who receives and reviews personnel monitoring reports in a health care facility

R. Apparent change in frequency of a light wave as an observer and light source move toward or away from each other

19. _____ Ionization chamber–type survey meter
20. _____ TLD

21. _____ Crystalline lattice structure

22. _____ Lithium fluoride (LiF)

23. _____ ALARA concept

24. _____ Fluoroscopy, surgery, and special procedures

25. _____ Thyroid shield and a protective lead apron

S. Sensing material found in TLDs
T. During high-level radiation procedures, imaging professionals are required to wear both of these items
U. Required whenever radiation workers are likely to risk receiving 10% or more of the annual EfD limit of 50 mSv (5 rem) in any single year as a consequence of their work-related activities
V. Areas of diagnostic radiology that produce the highest occupational radiation exposure for diagnostic imaging personnel
W. A weak, long-lived radioisotope located on one side of the external surface of a GM meter to verify its consistency daily
X. Keeping radiation exposure to personnel as low as reasonably achievable
Y. A graphic plot that demonstrates the relationship of light output, or emitted thermoluminescence intensity, to temperature variation

Exercise 2: Multiple Choice

Select the answer that *best* completes the following questions or statements.

1. In keeping with the ALARA concept, *most* health care facilities issue dosimetry devices when personnel could receive approximately _____ of the annual occupational EfD limit (50 mSv [5000 mrem]) in any month, or approximately 0.5 mSv (50 mrem).
   A. 25%
   B. 10%
   C. 5%
   D. 1%

2. What different filters are incorporated into the detector packet of the OSL dosimeter?
   1. Aluminum
   2. Tin
   3. Copper
   A. 1 and 2 only
   B. 1 and 3 only
   C. 2 and 3 only
   D. 1, 2, and 3

3. Diagnostic imaging personnel should wear a personnel dosimeter during routine operations in an imaging facility because the device provides:
   1. An indication of an individual's working habits
   2. An indication of working conditions in the facility
   3. A way for the employer to determine whether radiation workers are actively engaged in performing a specific number of x-ray procedures during a given period
   A. 1 and 2 only
   B. 1 and 3 only
   C. 2 and 3 only
   D. 1, 2, and 3

4. An OSL control monitor indicates:
   A. The sensitivity of the radiographic film in the dosimeter
   B. The presence of impurities in the lithium fluoride crystals
   C. Whether group dosimeters were exposed in transit
   D. Whether filters in group dosimeters are working correctly

5. Historically, which of the following personnel dosimeters allowed radiation workers to determine occupational exposure received as soon as a specific radiation procedure was completed?
   A. Film badge dosimeter
   B. OSL dosimeter
   C. Pocket ionization chamber (pocket dosimeter)
   D. TLD

6. Which of the following instruments should be used in a laboratory setting to detect alpha and beta radiation and small amounts of other types of low-level radioactive contamination?
   A. Ionization chamber–type survey meter
   B. Proportional counter
   C. GM detector
   D. Pocket ionization chamber

7. Which of the following devices is used to measure the amount of ionizing radiation to which a TLD badge has been exposed by first heating the crystals to free the trapped, highly energized electrons and then recording the amount of light emitted by the crystals (which is proportional to the TLD badge exposure)?
   A. Small ionization chamber
   B. Laser
   C. TLD analyzer
   D. Sensitometer

8. In a health care facility, a radiographer's deep, eye, and shallow occupational exposures, as measured by an exposure monitor, may be found on the:
   A. Compliance report
   B. Quality assurance report
   C. Personnel monitoring report
   D. Worker's yearly evaluation

9. When the negatively and positively charged electrodes in the pocket ionization chamber are exposed to ionizing radiation, the mechanism does which of the following?
   A. It charges in direct proportion to the amount of radiation to which it has been exposed.
   B. It discharges in direct proportion to the amount of radiation to which it has been exposed.
   C. It heats the central electrode.
   D. It heats the quartz fiber indicator.

10. Which of the following personnel monitoring devices resembles a flash drive in appearance?
    A. Personnel digital ionization dosimeter
    B. Optically stimulated luminescence dosimeter
    C. Thermoluminescent dosimeter
    D. Pocket ionization chamber (pocket dosimeter)

11. Radiation survey instruments measure which of the following?
    1. The total quantity of electrical charge resulting from ionization of the gas
    2. The rate at which an electrical charge is produced
    3. Luminescence
    A. 1 and 2 only
    B. 1 and 3 only
    C. 2 and 3 only
    D. 1, 2, and 3

12. What do ionization chamber–type survey meters, proportional counters, and GM meters have in common?
    A. They measure x-radiation and beta radiation only.
    B. They all can be used to calibrate radiographic and fluoroscopic x-ray equipment.
    C. They are all used to measure the only the radiation dose received outside of protective barriers.
    D. Each contains a gas-filled chamber.

13. Which of the following radiation monitors is currently the *most commonly* used dosimeter for monitoring occupational exposure in diagnostic imaging?
    A. Personnel digital ionization dosimeter
    B. Pocket ionization chamber
    C. TLD
    D. OSL

14. Which of the following are disadvantages of using a TLD as a personnel monitoring device?
    1. It can be read only once because the readout process destroys the stored information.
    2. It is necessary to use calibrated dosimeters with TLDs.
    3. The initial cost is higher than that for an OSL dosimeter service.
    4. Lithium fluoride is used as the sensing material in the TLD.
    A. 1 and 2 only
    B. 1 and 3 only
    C. 1 and 4 only
    D. 1, 2, and 3 only

15. Before a pocket ionization chamber (pocket dosimeter) is used to record radiation exposure, the quartz fiber indicator of the transparent reading scale should indicate which of the following?
    A. Zero (0)
    B. 100 mR
    C. 150 mR
    D. 200 mR

16. The OSL dosimeter uses:
    A. An Al_2O_3 detector
    B. LiF as a sensing material
    C. A miniature ionization chamber as a detector
    D. Radiation dosimetry film as a detector

17. A pocket ionization chamber resembles:
    A. A banana
    B. A flash drive
    C. An ordinary fountain pen
    D. A miniature cell phone

18. Monitoring companies send a control monitor to health care facilities along with each batch of dosimeters. The control monitor should be:
    A. Given as a monitor to a radiographer who has lost his or her original dosimeter
    B. Given as a second monitor to a pregnant radiographer
    C. Given as a second monitor to a nonpregnant radiographer working in the operating room
    D. Kept in a radiation-free area within the imaging facility

19. Dosimeter readings that exceed a trigger level set by the health care facility are investigated to:
    A. Ascertain the cause of the reading
    B. Determine whether wearing the dosimeter was actually necessary
    C. Find grounds to fire the radiographer
    D. Increase the workload of the RSO to justify his or her position

20. The TLD readout process:
    A. Destroys the information stored in the TLD
    B. Saves the information stored in the TLD for future use
    C. Transfers the information from the TLD to a computer, which reads the dosimeter
    D. Duplicates the stored information and sends a written report directly to the radiographer

21. An ionization chamber–type survey meter is also referred to as a:
    A. Cutie pie
    B. Flux capacitor
    C. Little rascal
    D. Warp drive

22. The increased sensitivity of the OSL dosimeter makes it ideal for monitoring employees working in low-radiation environments and for:
    A. Area monitoring of radioisotope storage facilities
    B. Monitoring of patients with a radioactive implant
    C. Monitoring of pregnant workers
    D. General patient and public monitoring

23. The RSO in a health care facility receives and reviews personnel monitoring reports to:
    A. Assess compliance with ALARA guidelines
    B. Assess compliance with National Academy of Sciences guidelines
    C. Gather information to compile a press report
    D. Meet guidelines established by the Health Insurance Portability and Accountability Act (HIPAA)

24. Wearing a personnel dosimeter in a consistent location is the responsibility of the:
    A. RSO
    B. Manager or director of the imaging department
    C. Chief radiologist
    D. Individual wearing the device

25. On termination of employment, a radiographer must receive a copy of:
    A. All personal health care records kept by the employer
    B. His or her occupational exposure report
    C. All employment records
    D. Incident reports in which the radiographer was involved

Exercise 3: True or False

Circle *T* if the statement is true; circle *F* if the statement is false.

1. T F Personnel dosimeters protect the wearer from exposure to ionizing radiation.

2. T F Wearing a personnel dosimeter in a consistent location is the responsibility of the individual wearing the device.

3. T F During lengthy interventional fluoroscopic procedures (e.g., cardiac catheterization), some health care facilities may prefer to have diagnostic imaging personnel wear two separate monitoring devices.

4. T F Cost is not a factor for health care facilities in selecting personnel dosimeters.

5. T F The personnel digital ionization dosimeter does not provide an instant readout of dose information when connected to a computer via a connector such as a USB.

6. T F An ionization chamber–type survey meter cannot be used to measure exposures produced by typical diagnostic procedures because the exposure times are too long to permit the meter to respond appropriately.

7. T F A disadvantage of the OSL dosimeter is that occupational exposure cannot be established on the day of occurrence because the dosimeter must be shipped to the monitoring company for reading and exposure determination unless the facility has an in-house reader.

8. T F Pocket ionization chambers are not commonly used in diagnostic imaging.

9. T F All radiation survey meters are equally sensitive in the detection of ionizing radiation.

10. T   F   The ionization chamber–type meter is used for radiation protection surveys.

11. T   F   A pocket dosimeter may be worn for up to 1 year.

12. T   F   In health care facilities that have a well-structured radiation safety program, personnel monitoring reports are received and reviewed by the RSO.

13. T   F   A personnel dosimeter must be able to detect and record both small and large exposures in a consistent and reliable manner.

14. T   F   The filters in an OSL dosimeter are made of lead, potassium iodide, and zinc.

15. T   F   Ionizing radiation causes some of the physical properties of the LiF crystals in the TLD to undergo changes.

16. T   F   When changing employment, the radiation worker must convey the data pertinent to his or her accumulated permanent equivalent dose to the new employer so that this information can be placed on file.

17. T   F   Although an OSL dosimeter can work for up to 10 years, it is commonly worn for 2 years.

18. T   F   Pocket dosimeters provide no permanent legal record of exposure.

19. T   F   Calibration is "the adjustment of a radiation survey instrument to accurately read the radiation level from a reference source."

20. T   F   A TLD can be read numerous times.

21. T   F   Humidity, pressure, and normal temperature changes do not affect TLDs.

22. T   F   The GM detector is likely to saturate or jam when placed in a pulsed very high intensity radiation area, thereby giving a false reading.

23. T   F   Health care facilities must maintain a record of exposure recorded by personnel dosimeters as part of each radiation worker's employment record.

24. T   F   Area monitoring can be accomplished through the use of radiation survey instruments.

25. T   F   In an OSL dosimeter each filter blocks a portion of the radiation-sensitive aluminum oxide and causes a different degree of attenuation for any radiation striking the dosimeter, depending on its energy.

Exercise 4: Fill in the Blank

Using the following Word Bank, fill in the blanks with the word or words that best complete the statements.

5	ionization	radiation output
40	laser light	reused
charged	lightweight	second
control	lost	sensitive
cost-effective	medical physicists	shallow
deep	occupational	thermoluminescent
electrometers	optically stimulated	thyroid
employment	periodically	trigger
equivalent	physical	usage
eyes	placement	worn
gestation	plastic	zero
inexpensive	radiation-free	

1. When a protective apron is worn and the personnel dosimeter is located at collar level, it provides a reading of approximate equivalent dose to the _____ gland and _____ of the occupationally exposed person.

2. Radiation survey instruments for area monitoring should be calibrated _____ to meet state and federal requirements.

3. Personnel dosimeters include _____ _____ luminescence dosimeters, pocket_____ chambers, _____ dosimeters, and personnel digital ionization dosimeters.

4. Because many employees in a health care facility may be required to wear radiation monitors, they should be reasonably _____ to purchase and maintain.

5. An OSL dosimeter is _____, durable, and easy to carry.

6. The control monitor should be kept in a _____ area in an imaging facility.

7. When changing employment, the radiation worker must convey those data pertinent to accumulated permanent _____ dose to the new employer.

8. Dosimeter readings that exceed a _____ level set by the health care facility are investigated to ascertain the cause of the reading.

9. Before use each pocket dosimeter must be _____ to a predetermined voltage so that the quartz fiber indicator shows a _____ reading.

10. _____ _____ use ionization chambers connected to _____ to perform the annual standard measurements required by state, federal, and health care accreditation organizations for radiographic and fluoroscopic devices.

11. Radiation survey instruments are not all equally _____ in detecting ionizing radiation.

12. Because the GM meter allows for rapid monitoring, it can be used to locate a _____ radioactive source or low-level radioactive contamination.

13. Ionization chambers can be used to measure the _____ _____ from both radiographic and fluoroscopic equipment.

14. Personnel monitoring ensures that _____ radiation exposure levels are kept well below the annual EfD limit.

15. The OSL dosimeter is "read out" by using _____ _____ at selected frequencies.

16. Pregnant diagnostic imaging personnel should be issued a _____ monitoring device to record the radiation dose to the abdomen during _____.

17. Monitoring reports list the _____, eye, and _____ occupational exposure of each person wearing the device in the facility as measured by the exposed monitor.

18. After a reading has been obtained, TLD crystals can be _____, thus making the device somewhat _____.

19. _____ monitors indicate whether group dosimeters were exposed in transit to or from a health care facility.

20. The front of the white paper packet of the OSL dosimeter may be color coded to facilitate correct _____ and _____ of the dosimeter on the body of occupationally exposed personnel.

21. A record of radiation exposure should be part of the _____ record of all radiation workers.

22. A TLD is not effective as a monitoring device if it is not _____.

23. Ionizing radiation causes the LiF crystals in the TLD to undergo changes in some of their _____ properties.

24. The OSL dosimeter provides an accurate reading as low as 10 μSv (1 mrem) for x-rays and gamma ray photons with energies ranging from _____ keV to greater than _____ MeV.

25. All components of an OSL dosimeter are sealed inside a tamperproof _____ blister packet.

Exercise 5: Labeling

Label the following illustration.

A. Pocket ionization chamber (pocket dosimeter).

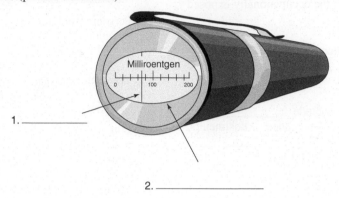

1. _____

2. _____

Exercise 6: Short Answer

Answer the following questions by providing a short answer.

1. How do personnel dosimeters determine occupational exposure?

   _____

   _____

2. If an OSL dosimeter is used as a radiation monitor, why can occupational exposure not be determined on the day of occurrence unless the facility has an in-house reader?

   _____

   _____

3. What does an extremity dosimeter measure?

   _____

   _____

4. In what areas of radiology are diagnostic imaging personnel subject to receiving the highest occupational radiation exposure?

   _____

   _____

5. If a pregnant radiographer wears a second monitoring device at abdominal level, what does this monitor provide?

   _____

   _____

6. List three radiation survey instruments that are used for area monitoring.

   _____

   _____

7. Where are proportional counters used? What do they detect?

_____

_____

8. List three disadvantages of a TLD.

_____

_____

9. What kind of detector is found in an OSL dosimeter?

_____

_____

10. A cutie pie can measure x-radiation and gamma radiation, and if equipped with a suitable window, what other type of radiation can this instrument measure?

_____

_____

11. Why does a GM tube have a "check source" of a weak, long-lived radioisotope located on one side of its external surface?

_____

12. When a protective lead apron is used during fluoroscopy or special procedures, why should the personnel dosimeter be worn outside the apron at collar level on the anterior surface of the body?

_____

_____

13. On a personnel monitoring report, what information is provided by the cumulative columns?

_____

_____

14. What does the letter *M* indicate when it appears under the current monitoring period or in the cumulative columns of a personnel monitoring report?

_____

_____

15. What must a radiation worker do when changing employment?

_____

_____

Exercise 7: General Discussion or Opinion Questions

The following questions are intended to allow students to express their knowledge and understanding of the subject matter or to present a personal opinion. The questions may be used to stimulate class discussion. Because answers to these questions may vary, determination of an answer's acceptability is left to the discretion of the course instructor.

1. How can the GM meter be used as an area radiation survey instrument?

2. What responsibilities does a radiation safety officer have in an imaging department?

3. Why is monitoring of radiation exposure important for occupationally exposed diagnostic imaging personnel?

4. How is the ionization chamber–type survey meter used for radiation protection surveys?

5. What requirements should radiation survey instruments used for area monitoring meet?

POST-TEST

The student should take this test after reading Chapter 5, finishing all accompanying textbook and workbook exercises, and completing any additional activities required by the course instructor. The student should complete the post-test with a score of 90% or higher before advancing to the next chapter. (Each of the following 20 questions are worth 5 points.)
Score = _____ %

1. Some means of monitoring personnel exposure must be employed to ensure that occupational radiation exposure levels are kept well below the annual _____ dose limit.

2. Define the term *optically stimulated luminescence dosimeter.*

   _____

   _____

3. How can the working habits and working conditions of diagnostic imaging personnel be assessed over a designated period?

   _____

   _____

4. To meet state and federal regulations, _____ from personnel monitoring programs must be recorded accurately and maintained for review.

5. When a protective apron is not being used, where should a radiation worker wear a personnel monitoring device during routine computed radiography, digital radiography, or conventional radiographic procedures to approximate the location of maximal radiation dose to the thyroid and the head and neck?

   _____

6. Which of the following devices are used for personnel monitoring?
     1. OSL dosimeter
     2. TLD
     3. Ionization chamber–type survey meter (cutie pie)
     4. Personnel digital ionization dosimeter
   A. 1, 2, and 4 only
   B. 1, 3, and 4 only
   C. 2, 3, and 4 only
   D. 1, 2, 3, and 4

7. LiF functions as the sensing material in which of the following devices?
   A. Film badge
   B. OSL dosimeter
   C. Pocket dosimeter
   D. TLD

8. In a health care facility, where can a radiographer's deep, eye, and shallow occupational exposure, as measured by an exposed monitor, be found?

_____

_____

9. What instrument should be used to locate a lost radioactive source or to detect low-level radioactive contamination?

_____

10. Before a pocket dosimeter is used to record radiation exposure, the quartz fiber indicator of the transparent reading scale should indicate a_____ reading.

11. In addition to a primary personnel dosimeter worn at collar level, pregnant imaging personnel should be issued a second monitoring device to record the radiation dose to the _____ during gestation to provide an estimate of the equivalent dose to the embryo-fetus.

12. When radiation workers change employment, what must they convey to the new employer?

_____

_____

13. Area monitoring can be accomplished through the use of radiation _____ instruments.

14. Health care facilities must maintain a record of exposure recorded by personnel dosimeters as part of each radiation worker's _____ record.

15. When are radiation workers required to wear personnel monitoring devices?

_____

_____

16. It is recommended that an extremity dosimeter, or TLD ring, be worn by an imaging professional as a second monitor whenever procedures are performed that require the hands to be near the _____ x-ray beam.

17. In a health care facility, who generally receives and reviews personnel monitoring reports?

_____

18. Although an OSL dosimeter can be worn for up to 1 year, it commonly is worn for _____ to _____ months.

19. What instrument is used by medical physicists to perform the annual standard measurements required by state, federal, and health care accreditation organizations for radiographic and fluoroscopic devices?

_____

20. In diagnostic imaging, the increased sensitivity of the OSL dosimeter makes it ideal for monitoring employees working in low-radiation environments and for _____ workers.

6 Overview of Cell Biology

OVERVIEW OF CELL BIOLOGY

Chapter 6 covers basic concepts of cell biology. The chapter begins with a discussion of the cell and continues with other related topics, such as the chemical composition of cells. It includes a discussion of organic and inorganic compounds, cell structure, and cell division. This material lays the foundation for radiation biology, which is covered in subsequent chapters. Before imaging professionals can understand the effects of ionizing radiation on the human body, they must acquire a basic knowledge of cell structure, composition, and function. This chapter is designed to provide an understanding of cellular biology that ultimately will help the learner in appreciating the effects of radiation in the body.

CHAPTER HIGHLIGHTS

- The cell is the fundamental component of structure, development, growth, and life processes in the human body.
- Cells are made of protoplasm, which consists of proteins, carbohydrates, lipids, nucleic acids, water, and mineral salts (electrolytes).
  - Proteins are essential to growth, the construction of new body tissue, and repair of injured or debilitated tissue; they may function as hormones and antibodies.
  - The primary purpose of carbohydrates is to provide fuel for cell metabolism.
  - Lipids act as a reservoir for long-term storage of energy, insulate and guard the body against the environment, and protect organs.
  - Nucleic acids (DNA and RNA) carry genetic information necessary for cell replication.
  - RNA has the nitrogenous base, uracil, as a component of its ladder steps, whereas DNA has thymine, instead, in its ladder steps.
  - Genes are the basic units of heredity.
  - The Human Genome Project has mapped the entire sequence of DNA base pairs on all 46 chromosomes. This project has led to the discovery of more than 1800 disease genes.
  - There are 2.9 billion base pairs arranged into approximately 30,000 genes.

- Water, the primary inorganic substance contained in the human body, comprises approximately 80% to 85% of the body's weight, is essential to sustaining life, and serves as the transport vehicle for material the cell uses and eliminates.
- Mineral salts keep the correct proportion of water in the cell, support proper cell function, assist in the creation of energy, aid in the conduction of impulses along nerves, and prevent muscle cramping.
- Cells have multiple components or subunits called organelles:
  - The cell membrane surrounds the human cell, functions as a barricade, and controls passage of water and other materials into and out of the cell.
  - Cytoplasm is the portion of a cell outside the nucleus in which all metabolic activity occurs.
  - The endoplasmic reticulum transports food and molecules from one part of the cell to another. It functions as the highway system of the cell.
  - The Golgi apparatus unites large carbohydrate molecules with proteins to form glycoproteins.
  - Mitochondria, the powerhouses of the cell, contain enzymes that produce energy for cellular activity.
  - Lysosomes break down unwanted large molecules; they may rupture when exposed to radiation, with resulting cell death.
  - Ribosomes synthesize the various proteins that cells require.
  - Centrosomes contain the centrioles.
  - The nucleus controls cell division, multiplication, and biochemical reactions.
- Somatic cells divide through the process of mitosis.
  - The cellular life cycle has four distinct phases: pre-DNA synthesis, actual DNA synthesis, post-DNA manufacturing, and division (mitosis).
  - Mitosis has four subphases: prophase, metaphase, anaphase, and telophase.
- Genetic cells divide through meiosis.
  - Meiosis is similar to mitosis except no DNA replication occurs in telophase; the number of chromosomes in the daughter cell is reduced to half the number of chromosomes in the parent cell.

Exercise 1: Matching

Match the following terms with their definitions or associated phrases.

1. ___D___ Electrolytes
2. ___M___ Antibodies

3. ___L___ Human genome

4. ___K___ Cytosine and thymine
5. ___F___ Mapping

6. ___C___ Enzymatic proteins

7. ___N___ Cell division
8. ___A___ Protoplasm
9. ___P___ Anaphase
10. ___G___ Protein synthesis
11. ___E___ Hormones
12. ___R___ Genes

13. ___H___ Sodium and potassium

14. ___T___ Cytoplasmic organelles

15. ___O___ Carbohydrates
16. ___J___ Adenine and guanine

17. ___U___ Inorganic compounds

18. ___I___ Deoxyribose

19. ___B___ Lipids

20. ___W___ Ribosomal RNA

21. ___Y___ Interphase
22. ___X___ Nucleic acid
23. ___V___ Organic compounds

24. ___S___ Lysosomes

25. ___Q___ Cell membrane

A. Chemical building material for all living things
B. Made up of a molecule of glycerin and three molecules of fatty acid
C. Moderate or control the cell's various physiologic activities
D. Mineral salts
E. Chemical secretions manufactured by various endocrine glands and carried by the bloodstream to influence the activities of other parts of the body
F. Process of locating and identifying genes in the genome
G. Protein production
H. Keep the correct proportion of water in the cell
I. A five-carbon sugar molecule
J. Compounds called *purines*
K. Compounds called *pyrimidines*
L. The total amount of genetic material (DNA) contained within the chromosomes of a human being
M. Protein molecules produced by specialized cells in the bone marrow called *B lymphocytes*
N. Multiplication process whereby one cell divides to form two or more cells
O. Saccharides
P. The phase of mitosis during which the duplicate centromeres are severed and the sister chromatids move apart and are subsequently pulled toward opposite poles of the mitotic spindle
Q. The frail, semipermeable, flexible structure encasing and surrounding the human cell that functions as a barricade to protect cellular contents from their outside environment and also controls the passage of water and other materials into and out of the cell
R. Segments of DNA that serve as the basic units of heredity
S. Small, pealike sacs or single-membrane spherical bodies that are of great importance for digestion within the cytoplasm
T. What all the miniature cellular components present in the cytoplasm of the cell are collectively called
U. Compounds that do not contain carbon
V. All carbon compounds, both natural and artificial
W. Functions to assist in the linking of messenger RNA to the ribosome to facilitate protein synthesis
X. Very large, complex macromolecules made up of nucleotides
Y. The period of cell growth that occurs before actual mitosis

Chapter **6** **Overview of Cell Biology**

Exercise 2: Multiple Choice

Select the answer that *best* completes the following questions or statements.

1. In humans, how many genes are contained in all 46 chromosomes?
   A. Approximately 300
   B. Approximately 3000
   C. Approximately 30,000
   D. Approximately 300,000

2. The nucleolus contains which of the following?
   A. Centrosomes and mitochondria
   B. Ribonucleic acid and proteins
   C. Ribosomes and Golgi bodies
   D. Lysosomes and endoplasmic reticulum

3. In the human cell, protein synthesis occurs in which of the following locations?
   A. Nucleus
   B. Mitochondria
   C. Ribosomes
   D. Endoplasmic reticulum

4. Interphase consists of which of the following phases?
   A. M, G_1, and S
   B. G_1, S, and G_2
   C. S, G_2, and M
   D. G_2, M, and G_1

5. Carbohydrates also may be referred to as:
   A. Lipids
   B. Nucleic acids
   C. Hormones
   D. Saccharides

6. DNA regulates cellular activity *indirectly* by reproducing itself in the form of _____ ____ to carry genetic information from the cell nucleus to ribosomes located in the cytoplasm.
   A. Messenger DNA
   B. Messenger RNA
   C. Messenger REM
   D. Transfer RNA

7. Human cells contain which four major organic compounds?
   A. Nucleic acids, water, protein, and mineral salts
   B. Mineral salts, carbohydrates, lipids, and proteins
   C. Carbohydrates, lipids, nucleic acids, and water
   D. Proteins, carbohydrates, lipids, and nucleic acids

8. Which of the following is a process of reduction cell division?
   A. Mitosis
   B. Meiosis
   C. Molecular synthesis
   D. Amniocentesis

9. Which of the following cellular organelles function(s) as a cellular garbage disposal?
   A. Endoplasmic reticulum
   B. Mitochondria
   C. Lysosomes
   D. Ribosomes

10. Which of the following describes the nuclear envelope that separates the nucleus from other parts of the cell?
    A. Single membrane
    B. Double-walled membrane
    C. Triple-walled membrane
    D. Quadruple-walled membrane

11. Which of the following are functions of the cell membrane?
    1. Protecting the contents of the cell from the outside environment
    2. Controlling the passage of water and other materials into and out of the cell
    3. Allowing penetration by all substances into the cell
    A. 1 and 2 only
    B. 1 and 3 only
    C. 2 and 3 only
    D. 1, 2, and 3

12. Lipids are also referred to as:
    A. Amino acids
    B. Carbohydrates
    C. Fats
    D. Sugars

13. The primary energy source for the cell is:
    A. Amino acids
    B. Glucose
    C. Protein
    D. Phosphate

14. Cytosine bonds *only* with which of the following nitrogenous organic bases?
    A. Adenine
    B. Guanine
    C. Thymine
    D. Uracil

15. Which of the following statements is *not* true?
    A. Lysosomes are sometimes referred to as "suicide bags."
    B. Adenosine triphosphate (ATP) is essential for sustaining life.
    C. The Golgi apparatus or complex is the powerhouse of the cell.
    D. The nucleus is the "heart" of the cell.

16. When ionizing radiation is used for therapeutic purposes to destroy malignant cells, a very significant effort using the latest advances in imaging and computer treatment planning algorithms is also made to spare healthy surrounding tissue. In radiation therapy, this concept is referred to as a(n):
    A. Enzyme repair effect
    B. Therapeutic ratio
    C. Tissue tolerance effect
    D. Malignant cell annihilation effect

17. Twenty-two different _____ _____ are involved in protein synthesis.
    A. Amino acids
    B. Antibodies
    C. Enzymes
    D. Hormones

18. The process of locating and identifying the genes in the human genome is called:
    A. Gene detecting
    B. Gene extrapolation
    C. Gene tracking
    D. Mapping

19. Approximately 80% to 85% of the weight of the human body is:
    A. Bone
    B. Fatlike substances
    C. Mineral salts
    D. Water

20. Meiosis is the process of:
    A. Converting inorganic substances into organic substances
    B. Identifying genes in the human genome
    C. Reduction cell division
    D. Repairing breaks in DNA

21. Water performs which of the following functions in the human body?
    1. Maintains a constant core temperature of 98.6°F (37°C)
    2. Acts as a solvent, keeping compounds dissolved so that they can more easily interact and their concentration may be regulated
    3. Lubricates both the digestive system and the skeletal articulations (joints)
    A. 1 and 2 only
    B. 1 and 3 only
    C. 2 and 3 only
    D. 1, 2, and 3

22. Which of the following is of primary importance in maintaining adequate amounts of intracellular fluid?
    A. Deoxyribose
    B. Glucose
    C. Potassium
    D. Ribose

23. The S phase of mitosis is the:
    A. Pre-DNA synthesis phase
    B. Actual DNA synthesis period
    C. Post-DNA synthesis phase
    D. Phase when DNA synthesis multiplies by a factor of 4

24. When a cell divides, the genetic-containing material contracts into tiny rod-shaped bodies called:
    A. Golgi apparatus
    B. Chromosomes
    C. Mitochondria
    D. Nucleotides

25. Nitrogenous base pairs form the:
    A. Hormones needed by various endocrine glands in the body
    B. Mitotic spindle
    C. Steps, or rungs, of the DNA ladderlike structure
    D. Sugars the body needs for energy

Exercise 3: True or False

Circle *T* if the statement is true; circle *F* if the statement is false.

1. T F Cells are engaged in an ongoing process of obtaining energy and converting it to support their vital functions.

2. T F Depending on the cell type, water normally accounts for 25% to 35% of protoplasm.

3. T F Proper cell functioning depends on enzymes.

4. T F The skin is the body's initial barrier to any outside invasion by pathogens; however, once the skin has been penetrated, the body's primary defense mechanism against infection and disease consists of the hormones that chemically attack any foreign invaders.

5. T F Lipids are organic macromolecules.

6. T F Oxygen bonds attach the nitrogenous bases to each other and join the two side rails of the DNA ladder.

7. T F A normal human being has 46 different chromosomes composed of 23 pairs in each somatic (non-reproductive) cell.

8. T F Taken as a whole, genes control the formation of proteins in every cell through the intricate process of parentally shared genetic coding.

9. T F All cellular metabolic functions occur in the nucleus.

10. T F Centrosomes are located in the center of the cell near the nucleus.

11. T F Chromosomes and genes organize the 22 different amino acids into certain sequences to form the different structural and enzymatic proteins.

12. T F Messenger RNA (mRNA) transfers its genetic code to another kind of RNA molecule, called *transfer RNA* (tRNA).

13. T F The cell membrane is a very thick structure encasing and surrounding the human cell.

14. T F Metabolism is the breaking down of large molecules into smaller ones.

15. T F Water is responsible for maintaining a constant body core temperature of 37°C.

16. T F Approximately 30,000 genes are contained in all 46 human chromosomes.

17. T F Radiation-induced damage to chromosomes may be evaluated during telophase.

18. T F Water lubricates the digestive system.

19. T F ATP is essential for sustaining life.

20. T F Sodium (Na) is the primary energy source for the human cell.

21. T F Protein characteristics determine cell characteristics, and cell characteristics ultimately determine the characteristics of the entire individual.

22. T F Cells are the basic units of all living matter, but they are not essential for life.

23. T F Proper cell function enables the body to maintain homeostasis, or equilibrium.

24. T F Lipids contain the most carbon of all the organic compounds.

25. T F Although carbohydrates are found throughout the body, they are most abundant in the spleen and nervous tissue.

Exercise 4: Fill in the Blank

Using the following Word Bank, fill in the blanks with the word or words that best complete the statement.

4	high	nucleus
amino acids	homeostasis	osmotic
catalytic	hormones	oxidative
cell	liver	repair
DNA (may be used more than once)	lysosomes	repair enzymes
electrolytes	macromolecules	replication
endoplasmic reticulum	metabolism (may be used more than once)	ribosomes
fluid		salts
fraternal	muscle	water

1. The _____ is the fundamental component of structure, development, growth, and life processes in the human body.

2. Proper cell function enables the body to maintain _____, or equilibrium.

3. The biomolecules that comprise protoplasm are formed from many elements, among which there are _____ primary elements.

4. Proteins are formed when organic compounds called _____ _____ combine into long, chainlike molecular complexes.

5. If radiation damage is excessive because of a large delivered equivalent dose, the damage will be too severe for _____ _____ to have a positive effect.

6. _____ regulate body functions such as growth and development.

7. Although carbohydrates are found throughout the body, they are most abundant in the _____ and in _____ tissue.

8. The arrangements of amino acids are determined by succession of adenine-thymine and cytosine-guanine base pairs in the _____ macromolecule.

9. By maintaining the correct proportion of water in the cell, _____ pressure is maintained.

10. Dizygotic twins are also known as _____ twins.

11. Chromosomes are composed of _____.

12. Water, a solvent, will preferentially move across cell surfaces or membranes into areas with a _____ concentration of ions.

13. By controlling its concentration of potassium ions (as well as the ever-present sodium [Na] and chlorine [Cl] ions resulting from the intake of table salt), the cell regulates the amount of _____ passing through its membrane and consequently the amount of _____ it contains.

14. _____ enables the cell to perform the vital functions of synthesizing proteins and producing energy.

15. The primary purpose of carbohydrates is to provide fuel for cell _____.

16. _____ manufacture (synthesize) the various proteins that cells require using the blueprints provided by mRNA.

17. Both the _____ and _____ capabilities of enzymes are of vital importance to the survival of the cell.

18. Lipids are organic _____, large molecules built from smaller chemical structures.

19. By directing protein synthesis, the _____ plays an essential role in active transport, metabolism, growth, and heredity.

20. The _____ _____ transports food and molecules from one part of the cell to another.

21. Nucleic acids (DNA, RNA) carry genetic information necessary for cell _____.

22. The primary function of _____ appears to be the breaking down of unwanted large molecules that either penetrate into the cell through microscopic channels or are drawn in by the cell membrane itself.

23. _____ metabolism is the oxidation of smaller molecules to release energy.

24. _____ are chemical compounds resulting from the action of an acid and a base on each other.

25. Salts are sometimes referred to as _____.

Exercise 5: Labeling

Label the following illustrations and box.

A. Typical cell.

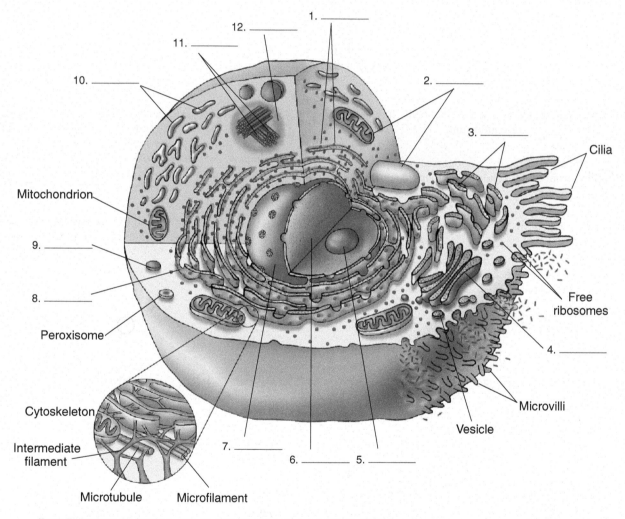

From Thibodeau A: *Anatomy and Physiology*, ed 9, St. Louis, 2016, Mosby.

B. Cellular life cycle.

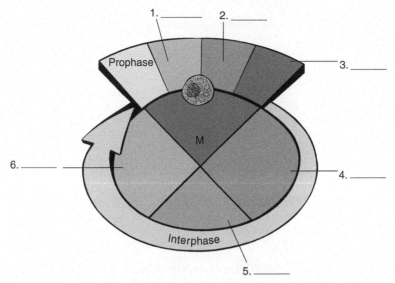

From Bushong SC: *Radiologic science for technologists: physics, biology and protection,* ed 10, St. Louis, 2013, Elsevier.

C. Summary of cell components.

Title	Site	Activity
1. _____	Cytoplasm	*Plastic storage bag*—Functions as a barricade to protect cellular contents from their environment and controls the passage of water and other materials into and out of the cell; performs many additional functions such as elimination of wastes and refining of material for energy through breakdown of the materials
2. _____	Cytoplasm	*The highway*—Enables the cell to communicate with the extracellular environment and transfers food from one part of the cell to another
3. _____	Cytoplasm	*Freight hauling*—Unites large carbohydrate molecules and combines them with proteins to form glycoproteins and transports enzymes and hormones through the cell membrane so that they can exit the cell, enter the bloodstream, and be carried to areas of the body in which they are required
4. _____	Cytoplasm	*Power-generating stations*—Produce energy for cellular activity by breaking down nutrients through a process of oxidation
5. _____	Cytoplasm	*Garbage bags with poison pills*—Dispose of large particles such as bacteria and food as well as smaller particles; also contain hydrolytic enzymes that can break down and digest proteins, certain carbohydrates, and the cell itself if the lysosome's surrounding membrane breaks
6. _____	Cytoplasm	*Manufacturing facilities*—Manufacture the various proteins that cells require
7. _____	Cytoplasm	*Spindle weaver*—Plays an important role in organizing the formation of the mitotic spindle during cell division
8. _____	Nucleus	*Information processing and administrative center of the cell*—Contains the genetic or hereditary material, DNA, and proteins. Also contains the nucleolus. The nucleus controls cell division and multiplication and the biochemical reactions that occur within the cell and also directs protein synthesis.
9. _____	Nucleus	*The blueprints*—Contain the genetic material; controls cell division and multiplication and also biochemical reactions that occur within the living cell
10. _____	Nucleus	*RNA copy center*—Holds a large amount of RNA and synthesizes ribosomes

Chapter **6** **Overview of Cell Biology**

Exercise 6: Short Answer

Answer the following questions by providing a short answer.

1. What must the human body do to ensure efficient cell operation?

   _____

   _____

2. What is destructive metabolism, or catabolism?

   _____

   _____

3. How are proteins formed? What determines the precise function of each protein molecule?

   _____

   _____

4. What functions do enzymatic proteins perform in the human body?

   _____

   _____

5. What are lipids? List six functions they perform for the human body.

   _____

   _____

6. What role do ribosomes play in the manufacture of protein by a cell?

   _____

   _____

7. Describe the function of water inside and outside the cells in the human body.

   _____

   _____

8. What does the nucleus in a human cell control?

   _____

   _____

9. List four distinct phases of the cellular life cycle.

   _____

   _____

10. How are a monosaccharide, a disaccharide, and a polysaccharide different?

    _____

    _____

11. List the four major classes of organic compounds found in the human body.

_____

_____

12. What is DNA?

_____

_____

13. What do structural proteins provide for the human body?

_____

_____

14. What is chromatin? What happens to this material when a cell divides?

_____

_____

15. What are hormones? What do the hormones that are produced in the thyroid gland control?

_____

_____

Exercise 7: General Discussion or Opinion Questions

The following questions are intended to allow students to express their knowledge and understanding of the subject matter or to present a personal opinion. The questions may be used to stimulate class discussion. Because answers to these questions may vary, determination of the answer's acceptability is left to the discretion of the course instructor.

1. Identify and describe the components of a typical human cell, and discuss how cells perform many diverse functions for the body.

2. What is the Human Genome Project? What advances have been achieved through this project, and what challenges still remain?

3. Explain the process of mitosis.

4. What is the significance of inorganic and organic compounds in the human body?

5. What are enzymes, and what functions do they perform for the human body?

POST-TEST

The student should take this test after reading Chapter 6, finishing all accompanying textbook and workbook exercises, and completing any additional activities required by the course instructor. The student should complete the post-test with a score of 90% or higher before advancing to the next chapter. (Each of the following 20 questions are worth 5 points.)
Score = _____ %

1. Cells are the basic units of all living _____ and are essential for life.

2. Proteins, carbohydrates, lipids, and nucleic acids are the four major classes of _____ compounds.

3. What type of enzymes can mend damaged molecules and therefore help the cell recover from a small amount of radiation-induced damage?

_____

4. In a DNA macromolecule, adenine (A), cytosine (C), guanine (G), and thymine (T) are the four _____ organic bases.

5. Approximately 80% to 85% of the weight of the human body is _____.

6. Describe a DNA macromolecule.

_____

_____

7. What is the process of locating and identifying genes in the human genome called?

_____

8. The large, double-membrane, oval or bean-shaped structures that function as the powerhouses of the cell are called:
   A. Endoplasmic reticulum
   B. Golgi apparatus
   C. Mitochondria
   D. Ribosomes

9. When somatic cells divide, they undergo:
   A. Centrosome removal
   B. Meiosis
   C. Mitosis
   D. Nuclear collapse

10. During which subphase of cell division can radiation-induced chromosomal damage be evaluated?

_____

11. What function do ribosomes perform in the cell?

_____

12. Approximately how many genes are contained in all 46 human chromosomes?

_____

13. If exposure to ionizing radiation damages the components involved in molecular synthesis beyond repair, what will happen to the affected cells?

_____

14. Protein synthesis involves _____ different amino acids.

15. What is formed from a nitrogen-containing organic base, a five-carbon sugar molecule, and a phosphate molecule?

_____

16. What serves as a prototype for mRNA?

_____

17. What is the protoplasm outside of the cell's nucleus called?

_____

18. _____ is the period of cell growth that occurs before actual mitosis.

19. _____ act as a reservoir for long-term storage of energy, insulate and guard the body against the environment, and support and protect organs such as the eyes and kidneys.

20. What is the function of the cell membrane?

_____

_____

7 Molecular and Cellular Radiation Biology

The human body is a complex, interconnected living system composed of very large numbers of various types of cells, most of which may be damaged by radiation. Because the potentially harmful effects of ionizing radiation on living systems occur primarily at the cellular level, the preceding chapter placed a strong emphasis on the basics of cell structure, composition, and function. Chapter 7 provides the reader with an introduction to those aspects of molecular and cellular radiation biology that are relevant to the subject of radiation protection.

CHAPTER HIGHLIGHTS

- Linear energy transfer (LET)
  - LET is the average energy deposited per unit length of track by ionizing radiation as it passes through and interacts with a medium along its path.
    - It is described in units of keV per micron (1 micron [μm] = 10^{-6} m).
  - The LET value of the radiation involved is a very important factor in assessing potential tissue and organ damage from exposure to that type of ionizing radiation.
  - Because of a property known as *wave-particle duality*, x-rays and gamma rays can also be referred to as a stream of particles called *photons*.
  - Low-LET radiation (x-rays and gamma rays) doses that are not excessive mainly cause indirect damage to biologic tissues that usually can be reversed by repair enzymes.
  - High-LET radiation (alpha particles, ions of heavy nuclei, and low-energy neutrons) can produce irreparable damage to DNA because of inducing multiple-strand breaks that cannot be undone by repair enzymes.
- Relative biologic effectiveness (RBE)
  - RBE of the type of radiation being used is the ratio of the dose of a reference radiation (conventionally 250-kVp x-rays) to the dose of radiation of the type in question that is necessary to produce the same biologic reaction in a given experiment. The reaction is what is produced by a dose of test radiation delivered under the same conditions.
  - As the LET of radiation increases, so do biologic effects; RBE quantitatively describes this relative effect.

- RBE describes the relative capabilities of radiation with differing LETs to produce a particular biologic reaction.
- The concept of RBE is not practical for specifying radiation protection dose levels in humans. Therefore to overcome this limitation, a radiation weighting factor (W_R) is used to calculate the equivalent dose (EqD) to determine the ability of a dose of any kind of ionizing radiation to cause biologic damage.
- Oxygen enhancement ratio (OER)
  - OER is a comparative measure used to obtain the amount of cellular injury for a species of ionizing radiation. It is the ratio of the radiation dose required to cause a particular biologic response of cells or organisms in an oxygen-deprived environment to the radiation dose required to cause an identical response under normal oxygenated conditions.
- Radiation-induced biologic damage in living systems is observed on molecular, cellular, and organic system levels.
- Radiation action on the cell is either direct or indirect, depending on the site of interaction.
  - If sufficient quantities of somatic cells are affected by exposure to ionizing radiation, entire body processes can be disrupted. Conversely, if radiation damages the germ cells, the damage may be passed on to future generations in the form of genetic mutations.
  - Action is direct when biologic damage occurs as a result of the ionization of atoms on essential molecules (e.g., DNA, RNA, proteins, enzymes) produced by straight interaction with the incident radiation.
  - Action is indirect when effects are produced by reactive free radicals created by the interaction of radiation with water molecules; these unstable, highly reactive molecules can cause substantial disruption to molecules such as DNA and result in cell death.
  - High-LET radiation is more likely to cause biologic damage through direct action than is low-LET radiation.
  - Because the human body is 80% water and less than 1% DNA, essentially all effects of low-LET irradiation in living cells result from indirect action.

- Point lesions commonly occur with low-LET radiation and are often reversible through the action of repair enzymes.
- Double-strand breaks of DNA happen more commonly with densely ionizing (high-LET) radiation and often are associated with the loss of one or more nitrogenous bases. Chance of repair from this type of damage is very low; the possibility of a lethal alteration of nitrogenous bases within the genetic sequence is far greater.
- When two interactions, one on each of the two sugar-phosphate chains, occur within the same rung of the DNA ladder-like configuration, the result is a cleaved or broken chromosome, with each new portion containing an unequal amount of genetic material. If this damaged chromosome divides, each new daughter cell will receive an incorrect amount of genetic material, resulting in either death or impaired functioning of the new daughter cell.
- Because the genetic information to be passed on to future generations is contained in the strict sequence of nitrogenous bases, the loss or change of a base in the DNA chain represents a mutation.
- Chromosome aberrations and chromatid aberrations are two types of chromosome anomalies that have been observed at metaphase.
- Consequences to the cell from structural changes within the nucleus can result in restitution, deletion, broken-end rearrangement, or broken-end rearrangement without visible damage to the chromatids. The last three types of consequences result in mutation because the position of the genes on the chromatids have been rearranged, thus altering the heritable characteristics of the cell.
- Target theory states that when cell DNA is directly or indirectly inactivated by exposure to radiation, the cell will die.
- When a cell nucleus is significantly damaged by exposure to ionizing radiation, the cell can die or experience reproductive death, apoptosis, mitotic death, mitotic delay, or interference with function.
- The cell survival curve is used to display the radiosensitivity of a particular type of cell, which helps determine the types of cancer cells that will respond to radiation therapy.
- The human body is composed of different types of cells and tissues, which vary in their degree of radiosensitivity.

- The law of Bergonié and Tribondeau states that the most pronounced radiation effects occur in cells with the least maturity and specialization or differentiation, the greatest reproductive activity, and the longest mitotic phases.
- The embryo-fetus is very susceptible to radiation damage, which can cause CNS anomalies, microcephaly, and intellectual disability.
- Lymphocytes are the most radiosensitive blood cells, and when they are damaged the body loses its natural ability to combat infection and becomes more susceptible to bacterial and viral antigens.
- Neither the blood nor the blood-forming organs of patients should undergo appreciable damage from radiation exposure received during diagnostic imaging procedures, but several studies have indicated some chromosome aberrations in circulating lymphocytes that have received radiation doses within the diagnostic radiology range. X-ray procedures responsible for these aberrations include high-level fluoroscopy or fluoroscopy with long exposure time such as cardiac catheterization and other specialized invasive procedures.
- Because the body constantly regenerates epithelial tissue, the cells comprising this tissue are highly radiosensitive.
- Muscle tissue is relatively insensitive to radiation.
- Nerve cells in the adult are highly specialized. If the cell nucleus has been damaged but not destroyed by exposure to radiation, the damaged nerve cell may still be able to function but in an impaired fashion. Radiation can cause temporary or permanent damage to a nerve's processes, thus disrupting communication with and control of some body areas.
- Developing nerve cells in the embryo-fetus are more radiosensitive than are the mature nerve cells of the adult. Studies indicate that the eighth to the fifteenth week after gestation is the time frame of maximal radiosensitivity. A lower but still significant level of risk remains until the twenty-fifth week after gestation.
- Human germ cells are relatively radiosensitive, although the exact responses of male and female germ cells to ionizing radiation differ because their courses of development from immature to mature status differ. For both males and females, temporary sterilization occurs at 2 Gy_t, and permanent sterilization occurs at 5 to 6 Gy_t.

Exercise 1: Matching

Match the following terms with their definitions or associated phrases.

1. _____ Direct action

2. _____ LET

3. _____ Covalent cross-links

4. _____ Radiation weighting factor (W_R)

5. _____ Mutation

6. _____ Cell survival curve

7. _____ Indirect action

8. _____ OER

9. _____ Apoptosis

10. _____ Chromosome aberrations

11. _____ Target theory

12. _____ RBE

13. _____ Chromatid aberrations

14. _____ Law of Bergonié and Tribondeau

15. _____ Free radicals

16. _____ Mitotic delay

17. _____ Chromosome breakage

18. _____ R^*

19. _____ Molecular damage

20. _____ HO_2^*

21. _____ Germ cells

22. _____ Radiation biology

23. _____ Hydrogen peroxide

24. _____ Point mutation

25. _____ H^* and OH^*

A. A multistage process that first involves the production of reactive free radicals that are created by the interaction of radiation with water molecules

B. Concept that the cell dies if the master, or key, molecule becomes inactivated as a consequence of exposure to ionizing radiation

C. Solitary atoms or most often a combination of atoms that behave as single entities and are very chemically reactive as a result of the presence of unpaired valence electrons

D. Used to calculate the equivalent dose to determine the ability of a dose of any kind of ionizing radiation to cause biologic damage

E. Loss or change of a nitrogenous base in the DNA chain

F. Results when irradiation occurs early in interphase, *before* DNA synthesis takes place

G. Describes the relative capabilities of radiation with differing LETs to produce a particular biologic reaction

H. Chemical unions created between atoms by the single sharing of one or more pairs of electrons

I. Programmed cell death

J. The radiosensitivity of cells is directly proportional to their reproductive activity and inversely proportional to their degree of differentiation

K. The ratio of the radiation dose required to cause a particular biologic response of cells or organisms in an oxygen-deprived environment to the radiation dose required to cause an identical response under normal oxygenated conditions

L. Classic method of displaying the sensitivity of a particular type of cell to radiation

M. Results when irradiation of individual chromatids occurs later in interphase, *after* DNA synthesis has taken place

N. Biologic damage that occurs as a result of ionization of atoms on essential molecules (e.g., DNA) produced by straight interaction with the incident radiation

O. The average energy deposited per unit length of track

P. The breaking of one or both of the sugar-phosphate chains of a DNA molecule that can be caused by exposure of the molecule to ionizing radiation

Q. Branch of biology concerned with the effects of ionizing radiation on living systems

R. Injury on the molecular level resulting from exposure to ionizing radiation

S. Female and male reproductive cells

T. A hydrogen radical and a hydroxyl radical

U. Can result when ionizing radiation interacts with a DNA macromolecule and the energy transferred in the process ruptures one of its chemical bonds and severs one of the sugar-phosphate chain side rails, or strands, of the ladderlike molecular structure

V. A hydroperoxyl radical

W. An organic neutral free radical

X. $OH^* + OH^* = H_2O_2$, a substance that is very poisonous to the cell

Y. Exposing a cell to as little as 0.01 Gy_t of ionizing radiation just before it begins dividing can result in the failure of the cell to start dividing on time

Exercise 2: Multiple Choice

Select the answer that *best* completes the following questions or statements.

1. Radiation damage is observed on which of the following three levels?
   A. Molecular, cellular, and inorganic systems
   B. Molecular, cellular, and organic systems
   C. Microscopic, molecular, and organic systems
   D. Organic, inorganic, and cellular systems

2. Molecular damage results in the formation of structurally:
   A. Changed molecules that permit cells to continue completing normal function
   B. Changed molecules that may impair cellular function
   C. Unchanged molecules that permit cells to continue functioning normally
   D. Unchanged molecules that may impair cellular function

3. According to the target theory, if only a few non-DNA cell molecules are made dysfunctional by radiation exposure, the cell will probably:
   A. Not show any evidence of injury after irradiation
   B. Show evidence of injury after irradiation
   C. Show evidence of severe impairment after irradiation
   D. Die

4. Each cell's function is governed and defined by the structures of its constituent molecules. If these structures are altered by radiation exposure, the following may result:
   1. Disturbance of the cell's chemical balance
   2. Disturbance of cell operation
   3. Failure of the cell to perform normal tasks
   A. 1 only
   B. 1 and 2 only
   C. 1 and 3 only
   D. 1, 2, and 3

5. Chromosome aberrations result when irradiation occurs:
   A. Early in interphase
   B. Late in prophase
   C. At the start of metaphase
   D. At the end of telophase

6. Which of the following are examples of distorted chromosomes?
   1. Anaphase bridges
   2. Dicentric chromosomes
   3. Ring chromosomes
   A. 1 and 2 only
   B. 1 and 3 only
   C. 2 and 3 only
   D. 1, 2, and 3

7. Which of the following is useful for explaining cell death and nonfatal cell abnormalities caused by exposure to radiation?
   A. Covalent cross-linking
   B. Bergonié-Tribondeau law
   C. Programmed cell death
   D. Target theory

8. X-rays and gamma rays can be referred to as "streams of particles" called *photons* because of a property known as:
   A. LET
   B. RBE
   C. Wave-particle duality
   D. Wave-particle fragmentation

9. The random interaction of x-rays with matter produces a variety of structural changes in biologic tissue, including:
   1. A single-strand break in one chromosome
   2. More than one break in the same chromosome
   3. Stickiness, or clumping together, of chromosomes
   A. 1 and 2 only
   B. 1 and 3 only
   C. 2 and 3 only
   D. 1, 2, and 3

10. Why are repair enzymes *usually* able to reverse the cellular damage generally caused by low-level ionizing radiation?
    A. Damage to DNA is sublethal.
    B. Irradiated cells are hypoxic.
    C. Only organic molecules are damaged.
    D. LET failed to occur.

11. What governs the radiation dose required to cause apoptosis?
    A. Changes in the cell protein content
    B. The phase of the cell cycle the individual cell is undergoing
    C. The radiosensitivity of the individual cell
    D. The number of cells irradiated

12. Which of the following describes the ratio of the radiation dose required to cause a particular biologic response of cells or organisms in an oxygen-deprived environment to the radiation dose required to cause an identical response under normal oxygenated conditions?
    A. OER
    B. Oxygen biologic effectiveness ratio
    C. Oxygen dose-response relationship
    D. Oxygen threshold ratio

13. Which of the following is a method of displaying the sensitivity of a particular type of cell to radiation?
    A. Cell survival curve
    B. Hypoxic cell measurement curve
    C. Radiolysis of water
    D. Radiation dose-response curve

14. Where are lymphocytes manufactured in the human body?
    A. Bone marrow
    B. Epithelial tissue
    C. Liver
    D. Pancreas

15. Which of the following defines the ratio of the dose of a reference radiation (conventionally 250-kVp x-rays) to the dose of radiation of the type in question that is necessary to produce the same biologic reaction in a given experiment?
    A. LET
    B. RBE
    C. W_R
    D. Low-level radiation effectiveness

16. A biologic reaction is produced by 6 Gy_t of a test radiation. It takes 36 Gy_t of 250-kVp x-ray radiation to produce the same biologic reaction. What is the RBE of the test radiation?
    A. 3
    B. 6
    C. 9
    D. 12

17. A hydroperoxyl radical (HO_2^*) is formed when a hydrogen free radical (H^*) combines with:
    A. A hydrogen ion (H^+)
    B. A hydroxyl ion (OH^-)
    C. Molecular oxygen (O_2)
    D. Another hydrogen free radical (H^*)

18. LET is an important factor for:
    A. Assessing potential tissue and organ damage from exposure to ionizing radiation
    B. Assessing the characteristics of ionizing radiation (e.g., charge, mass, and energy)
    C. Determining the OER
    D. Removing electrons from tissue exposed to ionizing radiation

19. Because high-LET types of radiation deposit more energy per unit length of biologic tissue traversed, they are:
    A. More destructive to biologic matter than low-LET radiation
    B. Significantly less destructive to biologic matter than low-LET radiation
    C. Slightly less destructive to biologic matter than low-LET radiation
    D. Not comparable to low-LET radiation because they do not deposit any energy per unit length of biologic tissue traversed

20. Ring chromosomes, dicentric chromosomes, and anaphase bridges are examples of:
    A. Normal chromosomes
    B. Chromosomes about to divide
    C. Distorted chromosomes
    D. Chromosomes that carry appropriate genetic information

Exercise 3: True or False

Circle *T* if the statement is true; circle *F* if the statement is false.

1. T F The human body is a living system composed of large numbers of various types of cells, most of which cannot be damaged by radiation.

2. T F Biologic damage begins with the ionization produced by various types of radiation.

3. T F The characteristics of ionizing radiation (e.g., charge, mass, and energy) are exactly the same from one type of radiation to another.

4. T F LET is an important factor in the assessment of potential tissue and organ damage from exposure to ionizing radiation.

5. T F For radiation protection purposes, low-LET radiation is of the greatest concern when internal contamination is possible.

6. T F A positive water molecule (HOH^+) and a negative water molecule (HOH^-) are basically stable.

7. T F A few hundred centigray (cGy) of radiation can kill very sensitive cells such as lymphocytes or spermatogonia.

8. T F The embryo-fetus contains large numbers of mature, specialized cells and therefore is relatively radioresistant.

9. T F A blood count is a relatively insensitive test that is unable to indicate doses of less than 10 cGy.

10. T F Because the ovaries of young women are less sensitive than those of older women, a higher dose of radiation is required to cause sterility in young women.

11. T F Experimental data strongly indicate that ribonucleic acid (RNA) is the irreplaceable master, or key, molecule in the human cell.

12. T F Reproductive death generally results from exposure of cells to doses of ionizing radiation in the range of 1 to 10 Gy_t.

13. T F Ionizing radiation cannot adversely affect cell division.

14. T F Although originally it was applied only to germ cells, the law of Bergonié and Tribondeau is true for all types of cells in the human body.

15. T F LD 50/60 is more practical for humans than is LD 50/30.

16. T F If radiation damages the germ cells, the damage may be passed on to future generations in the form of genetic mutations.

17. T F The presence of free radicals in tissue does not affect the amount of biologic damage that results from irradiation.

18. T F X-ray photons may interact with but do not ionize water molecules in the human body.

19. T F Because hydrogen and hydroxyl ions usually recombine to form a normal water molecule, the existence of these ions as free agents in the human body is insignificant in terms of biologic damage.

20. T F A cell survival curve is constructed from data obtained by a series of experiments.

21. T F The human body is composed of different types of cells and tissues, all of which have the same degree of radiosensitivity.

22. T F In radiation therapy the presence of oxygen is not significant in terms of radiosensitivity.

23. T F The more mature and specialized in performing functions a cell is, the more sensitive it is to radiation.

24. T F Radiation affects primarily the stem cells of the hematopoietic (blood-forming) system.

25. T F The higher the radiation dose to the bone marrow, the more severe is the resulting cell depletion.

Exercise 4: Fill in the Blank

Using the following Word Bank, fill in the blanks with the word or words that best complete the statements.

0.25	granulocytes	mitosis
2	hydroxyl	permanent
5	immature	platelets
6	infection	radiosensitive (may be
cellular	insensitive	used more than once)
charge	intellectual disability	radiosensitivity
decrease	internal	restored
dies	ionizing radiation	sublethal
energy	mass	susceptible
gene	microcephaly	

1. Potentially harmful effects of ionizing radiation on living systems occur primarily at the _____ level.

2. X-ray and gamma-ray photons can impart _____ _____ to orbital electrons in atoms if the photons happen to pass near the electrons.

3. Low-LET radiation generally causes _____ damage to DNA.

4. High-LET radiation includes particles with substantial _____ and _____.

5. High-LET radiation is of greatest concern when _____ contamination is possible.

6. The presence of oxygen in biologic tissues makes the damage produced by free radicals _____.

7. Approximately two-thirds of all radiation-induced damage is believed to be ultimately caused by the _____ free radical (OH*).

8. _____ mutations could result from a single alteration along the sequence of nitrogenous bases in DNA.

9. _____ of the individual cell governs the dose required to cause apoptosis.

10. When _____ _____ interacts with cell atoms and molecules, the amount of radiation energy transferred (absorbed by the tissues) plays a major role in determining the extent of the biologic response.

11. Neutrophils, a type of white blood cell, play an important role in fighting _____.

12. Thrombocytes, or _____, initiate blood clotting and prevent hemorrhage.

13. _____ initially respond to radiation by increasing in number.

14. A therapeutic dose of radiation causes a _____ in the blood count.

15. Epithelial tissue has no blood vessels and regenerates through the process of _____.

16. Because the body constantly regenerates epithelial tissue, the cells comprising this tissue are highly _____.

17. Developing nerve cells in the embryo-fetus are more _____ than the mature nerve cells of adults.

18. Irradiation of the embryo may lead to CNS anomalies, _____, and _____ _____.

19. Because mature spermatogonia are specialized and do not divide, they are relatively _____ to ionizing radiation.

20. Immature spermatogonia are unspecialized and divide rapidly; therefore these germ cells are extremely _____.

21. Nerve cells have a nucleus. If the nucleus of one of these cells is destroyed, the cell _____ and is never _____.

22. Temporary sterility usually results from a single dose of _____ Gy_t to the ovaries.

23. Permanent sterilization occurs at _____ to _____ Gy_t.

24. The embryo or fetus, which has a large number of _____, nonspecialized cells, is much more _____ to radiation damage than is a child or an adult.

25. A whole-body radiation dose of _____ Gy_t delivered within a few days produces a measurable hematologic depression.

Exercise 5: Labeling

Label the following illustrations and box.

A. Radiolysis of water.

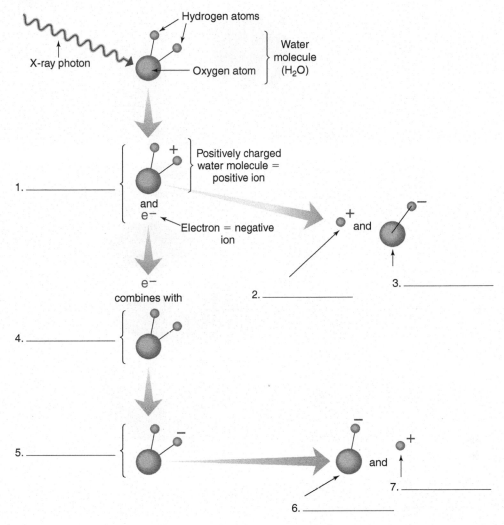

1. _____

2. _____

3. _____

4. _____

5. _____

6. _____

7. _____

Chapter **7 Molecular and Cellular Radiation Biology**

B. Indirect action of ionizing radiation on biologic molecules.

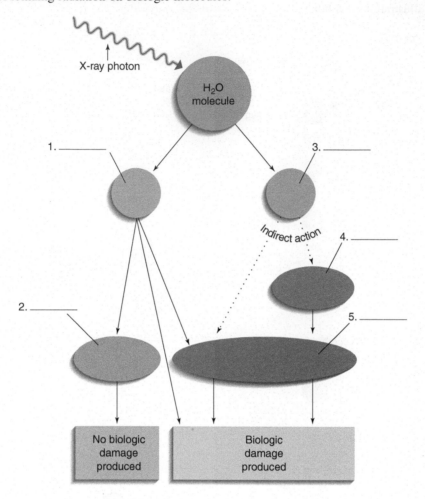

C. Examples of radiosensitive and radioinsensitive cells.

Radiosensitive Cells	Radioinsensitive Cells
1. _____	4. _____
2. _____	5. _____
3. _____	6. _____

Exercise 6: Short Answer

Answer the following questions by providing a short answer.

1. How can high-energy particles, such as alpha and beta particles and protons, ionize atoms?

_____

_____

2. What determines the extent to which different radiation modalities transfer energy into biologic tissue?

_____

_____

3. In what unit of measure is LET generally described?

_____

_____

4. Why can repair enzymes usually reverse the cellular damage caused by low-LET radiation?

_____

_____

5. What are free radicals?

_____

_____

6. Which cells in the human body are classified as somatic cells?

_____

_____

7. How does oxygen enhance the effects of ionizing radiation in biologic tissue?

_____

_____

8. List six ways in which damage to a cell's nucleus from ionizing radiation can reveal itself.

_____

_____

9. What is the difference between direct and indirect action of ionizing radiation on atoms or molecules in the human body?

_____

_____

10. If the nucleus in an adult human nerve cell is destroyed by exposure to ionizing radiation, what will happen to the cell?

_____

_____

11. How low a dose of ionizing radiation can cause menstrual irregularities, such as delay or suppression of menstruation?

_____

_____

12. List seven possible deleterious changes in biologic tissue caused by the random interaction of ionizing radiation with matter that can affect the cell nuclei.

_____

_____

13. On what three levels is radiation damage observed?

_____

_____

14. When does ionizing radiation cause complete chromosome breakage?

_____

_____

15. How was the law of Bergonié and Tribondeau established? What does it state?

_____

_____

Exercise 7: General Discussion or Opinion Questions

The following questions are intended to allow students to express their knowledge and understanding of the subject matter or to present a personal opinion. The questions may be used to stimulate class discussion. Because answers to these questions may vary, determination of the answer's acceptability is left to the discretion of the course instructor.

1. What events can occur when an x-ray photon interacts with and ionizes a water molecule in the human body?

2. What are the possible consequences of radiation exposure to the embryo-fetus throughout the entire period of gestation?

3. Contrast the differences between high-LET radiation and low-LET radiation.

4. What are the possible effects of ionizing radiation on DNA?

5. What factors govern cell radiosensitivity? What are the effects of ionizing radiation on various types of cells in the human body?

POST-TEST

The student should take this test after reading Chapter 7, finishing all accompanying textbook and workbook exercises, and completing any additional activities required by the course instructor. The student should complete the post-test with a score of 90% or higher before advancing to the next chapter. (Each of the following 20 questions is worth 5 points.)
Score = _____ %

1. A biologic reaction is produced by 7 Gy_t of a test radiation. It takes 21 Gy_t of 250-kVp x-rays to produce the same biologic reaction. What is the RBE of the test radiation?

_____

2. On what kinds of molecules in the human body does ionizing radiation most often act directly to produce molecular damage through an indirect action?

_____

3. Radiosensitivity of the individual cell governs the radiation dose required to cause _____.

4. Define LET, and identify how it is described.

_____

_____

5. What is the oxygen effect? What describes this effect numerically?

_____

_____

_____

6. The action of ionizing radiation is _____ when ionizing particles interact with a vital biologic macromole-cule such as DNA.

7. Because even low doses of ionizing radiation from diagnostic imaging procedures can cause chromosomal damage, which of the following should be done whenever possible?
   A. Avoid all x-ray procedures until age 60 years.
   B. Use a low-kVp and high-mAs technique.
   C. Shield the reproductive organs.
   D. Limit all radiographic procedures to just one projection per patient.

8. Immature ova are:
   A. Somewhat radioinsensitive
   B. Significantly radioinsensitive
   C. Slightly radiosensitive
   D. Very radiosensitive

9. The _____ theory concept is useful for explaining cell death and nonfatal cell abnormalities caused by expo-sure to radiation.

10. The action of ionizing radiation is _____ when ionizing particles interact with a water molecule, thus result-ing in the creation of ions and reactive free radicals that eventually produce toxic substances that can create biologic damage.

11. What types of blood cells are classified as most radiosensitive?

_____

12. What law states that the most pronounced radiation effects occur in cells with the least maturity and specialization, the greatest reproductive activity, and the longest mitotic phases?

_____

13. Changes in genes caused by the loss of or a change in a base in the DNA chain are called _____.

14. What is a cell survival curve used to display?

_____

_____

15. An ionized atom will not _____ properly in molecules.

16. What can result within a few days, if an adult receives a whole-body ionizing radiation dose of 0.25 Gy$_t$?

_____

17. If bone marrow cells have not been destroyed by exposure to ionizing radiation, they can _____ after a period of recovery.

18. A periodic _____ _____ is not recommended as a method of monitoring occupational radiation exposure because biologic damage already has been sustained when an irregularity is noted.

19. During the window of maximal sensitivity, a 0.1 Sv fetal equivalent dose is associated with as much as a 4% chance of _____ _____.

20. When does ionizing radiation cause complete chromosome breakage?

   _____

   _____

8 Early Tissue Reactions and Their Effects on Organ Systems

When biologic effects of radiation occur relatively soon after humans receive high doses of ionizing radiation, the biologic responses demonstrated are called *early effects*. Numerous laboratory animal studies and data from observation of some irradiated human populations provide substantial evidence of the consequences of such responses. Although early effects are not common in diagnostic imaging, they are discussed in Chapter 8 to provide the reader with a broader and more complete understanding of the impact of high radiation exposure on the human body.

CHAPTER HIGHLIGHTS

- Biologic effects that occur relatively soon after humans receive high doses of ionizing radiation are general referred to as *early effects*.
- Early tissue reactions are not common in diagnostic radiology.
- Somatic effects are *effects on the body* that was irradiated.
- Genetic effects are *effects on future generations* as a result of irradiation of germ cells in previous generations.
- Somatic tissue reactions include cell killing and are directly related to the dose of radiation received. As dose increases, so does the severity of these early tissue reactions.
    - Early tissue reactions vary depending on the duration of time after exposure to ionizing radiation. Subject to their nature, they may appear within minutes, hours, days, or weeks after receiving a high dose of ionizing radiation.
    - Possible high radiation dose consequences generally include nausea and fever, extreme fatigue, erythema, epilation, and blood and intestinal disorders. In addition, temporary or permanent sterility in the male and female and injury to the central nervous system (at extremely high radiation doses) can occur.
- Acute radiation syndrome (ARS) occurs in humans after whole-body reception of large doses of ionizing radiation delivered over a short period.
    - ARS can manifest as hematopoietic syndrome, gastrointestinal syndrome, and cerebrovascular syndrome.
    - ARS presents in four major response stages: prodromal, latent period, manifest illness, and recovery or death.
- Lethal dose (LD) 50/30 signifies the whole-body dose of ionizing radiation that can be lethal to 50% of an exposed population within 30 days.
    - LD 50/30 for adult humans is estimated to be 3 to 4 Gy_t without medical support.

- When cells are exposed to sublethal doses of ionizing radiation, repair and recovery are possible.
- After receiving a sublethal dose of radiation, surviving cells will be able to divide and thereby begin to repopulate in the irradiated region.
- Approximately 90% of radiation-induced damage may be repaired over time; 10% is irreparable.
- High radiation doses to any part of the human body can result in local tissue damage.
- Significant cell death usually results after a substantial radiation exposure, leading to potential atrophy of involved organs and tissues.
- Depending on the types of cells included and the dose of radiation received, recovery may be partial or complete, or it may fail to occur, resulting in death of the irradiated biologic structure.
- Factors such as radiosensitivity, reproductive characteristics, and growth rate govern organ and tissue response to radiation exposure.
- Many early radiologists and dentists developed radiodermatitis as a consequence of radiation exposure to the skin that eventually led to the development of cancerous lesions.
    - Human skin consists of three layers and several accessory structures, all of which are actively involved in the response of tissue to radiation exposure.
    - A single absorbed dose of 2 Gy_t can cause radiation-induced skin erythema within 24 to 48 hours after irradiation.
    - High radiation doses to the skin can cause moist and then dry desquamation.
    - Moderate radiation doses to the scalp can cause temporary hair loss, and large radiation doses can result in permanent hair loss.
    - Significant evidence of skin damage, as a consequence of exposure to orthovoltage radiation therapy, comes from oncology patients who underwent such treatments in earlier years for deep-seated tumors.
    - The use of high-level fluoroscopy for extended periods can result in radiation-induced skin injuries for patients.
- Human germ cells are relatively radiosensitive.
    - In males, a radiation dose of 0.1 Gy_t can depress the sperm population and possibly cause genetic mutations in future generations.
    - In females, a gonadal dose of 0.1 Gy_t may delay or suppress menstruation.
- Periodic blood counts have been replaced by personnel dosimeters as a means to monitor occupational radiation exposure.
    - Through the years, when predosimeter monitoring was employed, a whole-body dose of radiation as

low as 0.25 Gy$_t$ would produce measurable hematologic depression.

■ Mapping of chromosomes is called *karyotyping.*
  □ Karyotyping is done during metaphase, when each chromosome can be individually demonstrated and radiation-induced chromosome and chromatid aberrations can be observed.

□ Chromosomal damage can be caused by both low and high radiation doses.
□ Chromosome aberrations have been observed in individuals after completion of some imaging procedures in which high radiation dose rates were administered.

Exercise 1: Matching

Match the following terms with their definitions or associated phrases.

1. _____ Biologic dosimetry

2. _____ Skin

3. _____ LD 50/30

4. _____ Ovulation

5. _____ Spermatogonia

6. _____ Dermis

7. _____ Bone marrow syndrome

8. _____ Marshall Islanders

9. _____ Leukopenia

10. _____ Decrease

11. _____ Epilation

12. _____ Necrosis, or death

13. _____ Cerebrovascular syndrome

14. _____ Early tissue reactions

15. _____ ARS

16. _____ Oocytes

17. _____ 1920s and 1930s

18. _____ Pluripotential stem cell

19. _____ Prodromal stage

20. _____ Gastrointestinal syndrome

A. Stem cells of the testes that constantly reproduce

B. Early somatic effects on organ systems that result from high doses of radiation and appear within minutes, hours, days, or weeks after exposure

C. A single precursor cell from which all cells of the hematopoietic system develop

D. Form of ARS that occurs when people receive whole-body doses of ionizing radiation ranging from 1 to 10 Gy$_t$

E. Functions as an ongoing regeneration system for the human body; is relatively radiosensitive

F. Immature female germ cells

G. Population inadvertently subjected to high levels of fallout during an atomic bomb test in 1954

H. Result when an organ or tissue fails to recover from radiation exposure

I. What radiation exposure causes the number of red cells, white cells, and platelets in the circulating blood to do

J. An abnormal decrease in white blood corpuscles, usually below 5000/mm^3

K. Period during the female menstrual cycle when a mature follicle releases an ovum

L. Form of ARS that appears at a threshold dose of approximately 6 Gy$_t$

M. Signifies the whole-body dose of ionizing radiation that can be lethal to 50% of an exposed population within 30 days

N. Middle layer of skin composed of connective tissue

O. A method of dose assessment in which damaged biologic tissues are used to estimate radiation dose

P. Radiation sickness that occurs in humans after whole-body reception of large doses of ionizing radiation (1 Gy$_t$ or more) delivered over a short time

Q. Period when periodic blood counts were the only means of radiation exposure monitoring for radiation workers engaged in radiologic practices

R. Decrease in the number of blood cells in the circulating blood can result in a lack of vitality and this condition

S. The period after the initial stage of ARS during which no visible effects or symptoms of radiation exposure occur

T. Thermal trauma attributed to accumulated radiation exposure

21. _____ Manifest illness

U. After a period of about a week, during which no visible symptoms occur, symptoms again become visible during this stage of ARS

22. _____ Chromosome aberrations

V. The first stage of ARS, which occurs within hours after a whole-body absorbed dose of 1 Gy_t or more; characterized by nausea, vomiting, diarrhea, fatigue, and leukopenia

23. _____ Latent period

W. Deviation from normal development or growth

24. _____ Anemia

X. Form of ARS that results when the central nervous system and the cardiovascular system receive ionizing radiation doses of 50 Gy_t or more

25. _____ Burns

Y. Alopecia (loss of hair)

Exercise 2: Multiple Choice

Select the answer that *best* completes the following questions or statements.

1. After the reception of a high radiation dose, significant cell death usually results, leading to the shrinkage of organs and tissues. This process is referred to as:
   A. Atrophy
   B. Desquamation
   C. Erythema
   D. Radiodermatitis

2. Approximately what percentage of the human body's surface skin cells is replaced daily by stem cells from an underlying basal layer?
   A. 2%
   B. 12%
   C. 35%
   D. 50%

3. A cytogenetic analysis of chromosomes may be accomplished through the use of a chromosome map. This map is called a:
   A. Chromosomogram
   B. Karyograph
   C. Karyotype
   D. Photocytogenetic plot

4. How many mature ova are produced, matured, and made available for fertilization during a woman's reproductive life cycle?
   A. 50 to 100
   B. 100 to 200
   C. 300 to 400
   D. 400 to 500

5. Which of the following are parts of the hematopoietic system?
   1. Bone marrow
   2. Circulating blood
   3. Lymphoid organs
   A. 1 and 2 only
   B. 1 and 3 only
   C. 2 and 3 only
   D. 1, 2, and 3

6. Many early radiologists and dentists developed a significant reddening of the skin caused by exposure to ionizing radiation. This condition is called:
   A. Dermabrerration
   B. Desquamation
   C. Epidermatitis
   D. Radiodermatitis

7. Which of the following measures of lethality may be a more relevant indicator of outcome for humans?
   A. LD 10/30
   B. LD 50/30
   C. LD 50/60
   D. LD 100/60

8. Possible high radiation dose consequences that would result from exposure of the whole body to types of radiation other than x-ray include which of the following?
   1. Blood disorders
   2. Epilation
   3. Intestinal disorders
   A. 1 only
   B. 2 only
   C. 3 only
   D. 1, 2, and 3

9. In humans with the gastrointestinal form of ARS, the part of the body *most* severely affected is the:
   A. Brain
   B. Heart
   C. Large intestine
   D. Small intestine

10. After whole-body reception of large doses of ionizing radiation delivered over a short period, which of the following medical problems occurs in humans?
   A. Acute radiation syndrome
   B. Hypertension
   C. Multiple sclerosis
   D. Tuberculosis

11. The use of high-dose-rate fluoroscopy for extended periods can result in:
    A. A significant reduction in radiation-induced skin injuries for patients
    B. Minimal total-body radiation exposure for patients
    C. Radiation-induced skin injuries for patients
    D. The need for all patients to have periodic blood counts to monitor radiation dose received

12. What do the atomic bomb survivors of Hiroshima and Nagasaki, the Marshall Islanders inadvertently subjected to high levels of fallout during an atomic bomb test in 1954, and the nuclear radiation victims of the 1986 Chernobyl disaster have in common?
    A. All were exposed to low-level ionizing radiation.
    B. All were exposed to high levels of ionizing radiation, but no group members experienced any appreciable body damage.
    C. All were exposed to doses of ionizing radiation sufficient to cause ARS in many group members.
    D. These groups have nothing in common.

13. Which of the following factors govern organ and tissue response to radiation exposure?
    1. Growth rate
    2. Radiosensitivity
    3. Reproductive characteristics
    A. 1 and 2 only
    B. 1 and 3 only
    C. 2 and 3 only
    D. 1, 2, and 3

14. Which of the following *does not* generally cause early tissue reactions in humans exposed to radiation?
    A. Doses greater than 3 Gy_t
    B. Doses greater than 6 Gy_t
    C. Doses resulting from atomic bomb detonation
    D. Doses encountered in diagnostic radiology

15. The hematopoietic, gastrointestinal, and cerebrovascular syndromes are three separate dose-related syndromes that are part of the:
    A. Bone marrow syndrome
    B. Cytogenetic syndrome
    C. Prodromal syndrome
    D. Total-body syndrome

16. Without effective physical monitoring devices, what biologic criteria would play an important role in the identification of radiation casualties during the first 2 days after a nuclear disaster?
    A. Coma
    B. Edema in the cranial vault
    C. Meningitis
    D. Occurrence of nausea and excessive vomiting

17. Without medical support, the LD 50/30 for adult humans is estimated to be:
    A. 1.0 to 2.0 Gy_t
    B. 2.0 to 3.0 Gy_t
    C. 3.0 to 4.0 Gy_t
    D. 4.0 to 5.0 Gy_t

18. Infection, hemorrhage, and cardiovascular collapse are symptoms that can occur as part of acute radiation syndrome during the:
    1. Initial stage
    2. Latent period
    3. Stage called *manifest illness*
    A. 1 only
    B. 2 only
    C. 3 only
    D. 1, 2, and 3

19. Which of the following local tissues will experience immediate consequences from high radiation doses?
    1. Bone marrow
    2. Male and female reproductive organs
    3. Skin
    A. 1 and 2 only
    B. 1 and 3 only
    C. 2 and 3 only
    D. 1, 2, and 3

20. Imaging procedures generally result in:
    A. Relatively low doses of gonadal radiation for the patient and for imaging personnel
    B. Moderate doses of gonadal radiation for the patient and for imaging personnel
    C. High doses of gonadal radiation for the patient and for imaging personnel
    D. Relatively low doses of gonadal radiation for the patient and very high gonadal doses for imaging personnel

21. Which of the following are accessory structures of the skin?
    1. Hair follicles
    2. Sebaceous glands
    3. Sweat glands
    A. 1 and 2 only
    B. 1 and 3 only
    C. 2 and 3 only
    D. 1, 2, and 3

22. When cells are exposed to sublethal doses of ionizing radiation, repair and recovery may occur because cells:
    A. Are completely insensitive to radiation exposure
    B. Contain a repair mechanism inherent in their biochemistry (repair enzymes)
    C. Exposed to sublethal doses become hypoxic and recover more efficiently
    D. Mutate and become radioresistant

23. The testes of the human male and the ovaries of the female do *not* respond the same way to irradiation because:
    A. The oogonia, the ovarian stem cells of the female, constantly reproduce throughout life.
    B. There is a difference in the way in which male and female germ cells are produced and progress from elementary stem cells to mature cells.
    C. The oogonia become encapsulated by numerous primordial follicles during development.
    D. The spermatogonia of the male never mature.

24. When are human ovaries *most* radiosensitive?
    A. During the fetal stages of life and during early childhood
    B. After puberty and the onset of menstruation
    C. From 20 to 30 years of age
    D. During pregnancy

25. ARS is actually a collection of symptoms associated with:
    A. Exposure to low-level radiation
    B. Exposure to moderate-level radiation
    C. Exposure to high-level radiation
    D. Exposure to nonionizing radiation

Exercise 3: True or False

Circle *T* if the statement is true; circle *F* if the statement is false.

1. T F Current radiation protection programs rely on hematologic depression as a means for monitoring imaging personnel to assess if they have sustained any degree of radiation damage from occupational exposure.

2. T F If cells that are needed to clot blood are depleted, the risk of hemorrhage decreases.

3. T F Telophase is the phase of cell division in which chromosomal damage caused by radiation exposure can be evaluated.

4. T F If the effects of ionizing radiation are cell killing and directly related to the dose received, they are called *somatic tissue reactions*.

5. T F A person who has received a radiation exposure sufficient to cause radiation sickness will experience the initial stage of the syndrome within hours after the whole-body absorbed dose. After this stage, no visible symptoms occur for about 1 week.

6. T F Radiation exposure causes an increase in the number of red cells, white cells, and platelets in the circulating blood.

7. T F The LD 50/30 for adult humans is estimated to be 8 to 9 Gy_t.

8. T F The Japanese atomic bomb survivors of Hiroshima and Nagasaki are examples of a human population with ARS as a consequence of war.

9. T F Patients who underwent radiation therapy and who received orthovoltage radiation therapy treatments provide significant evidence of skin damage caused by radiation exposure.

10. T F Early tissue reactions occur within a long period after exposure to ionizing radiation.

11. T F Ionizing radiation produces the greatest amount of biologic damage in the human body when a small dose of sparsely ionizing (low-LET) radiation is delivered to a small or radiosensitive area of the body.

12. T F ARS actually is a collection of symptoms associated with low-LET radiation exposure.

13. T F Intestinal disorders are caused by radiation damage to the sensitive epithelial tissue lining the intestines.

14. T F Radiation doses ranging from 1 to 10 Gy_t produce an increase in the number of bone marrow stem cells.

15. T F In the human female, a gonadal dose of 0.1 Gy_t may delay or suppress menstruation.

16. T F Whole-body equivalent doses greater than 1 Gy_t are considered fatal regardless of medical treatment.

17. T F Moderate radiation doses can cause temporary hair loss, and large radiation doses can result in permanent hair loss.

18. T F Chromosomal damage can be caused by both low and high radiation doses.

19. T F Karyotyping is done during anaphase, when each chromosome can be individually demonstrated and radiation-induced chromosome and chromatid aberrations can be observed.

20. T F As a result of the effects of the atomic bomb in Japan and the nuclear accident at Chernobyl, the medical community has recognized the need for a thorough understanding of ARS and appropriate medical support of victims.

21. T F The massive explosion at the Chernobyl nuclear power plant on April 26, 1986, ejected several tons of burning graphite, uranium dioxide fuel, and other contaminants (e.g., cesium-137, iodine-131, and plutonium-239) vertically into the atmosphere in a 3-mile-high, radioactive plume of intense heat.

22. T F LD 50/30 for humans may be more accurate than LD 50/60.

23. T F The workers and firefighters at Chernobyl are examples of humans who died as a result of the gastrointestinal syndrome.

24. T F Only some layers of the skin and its accessory structures are actively involved in the response of the tissue to radiation exposure.

25. T F Highly specialized, nondividing cells in the circulating blood with the exception of lymphocytes are relatively insensitive to radiation.

Exercise 4: Fill in the Blank

Using the following Word Bank, fill in the blanks with the word or words that best complete the statements.

0.25	dose	neutrophils
1	early	photograph
2	functional	photomicrograph
100	grenz rays	platelets
200	high	radiation sickness
anemia	impaired fertility	radiosensitive
atrophy	indirect action	repair
biologic criteria	ionizing radiation	repopulation
chromosomal abnormalities	late	substantial dose
death	menstruation	William Herbert Rollins

1. A _____ _____ of ionizing radiation is required to produce biologic effects soon after irradiation, and the severity of these changes is _____ related.

2. Acute radiation syndrome (ARS) occurs when the whole body is exposed to _____ Gy_t or more.

3. _____ _____ is another term for *acute radiation syndrome* (ARS).

4. Depending on the length of time from the moment of irradiation to the first appearance of symptoms of radiation damage, the effects are classified as either _____ or _____ somatic effects.

5. Because the number of _____ decreases with loss of bone marrow function, the body loses a corresponding amount of its blood-clotting ability.

6. During the accident at the Chernobyl nuclear power plant in 1986, dose assessment was determined from _____ _____.

7. Whole-body radiation doses greater than 6 Gy_t may cause _____ of the entire population in 30 days without medical support.

8. When the processes of _____ and _____ work together, they aid in healing the body from radiation injury and promote recovery.

9. The amount of _____ damage sustained determines an organ's potential for recovery.

10. A response in biologic tissue can occur when any part of the human body receives a _____ radiation dose.

11. Safety practices such as wearing radiopaque glasses, enclosing the x-ray tube in a protective housing, irradiating only areas of interest on the patient, and covering the adjacent areas with radiopaque materials,[1] were recommendations made by _____ _____ _____.

12. A single absorbed dose of _____ Gy_t can cause radiation-induced skin erythema within 24 to 48 hours after irradiation.

13. During cardiovascular or therapeutic interventional procedures that use high-level fluoroscopy for extended periods, patient exposure rates have been estimated to range from _____ to _____ MGy$_a$/min and sometimes even greater.

14. Human germ cells are relatively_____.

15. If an ovum is not fertilized by a male sperm, it will be lost during _____ and not replaced.

16. High radiation doses to the testes can result in _____.

17. Because any dose of radiation to the gonads could cause _____ _____, the testes should be protected with lead shielding whenever possible.

18. In the years when periodic blood counts were used for radiation monitoring purposes, a whole-body dose as low as _____ Gy$_t$ would produce a measurable hematologic depression.

19. A decrease in the number of red blood cells in the circulating blood can result in a lack of vitality and a condition known as _____.

20. Most chromosomal damage results from the process of _____ _____ of ionizing radiation on vital biologic macromolecules.

21. A chromosome may consist of a _____ or _____.

22. Historically, skin diseases, such as ringworm, were treated and successfully cured by irradiating the affected area with _____ _____.

23. Almost every type of chromosome aberration can be caused by exposure to _____ _____.

24. A radiation dose of 0.5 Gy$_t$ causes a decrease in _____.

25. For the female, _____ _____ may not be the only consequence of gonadal irradiation.

Exercise 5: Labeling

Label the following table and illustrations.

A. Overview of acute radiation lethality.

Stage	Dose (Gy$_t$	Average Survival Time	Signs and Symptoms
1. _____	1	—	Nausea, vomiting, diarrhea, fatigue, leukopenia
2. _____	1-100	—	None
3. _____	1-10	6-8 wk (doses >2 Gy)	Nausea; vomiting; diarrhea; decrease in number of red blood cells, white blood cells, and platelets in the circulating blood; hemorrhage; infection
4. _____	6-10	3-10 days	Severe nausea, vomiting, diarrhea, fever, fatigue, loss of appetite, lethargy, anemia, leukopenia, hemorrhage, infection, electrolytic imbalance, and emaciation
5. _____	≥50	Several hours to 2 or 3 days	Same as hematopoietic and gastrointestinal, excessive nervousness, confusion, lack of coordination, loss of vision, a burning sensation of the skin, loss of consciousness, disorientation, shock, periods of agitation alternating with stupor, edema, loss of equilibrium, meningitis, prostration, respiratory distress, vasculitis, coma

B. Development of the germ cell from stem cell phase to the mature cell.

Male:

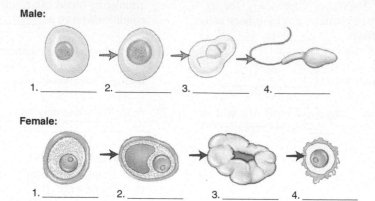

1._____ 2._____ 3._____ 4._____

Female:

1._____ 2._____ 3._____ 4._____

C. Progressive development of various cells from a single pluripotential stem cell.

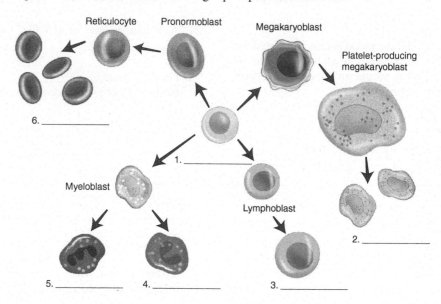

Exercise 6: Short Answer

Answer the following questions by providing a short answer.

1. What has provided substantial evidence of the consequences of early biologic responses to high doses of ionizing radiation?

_____

_____

2. During the explosion at the Chernobyl nuclear power plant in 1986, what are some of the radioactive materials that were ejected vertically into the atmosphere in a 3-mile-high radioactive plume of intense heat?

_____

_____

3. Name the four major response stages of ARS.

_____

_____

4. Name the three separate dose-related syndromes that occur as part of the total-body syndrome.

_____

_____

5. What happens to the human body when bone marrow cells are being destroyed by radiation exposure?

_____

_____

6. Why is a bone marrow transplant not an absolute cure for patients with the hematopoietic syndrome?

_____

_____

7. What are some symptoms of the cerebrovascular syndrome?

_____

_____

8. To what have the techniques used to study and observe the chromosomes of each human cell contributed?

_____

_____

9. What is the origin of the term *somatic*?

_____

_____

10. If both oxygenated and hypoxic cells receive a comparable dose of low-LET radiation, what impact will the radiation dose have on each of these types of cells?

_____

_____

11. What are the most important measures used to quantify human radiation lethality?

_____

_____

12. When the number of lymphocytes in the blood is decreased by exposure to ionizing radiation, what is the consequence to the human body?

_____

_____

13. When shedding of the outer layer of skin occurs after reception of higher radiation doses, how does it generally manifest?

_____

_____

14. What was the overall goal of radiation therapeutic treatment?

_____

_____

15. Why is LD 50/60 a more relevant indicator of outcome than LD 50/30 for humans who have received a substantial dose of ionizing radiation?

_____

_____

Exercise 7: General Discussion or Opinion Questions

The following questions are intended to allow students to express their knowledge and understanding of the subject matter or to present a personal opinion. The questions may be used to stimulate class discussion. Because answers to these questions may vary, determination of the answer's acceptability is left to the discretion of the course instructor.

1. What has been the mental and physical impact on the exposed population of the 1986 accident at the Chernobyl nuclear power plant?

2. What knowledge of early effects of high-dose radiation exposure has been gained from pioneers in the radiation field and from exposed populations?

3. How do human male and female germ cells differ in their development?

4. What type of local tissue damage can occur from high radiation exposure?

5. What is the potential for recovery for humans who receive nonlethal doses of radiation in the range of 1 to 2 Gy_t? On what factors does recovery depend? If death does occur, from what does it result?

POST-TEST

The student should take this test after reading Chapter 8, finishing all accompanying textbook and workbook exercises, and completing any additional activities required by the course instructor. The student should complete the post-test with a score of 90% or higher before advancing to the next chapter. (Each of the following 20 questions is worth 5 points.)
Score = _____ %

1. When biologic effects of radiation occur relatively soon after humans receive high doses of ionizing radiation, the biologic responses demonstrated are called _____ _____.

2. What are the three separate dose-related syndromes that occur as part of the total body syndrome?

_____

3. Acute radiation syndrome presents in four major response stages: _____, _____ _____, _____ _____, and _____ or _____.

4. When cells of the lymphatic system are damaged, the body:
   A. Increases its ability to combat infection
   B. Loses some of its ability to combat infection
   C. Manufactures large numbers of platelets to compensate for the damage
   D. Responds by repopulating mature erythrocytes in the circulating blood

100

5. What term is used to signify the whole-body dose of radiation that can be lethal to 50% of an exposed population within 30 days?

_____

6. Research has shown that repeated radiation injuries have a(n) _____ effect.

7. Some local tissues experience immediate consequences from high radiation doses. Which of the following are examples of such tissues?
   1. Bone marrow
   2. Male and female reproductive organs
   3. Skin
   A. 1 and 2 only
   B. 1 and 3 only
   C. 2 and 3 only
   D. 1, 2, and 3

8. *Epilation* is another term for:
   A. Decrease of red blood cells
   B. Increase of white blood cells
   C. Hair loss
   D. Shedding of the outer layer of skin

9. The use of high-level fluoroscopy for extended periods can result in which of the following in patients?
   1. Acute radiation syndrome
   2. Repair of damaged chromosomes
   3. Radiation-induced skin injuries
   A. 1 only
   B. 2 only
   C. 3 only
   D. 1, 2, and 3

10. Define the term *early tissue reactions.*

_____

_____

11. In which phase of cell division can chromosomal damage caused by radiation exposure be evaluated?

_____

12. Without effective physical monitoring devices, what played an important role in the identification of radiation casualties in the first 2 days after the 1986 accident at the Chernobyl nuclear power plant?

_____

_____

13. The workers and firefighters at Chernobyl are examples of humans who died as a result of the _____ syndrome.

14. What is the estimated LD 50/30 for adult humans if medical support is unavailable?

_____

15. A cytogenetic analysis of chromosomes may be accomplished through the use of a chromosome map called a _____.

Chapter **8** Early Tissue Reactions and Their Effects on Organ Systems

16. In females, a gonadal dose of _____ Gy$_t$ may delay or suppress menstruation. A single dose of _____ Gy$_t$ to the ovaries can result in temporary sterility, and a dose of _____ to _____ Gy$_t$ to the ovaries can result in permanent sterility.

17. In males, a radiation dose of _____ Gy$_t$ can depress the sperm population and possibly cause genetic mutations in future generations.

18. How do cells of the hematopoietic system develop?

_____

19. The cerebrovascular form of ARS results when the central nervous and cardiovascular systems receive doses of ionizing radiation of _____ Gy$_t$ or more.

20. The hematopoietic form of ARS is also called the _____ _____ _____.

Reference

1. Hidden giants, *ASRT Scanner* 41:1, 2008.

9 Stochastic Effects and Late Tissue Reactions of Radiation in Organ Systems

Radiation-induced damage at the cellular level may lead to measurable somatic and hereditary damage in the living organism as a whole further on in life. These *late effects* are the long-term results of radiation exposure. Some examples of measurable delayed biologic damage are cataracts, leukemia, and genetic mutations. Chapter 9 focuses on late tissue reactions and stochastic radiation effects in organ systems that occur months or years after radiation exposure.

CHAPTER HIGHLIGHTS

- Scientists use the information from epidemiologic studies to formulate dose-response graphic relationships to predict the risk of cancer in human populations exposed to low doses of ionizing radiation.
  - Curves that demonstrate radiation dose-response relationships can be either linear or nonlinear and depict either a threshold or a nonthreshold dose.
  - A linear nonthreshold (LNT) curve currently is used for most types of cancers.
  - Risk associated with low-level radiation other than cancer is usually estimated with the linear-quadratic nonthreshold curve (LQNT).
  - Late tissue reactions may be demonstrated graphically through the use of a linear threshold (LT) curve of radiation dose-response.
  - High-dose cellular response may be demonstrated through the use of a sigmoid threshold curve.
- Late effects include carcinogenesis, cataractogenesis, and embryologic (birth) defects.
- Effects that have no threshold, that occur arbitrarily, that have a severity that does not depend on dose, and that occur months or years after exposure are called *stochastic effects*.
- Cancer is the most important stochastic somatic effect caused by exposure to ionizing radiation.

- Risk estimates are given in terms of *absolute risk* or *relative risk*.
  - The absolute risk model forecasts that a specific number of malignancies will occur as a result of radiation exposure.
  - The relative risk model predicts that the number of excess cancers rises as the natural incidence of cancer increases with advancing age in a population.
  - Linear and linear-quadratic models are used for extrapolation of risk from high-dose to low-dose data.
- The first trimester of pregnancy is the most critical period for radiation exposure of the embryo-fetus.
  - Radiation-induced congenital abnormalities can occur approximately 10 days to 12 weeks after conception.
  - Skeletal abnormalities most frequently occur from weeks 3 to 20.
- Radiation exposure even in the second and third trimesters can potentially cause congenital abnormalities, functional disorders, and a predisposition to the development of childhood cancer.
- Genetic effects of ionizing radiation are biologic effects on generations yet unborn.
  - Radiation-induced abnormalities are caused by unrepaired damage to DNA molecules in the sperm or ova of an adult.
  - There is no 100% safe gonadal radiation dose; even the smallest radiation dose could cause some hereditary damage.
  - Doubling dose measures the effectiveness of ionizing radiation in causing mutations; it is the radiation dose that causes the number of spontaneous mutations in a given generation to increase to two times their original number.
  - For humans, the doubling dose is estimated to have a mean value of 1.56 Sv.

103

Exercise 1: Matching

Match the following terms with their definitions or associated phrases.

1. _____ Female Japanese atomic bomb survivors

2. _____ Mutagens

3. _____ Fetal radiosensitivity

4. _____ Radon

5. _____ Linear nonthreshold dose-response curve

6. _____ Relative risk model

7. _____ Cancer and genetic effects

8. _____ Cataracts

9. _____ Linear quadratic nonthreshold dose-response curve

10. _____ Thorotrast

11. _____ Mutant genes

12. _____ Thyroid cancer

13. _____ Point mutations

14. _____ Skeletal damage

15. _____ Radiobiologists

16. _____ Absolute risk model

17. _____ Doubling dose

18. _____ Linear

19. _____ Dominant mutations

20. _____ Recessive mutations

21. _____ Nonlinear

22. _____ Embryologic effects (birth effects or defects)

23. _____ Uranium

24. _____ Carcinogenesis

25. _____ Zero

A. Implies that the biologic response to ionizing radiation is directly proportional to the dose

B. A dose-response curve that is curved to some degree

C. Radioactive element with a half-life of 4.5 billion years

D. Example of stochastic effects that probably do not have a threshold

E. Certain agents such as ionizing radiation, viruses, and specific chemicals that can increase the frequency of mutations

F. Forecasts that a specific number of malignancies will occur as a result of exposure to ionizing radiation

G. Considered to be a late tissue reaction that is nonrandom

H. As of April 1996, more than 700 cases of this disease were diagnosed among children and adolescents residing near the Chernobyl nuclear power plant

I. Radioactive contrast agent used from 1925 to 1945 for diagnostic angiography that caused liver and spleen cancer in many patients after a latent period of 15 to 20 years

J. Estimates the risk associated with low-level radiation

K. Gas that emanates through tiny gaps in the rocks and creates an insidious airborne hazard to uranium miners

L. Group of people who provide strong evidence that ionizing radiation can induce breast cancer

M. Safe gonadal dose of ionizing radiation for humans

N. Predicts that the number of excess cancers will increase as the natural incidence of cancer increases with advancing age in a population

O. Genetic mutations at the molecular level

P. Mutations probably expressed in the offspring

Q. The radiation dose that causes the number of spontaneous mutations occurring in a given generation to increase to two times their original number

R. The production or origin of cancer

S. Decreases as gestation progresses

T. Mutations probably not expressed for several generations

U. These cannot properly govern the cell's normal chemical reactions or properly control the sequence of amino acids in the formation of specific proteins

V. People who engage in research by using information from epidemiologic studies to formulate dose-response estimates for making predictions on the risk of cancer in human populations from low doses of ionizing radiation

W. Damage to an organism that occurs as a result of exposure to ionizing radiation during the embryonic stage of development

X. A dose-response curve that exists as a straight line

Y. Abnormalities that most frequently occur from weeks 3 to 20 of gestation in humans

Exercise 2: Multiple Choice

Select the answer that *best* completes the following questions or statements.

1. Epidemiologic studies are of significant value to scientists who use the information from these studies to formulate dose-response estimates to predict the risk of:
   A. Cancer in human populations exposed to low doses of ionizing radiation
   B. Cataract formation in humans exposed to low doses of ionizing radiation
   C. Radiodermatitis in radiologic technologists working in the field between 1970 and 1990
   D. Radiodermatitis in radiologic technologists working in the field from 1990 to the present

2. Which of the following measures the effectiveness of ionizing radiation in causing mutations?
   A. Lethal dose (LD) 50/30
   B. Doubling dose
   C. Relative biologic effectiveness (RBE)
   D. Dose-response curve

3. Recent studies of atomic bomb survivors tend to support the _____ risk model over the _____ risk model.
   A. Absolute, relative
   B. Relative, absolute
   C. Stochastic, nonstochastic
   D. Nonstochastic, stochastic

4. The linear dose-response model is used to establish radiation protection standards because it accurately reflects the effects of:
   A. Both high–linear energy transfer (LET) and low-LET types of radiation at higher doses
   B. Both high-LET and low-LET types of radiation at lower doses
   C. High-LET radiation at higher doses
   D. Low-LET radiation at lower doses

5. The number of excess cancers, or cancers that would *not* have occurred in a given population in question without exposure to ionizing radiation, may be predicted by which of the following?
   1. Absolute risk model
   2. Nonstochastic risk model
   3. Relative risk model
   A. 1 and 2 only
   B. 1 and 3 only
   C. 2 and 3 only
   D. 1, 2, and 3

6. After the radiation accident at the Chernobyl nuclear power plant in 1986, many children in Poland and some other countries were given potassium iodide in an attempt to prevent:
   A. Breast cancer
   B. Bone cancer
   C. Leukemia
   D. Thyroid cancer

7. *Most* radiation-induced genetic mutations are:
   A. Dominant mutations
   B. Expressed in first-generation offspring
   C. Spontaneous mutations unique to radiation
   D. Recessive mutations

8. Spontaneous mutations in human genetic material cause a wide variety of diseases, including:
   1. Down syndrome
   2. Hemophilia
   3. Sickle cell anemia
   A. 1 only
   B. 2 only
   C. 3 only
   D. 1, 2, and 3

9. When exposure to ionizing radiation causes proliferation of the white blood cells, the radiation-induced disease that occurs is:
   A. Anemia
   B. Erythroleukosis
   C. Granulocytopenia
   D. Leukemia

10. Radiation can induce genetic damage by which of the following means?
    A. Interacting with somatic cells of only one parent
    B. Interacting with somatic cells of both parents
    C. Altering the essential base coding sequence of DNA
    D. None of the above; radiation cannot induce genetic damage

11. Using the doubling dose concept to measure the effectiveness of ionizing radiation at causing mutations, if 9% of the offspring in each generation are born with mutations in the absence of radiation other than background levels, administration of the doubling dose to all members of the population eventually would increase the number of mutations to:
    A. 18%
    B. 36%
    C. 72%
    D. 100%

12. Which of the following groups of individuals received radiation treatment that indicated radiation can cause breast cancer when healthy breast tissue was exposed to radiation?
    A. Female patients treated for malignant breast disease
    B. Male patients treated for malignant breast disease
    C. Patients treated for benign postpartum mastitis
    D. Radiologic technologists currently working in diagnostic imaging

13. For a recessive mutation to appear in an offspring:
    A. Both parents must have the same genetic defect.
    B. Both parents must have only dominant genes.
    C. Neither parent needs to have a genetic defect.
    D. Only one parent must have a genetic defect.

14. Based on revised atomic bomb data from Hiroshima and Nagasaki, radiation-induced leukemias and solid tumors in the survivors may be attributed predominantly to:
    A. Alpha particle exposure
    B. Beta particle exposure
    C. Gamma radiation exposure
    D. X-radiation exposure

15. Following the Chernobyl nuclear power plant accident, what health effect was found to have increased beyond normal incidence in a human population in the vicinity of the power plant?
    A. Bone tumors in adult females
    B. Lung cancers in smokers
    C. Thyroid cancer in children
    D. Skin cancers in males

16. Which of the following are examples of stochastic effects?
    A. Nausea and vomiting
    B. Epilation and fatigue
    C. Diarrhea and leukopenia
    D. Cancer and genetic defects

17. During the embryonic stage of development:
    A. All life forms seem to be most vulnerable to radiation exposure.
    B. Only a very small percentage of life forms seem to be vulnerable to radiation exposure.
    C. A significant percentage of life forms seem to be vulnerable to radiation exposure.
    D. Exposure to radiation cannot damage any life form.

18. Young women who painted watch dials with radium in some factories in New Jersey in the 1920s and 1930s eventually developed which of the following conditions as a consequence of their exposure to radiation?
    1. Osteoporosis
    2. Osteogenic sarcoma
    3. Carcinomas of the epithelial lining of the nasopharynx and paranasal sinuses
    A. 1 only
    B. 2 only
    C. 3 only
    D. 1, 2, and 3

19. Radium decays with a half-life of 1622 years by alpha particle emission to the radioactive element:
    A. Uranium
    B. Radon
    C. Plutonium
    D. Americium

20. Mutant genes cannot properly govern the cell's normal chemical reactions or properly control the sequence of _____ in the formation of specific proteins.
    A. Amino acids
    B. Enzymes
    C. Hormones
    D. Peptic acids

21. Which of the following are mutagens?
    1. Elevated temperatures
    2. Ionizing radiation
    3. Viruses
    A. 1 and 2 only
    B. 1 and 3 only
    C. 2 and 3 only
    D. 1, 2, and 3

22. The only concrete evidence that ionizing radiation causes genetic effects comes from:
    A. Human populations exposed to low radiation doses
    B. Human populations exposed to moderate radiation doses
    C. Human populations exposed to high radiation doses
    D. Extensive experiments with fruit flies and mice at high radiation doses

23. Which of the following led to the development of the doubling dose concept?
    A. Animal studies of radiation-induced genetic effects
    B. Human studies of radiation-induced genetic effects
    C. Animal studies of radiation-induced somatic effects
    D. Human studies of radiation-induced somatic effects

24. Cataracts, leukemia, and genetic mutations are examples of:
    A. Diseases that are not caused by ionizing radiation
    B. Measurable radiation-induced biologic damage
    C. Diseases caused by nonionizing radiation
    D. Radiation-induced biologic damage that cannot be measured

25. Members of which of the following groups of radiologic technologists have demonstrated the *greatest* risk of dying of breast cancer as a consequence of their occupation?
    A. Technologists who began working before 1940
    B. Technologists who began working after 1950
    C. Women employed as technologists after 1960
    D. Women employed as technologists after 2000

Exercise 3: True or False

Circle *T* if the statement is true; circle *F* if the statement is false.

1. T F Cataracts, leukemia, and genetic mutations are examples of measurable radiation-induced biologic damage.

2. T F If a threshold relationship exists between a radiation dose and a biologic response, even the smallest dose of ionizing radiation will have some biologic effect on a living organism.

3. T F The Biological Effects on Ionizing Radiation (BEIR) Committee believes that the linear-quadratic threshold curve of radiation dose-response is a more accurate reflection of stochastic and genetic effects at low-dose levels from low-LET radiation.

4. T F Effects of radiation exposure that have no threshold, that occur arbitrarily, that have a severity that does not depend on dose, and that occur months or years after exposure are called *stochastic effects*.

5. T F Low-level doses are a consideration for patients and personnel exposed to ionizing radiation as a result of diagnostic imaging procedures.

6. T F Distinguishing radiation-induced cancer by its physical appearance is relatively easy because it looks very different from cancers initiated by other agents.

7. T F Any nonlethal radiation dose received by the germ cells can cause chromosome mutations that may be transmitted to successive generations.

8. T F Hereditary disorders are present in approximately 50% of all living newborns in the United States.

9. T F The impact of the atomic bomb dosimetry revision is a significant increase in cancer risk estimates.

10. T F Radium watch dial painters of the 1920s and 1930s provide proof of radiation cataractogenesis.

11. T F Many cases of radiation-induced skin cancer among radiation workers have been documented in recent years.

12. T F The term *linear-quadratic* implies that the equation that best fits the data has components that depend on dose to the first power (linear or straightline behavior) and also on dose squared (quadratic or curved behavior).

13. T F Technologists who entered the medical radiation industry in 1950 or later have demonstrated a somewhat higher risk of dying from leukemia compared with individuals who entered the workforce before 1950.

14. T F Conclusive proof exists that low-level ionizing radiation doses (i.e., those below 0.1 Gy) cause a significant increase in the risk of malignancy.

15. T F Currently, evidence of radiation-induced hereditary effects has not been observed in persons employed in diagnostic imaging or in patients undergoing radiologic examinations.

16. T F Irradiation of the embryo-fetus during the first 12 weeks of development to equivalent doses in excess of 200 mSv often may result in death or severe congenital abnormalities.

17. T F The effect of low-level ionizing radiation on the embryo-fetus can only be estimated.

18. T F Genetic (hereditary) effects occur as a result of radiation-induced damage to the DNA molecule in the sperm or ova of an adult.

107

19. T F Follow-up studies of the Japanese atomic bomb survivors of Hiroshima and Nagasaki who did not die of acute radiation syndrome (ARS) have not demonstrated late tissue reactions and stochastic effects of ionizing radiation.

20. T F For humans, the doubling dose is estimated to have a mean value of 1.56 Sv.

21. T F Information obtained from a radiation dose-response curve can be used to predict the risk of malignancy in human populations exposed to low levels of ionizing radiation.

22. T F The lens of the eye contains opaque fibers that transmit light.

23. T F Organ atrophy is the most important late stochastic somatic effect caused by exposure to ionizing radiation.

24. T F The 1989 BEIR V Report supported use of the linear-quadratic model of radiation dose response for leukemia only.

25. T F During the 1940s and early 1950s, to reduce an enlarged thymus gland in infants with respiratory disorders, physicians treated the babies with therapeutic doses of x-radiation (1.2-60 Gy$_t$), resulting in a substantial dose to the nearby thyroid gland; this caused thyroid nodules and carcinomas some 20 years later.

Exercise 4: Fill in the Blank

Using the following Word Bank, fill in the blanks with the word or words that *best* complete the statements.

1.56	hereditary (genetic)	radiosensitive
4:1	iodine	reticuloendothelial
10:1	irradiated	risk
breast	lens	somatic
calcium	leukemia (may be used more	stem
cancer-causing	than once)	threshold
cancers	linear	Thorotrast
cellular	low	thyroid (may be used more
damaged	malignancy	than once)
death	months	time
first	natural	underestimate
follow-up studies	overestimate	years

1. Radiation-induced damage at the cellular level may lead to measurable _____ and _____ damage in the living organism as a whole further on in life.

2. A radiation dose-response curve is either _____ or nonlinear and depicts either a _____ dose or a nonthreshold dose.

3. In establishing radiation protection standards, the regulatory agencies have chosen to be conservative and use a model that could _____ risk but is not expected to _____ risk.

4. The incident rates at which malignancies occur as a consequence of irradiation are determined by comparing the _____ incidence of cancer occurring in a human population with the incidence of cancer occurring in an _____ population.

5. The _____ for radiation-induced cancer in radiation workers is not really measurable at _____ doses encountered in diagnostic imaging.

6. Late somatic effects are effects that appear _____ or _____ after exposure to ionizing radiation.

7. In humans, radiation-induced _____ may take 5 or more years to develop.

8. Because radium is chemically similar to _____, it was incorporated into the bone tissue of many radium watch dial painters in the early 1920s and 1930s who placed the radium-containing paint-saturated brush tip on their lips to draw the bristles of the brush to a fine point before painting the watch dial.

9. Possessing high-LET radiation, alpha particles passing through a person's lungs have a high probability of producing a great deal of _____ damage.

10. According to a study of 146,000 U.S. radiologic technologists, those who began working before 1940 had the greatest risk of dying of _____ cancer.

11. The mean value of the radiation doubling equivalent dose for humans, as determined from children of the atomic bomb survivors of Hiroshima and Nagasaki, is _____ Sv.

12. From 1925 to 1945, when used as a contrast agent and administered by an intravascular injection, _____, a radioactive material, emitted alpha particles that were deposited in the patient's _____ system.

13. Radiation dose-response curves can be used to attempt to predict the risk of _____ in human populations exposed to low levels of ionizing radiation.

14. The _____ gland is adjacent to the thymus gland.

15. Numerous studies of Japanese female atomic bomb survivors have indicated a relative risk for breast cancer ranging from _____ to as high as _____.

16. Epidemiologic data on the Hiroshima atomic bomb survivors indicate that a linear relationship exists between radiation dose and radiation-induced _____.

17. Radiation actually is not a highly effective _____ agent.

18. The 1986 radiation accident at the Chernobyl nuclear power station necessitates long-term _____ _____ to assess the magnitude and severity of late effects on the exposed population.

19. During the first 10 years after the Chernobyl disaster, the incidence of _____ cancer increased dramatically among children living in the regions of Belarus, Ukraine, and Russia, where the heaviest radioactive _____ contamination occurred.

20. Latent period refers to the _____ between a radiation event and the occurrence of a radiation bioeffect.

21. Early studies of the Chernobyl victims did not demonstrate a significant increase in the incidence of _____.

22. The _____ of the eye contains transparent fibers that transmit light.

23. Because embryonic cells begin dividing and differentiating after conception, they are extremely _____ and therefore may easily be _____ by exposure to ionizing radiation.

24. The _____ trimester of pregnancy seems to be the most crucial period with regard to irradiation of the embryo-fetus because the embryo-fetus contains a large number of _____ cells during this period of gestation.

25. During the preimplantation period (approximately 0 to 9 days after conception), the fertilized ovum divides and forms a ball-like structure containing undifferentiated cells. If this structure is irradiated with a dose in the range of 0.05 to 0.15 Gy_t, embryonic _____ occurs.

Exercise 5: Labeling

Label the following illustrations and list.

A. Radiation dose-response curves. (Hint: The terms are included in the figure legend in the textbook.)

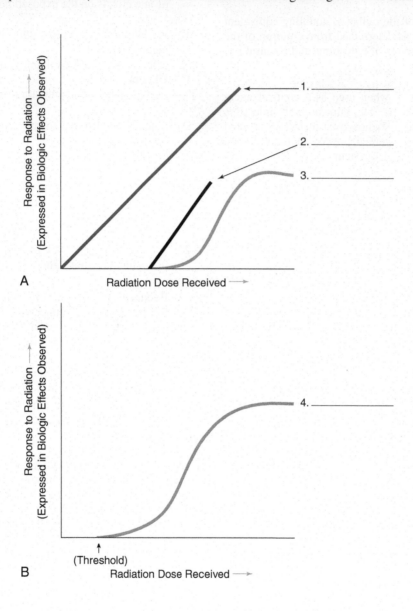

B. Radiation dose-response curve.

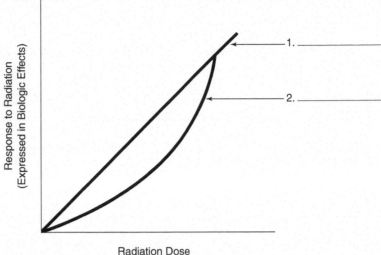

C. Late somatic effects.

Late Tissue Reactions

1. _____

2. _____

3. _____

4. _____

5. _____

6. _____

Stochastic Effects

1. _____

2. _____

Exercise 6: Short Answer
Answer the following questions by providing a short answer.

1. With reference to ionizing radiation, how do threshold and nonthreshold relationships differ in terms of radiation dose and biologic response?

_____

_____

2. What type of experiments and data provide the foundation for a linear, threshold curve of radiation dose-response?

_____

_____

3. Of what do epidemiologic studies consist, and how is the risk of radiation-induced cancer determined?

_____

_____

4. To minimize the possibility of genetic effects in those persons engaged in the practice of medical imaging, and in patients, what precautions must be taken?

_____

_____

5. According to members of the scientific and medical communities, what three categories of health consequences related to low-level radiation dose require further study?

_____

_____

6. Name three major types of late effects, and state how each type of effect is regarded.

_____

_____

7. What human evidence exists for radiation cataractogenesis?

_____

_____

8. What happens to fetal radiosensitivity as gestation progresses? What are the possible consequences to the developing human fetus of irradiation during the second and third trimesters of pregnancy?

_____

_____

9. What impact do mutagens such as ionizing radiation have on genetic mutations that occur as part of the natural order of events?

_____

_____

10. Name two models that researchers commonly use for extrapolation of the risk of ionizing radiation from high-dose data to low-dose data.

_____

_____

11. What evidence exists that ionizing radiation causes genetic effects?

_____

_____

12. What types of point mutations is radiation thought to cause?

_____

_____

13. What has led to the development of the doubling dose concept?

_____

_____

14. List the three stages of gestation in human beings, and identify the period in the pregnancy to which they correspond.

_____

_____

15. Why were the immediate families of uranium miners extremely vulnerable to radiation-induced cancers?

_____

_____

Exercise 7: General Discussion or Opinion Questions

The following questions are intended to allow students to express their knowledge and understanding of the subject matter or to present a personal opinion. The questions may be used to stimulate class discussion. Because answers to these questions may vary, determination of an answer's acceptability is left to the discretion of the course instructor.

1. What is the long-range global impact of the 1986 Chernobyl nuclear power plant accident?

2. How does the radiosensitivity of the fetus during the third trimester of pregnancy compare with fetal radiosensitivity during the first trimester? What protective measures can be taken during each trimester to protect the fetus from unnecessary radiation exposure?

3. What human evidence exists that proves ionizing radiation induces cancer?

4. How is the concept of risk used to predict cancer incidence for populations exposed to ionizing radiation?

5. Identify populations with significant rates of radiation-induced cancer, and explain the circumstances that led to such an occurrence.

POST-TEST

The student should take this test after reading Chapter 9, finishing all accompanying textbook and workbook exercises, and completing any additional activities required by the course instructor. The student should complete the post-test with a score of 90% or higher before advancing to the next chapter. (Each of the following 20 questions is worth 5 points.)
Score = _____ %

1. What is the period of gestation in humans that approximately corresponds with 10 days to 12 weeks after conception?

_____

2. What is the most important stochastic effect of exposure to ionizing radiation?

_____

3. When are all life forms most vulnerable to radiation exposure?

_____

4. Using the doubling dose concept to measure the effectiveness of ionizing radiation at causing mutations, if 4% of the offspring in each generation are born with mutations in the absence of radiation other than background levels, administration of the doubling dose to all members of the population eventually would increase the number of mutations to _____%.

113

5. Which risk model is used to forecast that a specific number of malignancies will occur as a result of exposure to ionizing radiation?

_____

6. How can late tissue reactions be demonstrated graphically?

_____

7. Which radiation dose-response curve model implies that the biologic response to ionizing radiation is directly proportional to the dose?

_____

8. Revised atomic bomb data for Hiroshima and Nagasaki suggest that radiation-induced leukemias and solid tumors in the survivors may be attributed predominantly to exposure to which of the following types of radiation?
   A. Alpha particles
   B. Beta particles
   C. Gamma rays
   D. Neutrons

9. Which of the following groups provide evidence for radiation carcinogenesis?
   1. Radium watch dial painters (1920s and 1930s)
   2. Early medical radiation workers (1896-1910)
   3. Japanese atomic bomb survivors (1945)
   A. 1 and 2 only
   B. 1 and 3 only
   C. 2 and 3 only
   D. 1, 2, and 3

10. How may risk estimates to predict cancer incidence in a population be given?

_____

_____

11. Where is the sigmoid, or S-shaped (nonlinear), threshold curve of the radiation dose-response relationship generally employed?

_____

_____

12. What incapacities are associated with mutant genes?

_____

_____

13. What disease occurred in the children of the Marshall Islanders who were inadvertently subjected to high levels of fallout during an atomic bomb test on March 1, 1954?

_____

14. What does the term *linear-quadratic* mean?

_____

_____

15. How can ionizing radiation induce genetic damage?

_____

_____

16. What are mutations in genes and DNA that occur at random as a natural phenomenon known as?

_____

17. According to a study of 146,000 U.S. radiologic technologists, those who began working before 1940 had the _____ risk of dying of breast cancer.

18. With reference to ionizing radiation, what does the term *threshold* mean?

_____

_____

19. The probability that a single dose of ionizing radiation of approximately _____ Gy_t will induce the formation of cataracts is high.

20. What currently is considered the most pronounced health consequence of the radiation accident at the Chernobyl nuclear power plant?

_____

_____

10 Dose Limits for Exposure to Ionizing Radiation

Exposure of the general public, patients, and radiation workers to ionizing radiation must be limited to minimize the risk of harmful biologic effects. To this end, scientists have developed occupational and nonoccupational effective dose (EfD) limits and equivalent dose (EqD) limits for tissues and organs such as the lens of the eye, skin, hands, and feet. This information is discussed in Chapter 10, which also covers the EfD limiting system that has been incorporated into Title 10 of the Code of Federal Regulations, Part 20, a document prepared and distributed by the U.S. Office of the Federal Register. The rules and regulations of the Nuclear Regulatory Commission (NRC) and fundamental radiation protection standards governing occupational radiation exposure are included in this document.

CHAPTER HIGHLIGHTS

- Effective dose limiting system:
  - Adherence to occupational and nonoccupational EfD limits helps prevent harmful biologic effects of radiation exposure.
  - The concept of radiation exposure and the associated risk of radiation-induced malignancy is the basis of the EfD limiting system.
  - The sum of both external and internal whole-body exposures is considered when establishing the cumulative EfD (CumEfD) limit.
  - Accounting for tissue weighting factors is important because various tissues and organs do not have the same degree of sensitivity.
  - Different biologic threats posed by different types of ionizing radiation must be taken into consideration even when the absorbed dose is the same.
- Radiation hormesis is the hypothesis that a positive effect exists for certain populations that are continuously exposed to moderately higher levels of radiation.
- Major organizations involved in regulating radiation exposure include the following:
  - The United Nations Scientific Committee on the Effects of Atomic Radiation (UNSCEAR) and the National Academy of Sciences/National Research Council Committee on the Biological Effects of Ionizing Radiation (NAS/NRC-BEIR) supply information to the International Commission on Radiological Protection (ICRP).
  - The ICRP makes recommendations on occupational and public dose limits.
- The National Council on Radiation Protection and Measurements (NCRP) reviews ICRP recommendations and may adopt them into recommendations for U.S. radiation protection policy.
  - The NRC is the watchdog of the nuclear energy industry; it controls the manufacture and use of radioactive substances.
  - The Environmental Protection Agency (EPA) develops and enforces regulations pertaining to the control of environmental radiation.
  - The U.S. Food and Drug Administration (FDA) regulates the design and manufacture of products used in the radiation industry.
  - The Occupational Safety and Health Administration (OSHA) monitors the workplace and regulates occupational exposure to radiation.
- Individual health care facilities establish a radiation safety committee (RSC) and designate a radiation safety officer (RSO).
  - The RSO is responsible for developing a radiation safety program for the health care facility; he or she maintains personnel radiation-monitoring records and provides counseling in radiation safety.
- The ALARA concept (optimization) states that radiation exposure should be kept "as low as reasonably achievable."
- Serious radiation-induced responses may be classified as having either tissue reactions or stochastic effects.
  - Tissue reactions are those biologic somatic effects of ionizing radiation that exhibit a threshold dose below which the effect does not normally occur and above which the severity of the biologic damage increases as the dose increases.
  - Stochastic effects are nonthreshold, randomly occurring biologic somatic changes in which the chance of occurrence of the effect rather than the severity of the effect is proportional to the dose of ionizing radiation.
- EfD limits for occupationally exposed personnel:
  - The NCRP has established an annual occupational EfD limit of 50 mSv and a lifetime EfD that does not exceed 10 times the occupationally exposed person's age in years.
  - Internal action limits are established by health care facilities to trigger an investigation to uncover the reasons for any unusual high exposures received by individual staff members.

Exercise 1: Matching

Match the following terms with their definitions or associated phrases.

1. _____ NCRP reports

2. _____ EfD limiting system

3. _____ EfD

4. _____ ICRP

5. _____ RSO

6. _____ UNSCEAR

7. _____ Negligible individual dose (NID)

8. _____ Annual occupational EfD limit

9. _____ ALARA concept

10. _____ NARM

11. _____ §10 CFR 35.50 and §10 CFR 35.900 of the *Code of Federal Regulations*

12. _____ *Annals of ICRP*

13. _____ Action limits

14. _____ Radiation Control for Health and Safety Act of 1968 (Public Law 90-602)

15. _____ OSHA

16. _____ BEIR reports

17. _____ FDA

18. _____ EfD limit

19. _____ NRC

A. Cancerous neoplasms caused by exposure to ionizing radiation

B. Optimization for radiation protection

C. Documents that identify the necessary training and experience for an RSO

D. Strictly an equipment performance standard in which diagnostic x-ray equipment was included

E. Agency that has the power to enforce radiation protection standards

F. "Indicates the ratio of the risk of stochastic effects attributable to irradiation of a given organ or tissue *(T)* to the total risk when the whole body is uniformly irradiated"[1]

G. International authority on the safe use of sources of ionizing radiation. Responsible for providing clear and consistent radiation guidance through its recommendations for occupational and public dose limits

H. Lifetime EfD limit

I. Naturally occurring and/or accelerator-produced materials

J. Evaluates human and environmental ionizing radiation exposures from a variety of sources, including radioactive materials, radiation-producing machines, and radiation accidents

K. Responsible for regulations concerning an employee's "right to know" with regard to hazards that may be present in the workplace

L. Federal legislation requiring the establishment of minimal standards for the accreditation of educational programs for persons who perform radiologic procedures and the certification of such persons

M. Established by health care facilities to trigger an investigation to uncover the reason for any abnormal exposure received by individual staff members

N. Set of numeric dose limits that are based on calculations of the various risks of cancer and genetic (hereditary) effects to tissues or organs exposed to radiation

O. Conducts an ongoing product radiation control program, regulating the design and manufacture of electronic products, including diagnostic x-ray equipment

P. An upper boundary limit for radiation workers for yearly whole-body exposure (excluding personal medical and natural background exposure) of 50 mSv/yr

Q. An annual EfD that provides a low-exposure cutoff level so that regulatory agencies may consider a level of effective dose as being of negligible risk

R. Normally a medical physicist, health physicist, radiologist, or other individual qualified through adequate training and experience. This person has been designated by a health care facility and approved by the NRC and the state

S. Scientific journals published by the ICRP

20. _____ Cumulative effective dose (CumEfD) limit

21. _____ EqD limit

22. _____ Tissue weighting factor (W_T)

23. _____ Radiation-induced malignancy

24. _____ Consumer-Patient Radiation Health and Safety Act of 1981 (Title IX of Public Law 97-35)

25. _____ Code of standards for diagnostic x-ray equipment

T. The sum of both external and internal whole-body exposures is considered when establishing this limit

U. Publications that list studies of biologic effects and associated risk of groups of people who were either routinely or accidentally exposed to ionizing radiation

V. Concerns the upper boundary dose of ionizing radiation that results in a negligible risk of body injury or hereditary damage

W. Applies to complete x-ray systems and major components manufactured after August 1, 1974

X. Publications that provide the most recent guidance on radiation protection

Y. A radiation quantity used for radiation protection purposes when a person receives exposure from various types of ionizing radiation

Exercise 2: Multiple Choice

Select the answer that *best* completes the following questions or statements.

1. Why have scientists developed occupational and non-occupational effective dose limits for exposure to ionizing radiation?
   A. To eliminate all harmful effects of low-level ionizing radiation exposure
   B. To minimize the risk of harmful biologic effects to the general public, patients, and radiation workers
   C. To promote radiation hormesis
   D. To be comparable to the risk occurring in both nonsafe and safe industries

2. Which of the following concerns the upper boundary dose of ionizing radiation that results in a *negligible risk* of body injury or genetic damage?
   A. Skin erythema dose
   B. Dose limits
   C. NARM
   D. EfD limit

3. Fundamental radiation protection standards governing occupational radiation exposure may be found in which of the following documents?
   A. 5 CFR 10
   B. 10 CFR 20
   C. *The ALARA Manual*
   D. Public Law 90-602

4. Which of the following groups are radiation protection standards organizations?
   1. ICRP
   2. NCRP
   3. UNSCEAR
   A. 1 and 2 only
   B. 1 and 3 only
   C. 2 and 3 only
   D. 1, 2, and 3

5. The NCRP recommends that radiation exposure be kept at which of the following levels?
   A. As low as reasonably achievable
   B. At threshold levels
   C. Slightly above upper boundary levels
   D. At 0.01 mSv/yr

6. Which of the following concepts is behind the establishment of the effective dose limiting system?
   A. Negligible risk
   B. Organ and tissue radiosensitivity
   C. Radiation hormesis
   D. Radiation exposure and associated risk of possible radiation-induced malignancy

7. The term *mutagenesis* refers to which of the following?
   A. Irradiation of DNA of somatic cells leading to abnormalities in new cells as they divide in that individual
   B. Birth defects from irradiation of the unborn child in utero
   C. Cancer caused by ionizing radiation exposure
   D. Somatic and hereditary effects of ionizing radiation caused by low-level exposure

8. Biologic somatic effects of ionizing radiation that can be directly related to the dose received, exhibit a threshold dose *below* which the response does not normally occur, and *above* which the severity of the biologic damage *increases* as the dose *increases,* are classified as which of the following?
   A. Tissue reactions
   B. Epidemiologic effects
   C. Probabilistic effects
   D. Stochastic effects

9. Congress passed the Radiation Control for Health and Safety Act (Public Law 90-602) in 1968 to protect the public from the hazards of unnecessary radiation exposure resulting from which of the following?
   A. Diagnostic x-ray equipment only
   B. Therapeutic x-ray equipment only
   C. Electronic products, excluding diagnostic x-ray equipment
   D. Electronic products, including diagnostic x-ray equipment

10. Which of the following are classified as *late* tissue reactions caused by high-level radiation exposure that occur months or more after that exposure?
   1. Cataract formation
   2. Organ atrophy
   3. Radiation-induced malignancy
   A. 1 and 2 only
   B. 1 and 3 only
   C. 2 and 3 only
   D. 1, 2, and 3

11. What term is used for a beneficial aspect or result of radiation to a group of individuals from continuing exposure to small amounts of radiation?
   A. Nonoccupational EqD effect
   B. Radiation negligible risk level effect
   C. Radiation hormesis effect
   D. Radiation benevolent effect

12. In addition to the annual occupational effective dose limit established for radiation workers, the NCRP recommends a lifetime effective dose limit, which is found by multiplying a person's age in years by which of the following subunits?
   A. 1 mSv
   B. 10 mSv
   C. 100 mSv
   D. 1000 mSv

13. For individual members of the general public not occupationally exposed, the NCRP recommended an annual effective dose limit of _____ for continuous (or frequent) exposures from artificial sources of ionizing radiation other than medical irradiation and natural background and a limit of _____ annually for infrequent exposures.
   A. 1 mSv, 5 mSv
   B. 3 mSv, 8 mSv
   C. 10 mSv, 20 mSv
   D. 50 mSv, 75 mSv

14. Current radiation protection philosophy is based on the:
   A. Assumption that a linear-quadratic threshold relationship exists between radiation dose and biologic response
   B. Occupational risk factor
   C. Assumption that a linear nonthreshold relationship exists between radiation dose and biologic response
   D. Sum of both external and internal whole-body occupational exposures

15. A set of numeric dose limits that are based on calculations of the various risks of cancer and genetic (hereditary) effects to tissues or organs exposed to radiation defines:
   A. ALARA concept
   B. Effective dose limiting system
   C. Investigational levels
   D. Risk protocol

16. Previously, the NRC was known as the:
   A. AEC
   B. EPA
   C. FDA
   D. OSHA

17. The Radiation Effects Research Foundation is a group run by the government of:
   A. The United States, to study the effects of low-level ionizing radiation on populations
   B. Germany, to study the effects of ionizing radiation on the population
   C. Japan, primarily to study the atomic bomb survivors of Hiroshima and Nagasaki
   D. England, to study the development of childhood cancer in children exposed in utero to ionizing radiation

18. In 1991 the ICRP recommended that the annual effective dose limit for occupationally exposed persons:
   A. Remain at 50 mSv indefinitely
   B. Be reduced from 50 mSv to 20 mSv
   C. Be raised from 50 mSv to 75 mSv
   D. Be permanently eliminated

19. Which agency is responsible for regulations regarding am employee's "right to know" with regard to hazards that may be present in the workplace?
   A. NRC
   B. All NRC agreement states
   C. EPA
   D. OSHA

20. The risk to a radiographer from radiation exposure may be equated with:
  A. Lifetime fatal risk in hazardous occupations such as logging
  B. Lifetime fatal risk in hazardous occupations such as deep sea fishing
  C. Occupational risk in some industries that are generally considered to be somewhat unsafe
  D. Occupational risk in other industries that are generally considered reasonably safe

21. Because the tissue weighting factors (W_T) used to calculate effective dose are so small for some organs, an organ associated with a low weighting factor may receive an unreasonably large dose, whereas the effective dose remains within the allowable total limit. Therefore special limits are set for the crystalline lens of the eye and localized areas of the skin, hands, and feet to prevent:
    1. Tissue reactions
    2. Stochastic effects
    3. Probabilistic effects
  A. 1 only
  B. 2 only
  C. 3 only
  D. 1, 2, and 3

22. Late tissue reactions (i.e., cataract formation) have a high probability of occurring when entrance radiation doses exceed:
  A. 0.05 Gy
  B. 0.5 Gy
  C. 1 Gy
  D. 2 Gy

23. Established organ or tissue weighting factors for calculating the effective dose include a "remainder" that takes into account additional tissues and organs, some of which are the:
    1. Brain
    2. Small intestine and large intestine
    3. Uterus
  A. 1 and 2 only
  B. 1 and 3 only
  C. 2 and 3 only
  D. 1, 2, and 3

24. In International System (SI) units, the cumulative effective dose limit for the whole body of an occupationally exposed person who is 26 years old is:
  A. 26 mSv
  B. 260 mSv
  C. 2600 mSv
  D. 26,000 mSv

25. NARM stands for:
  A. Natural atomic radioactive material
  B. Naturally occurring and/or accelerator-produced materials
  C. Negligible accelerator-produced materials
  D. Negligible atomic radioactive material

Exercise 3: True or False

Circle *T* if the statement is true; circle *F* if the statement is false.

1. T F The ICRP functions as an enforcement agency for radiation protection purposes.

2. T F Future radiation protection standards are expected to continue to be based on risk.

3. T F The Radiation Effects Research Foundation is a group run by the government of Japan primarily for the purpose of studying the atomic bomb survivors.

4. T F The NRC regulates and inspects x-ray imaging facilities.

5. T F In 1991 the ICRP recommended that the annual EfD limit for occupationally exposed persons be reduced from 50 mSv to 20 mSv as a result of newer information obtained regarding the Japanese atomic bomb survivors in whom the risk of radiation from the atomic bomb detonations was estimated to be approximately three to four times greater (more damaging) than previously estimated.

6. T F Health care facilities that provide imaging services do not need to have an effective radiation safety program.

7. T F Effective dose limits may be specified for whole-body exposure, partial-body exposure, and exposure of individual organs.

8. T   F   Quantitative values for radiation risks are derived from the complete injury caused by radiation exposure.

9. T   F   The Center for Devices and Radiological Health (CDRH) is responsible for credentialing radiographers.

10. T   F   Late tissue reactions may occur months or years after high-level radiation exposure.

11. T   F   The ICRP is considered the international authority on the safe use of sources of ionizing radiation.

12. T   F   The NRC publishes rules and regulations in Title X of the *Code of Federal Regulations.*

13. T   F   The FDA facilitates the development and enforcement of regulations pertaining to the control of radiation in the environment.

14. T   F   For high–dose-rate fluoroscopic procedures, entrance exposure rates as great as 200 mGy_a/min are possible.

15. T   F   Health care facilities, such as hospitals, set their own internal action limits.

16. T   F   Because a stochastic event is an all-or-none random effect, ionizing radiation could induce cancers within a general large population, but determining beforehand which members of that population will develop cancer is not possible.

17. T   F   The embryo-fetus is particularly insensitive to radiation exposure.

18. T   F   EfD limits include radiation exposure from natural background radiation and exposure acquired when a worker undergoes medical imaging procedures.

19. T   F   To reduce exposure for pregnant radiation workers and control exposure to the unborn during potentially sensitive periods of gestation, the NCRP now "recommends" a monthly EqD limit not exceeding 0.5 mSv per month to the embryo-fetus and a limit during the entire pregnancy not to exceed 5.0 mSv after declaration of the pregnancy.

20. T   F   The NRC does not require the name of the RSO on a health care facility's radioactive materials license.

21. T   F   Lifetime survival data possibly appear to indicate that Japanese atomic bomb survivors with moderate radiation exposure of 5 mSv to 50 mSv, the equivalent of 1.5 to 15 years of natural radiation, have a reduced cancer death rate compared with a normally exposed control population.

22. T   F   Employers are not required by law to evaluate their workplace for hazardous agents or to provide training and written information to their employees.

23. T   F   The CDRH falls under the jurisdiction of the FDA.

24. T   F   Radiation hormesis is a beneficial aspect or result to groups of individuals from continuing exposure to small amounts of radiation.

25. T   F   All imaging personnel should be familiar with NCRP recommendations.

Exercise 4: Fill in the Blank

Using the following Word Bank, fill in the blanks with the word or words that best complete the statements.

0.4	external	optimization
1	greater	previous
8	hereditary	radiation safety
10	internal	radioactive
15	linear	radon
50	linear-quadratic	random
biologic	mutations	risk (may be used more than once)
cancer	new	
dose limits (may be used more than once)	nongovernmental	same
	nonoccupationally	stochastic
existing	nonprofit	whole body

1. Because medical imaging professionals share the responsibility for patient safety from radiation exposure and are subject themselves to such exposure in the performance of their duties, they must be familiar with _____, _____, and _____ guidelines.

2. Since its inception in 1928, the ICRP has been the leading international organization responsible for providing clear and consistent radiation protection guidance through its recommendations for occupational and public _____ _____.

3. In the United States the NCRP is a _____, _____, private corporation.

4. NAS/NRC-BEIR is an advisory group that reviews studies of _____ effects of ionizing radiation and _____ assessment.

5. The EPA has the authority for determining the action level for _____.

6. The NRC licenses users of _____ materials.

7. The NRC mandates that a _____ _____ committee be established for a facility.

8. Separate _____ _____ are set for occupationally exposed individuals and for the general public.

9. ALARA may also be referred to as _____.

10. Cancer and genetic alterations are examples of _____ effects.

11. The limit for any education and training exposures of individuals younger than age 18 years is an EfD of _____ mSv annually.

12. The ALARA concept adopts an extremely conservative model with respect to the relationship between ionizing radiation and potential _____.

13. Because stochastic effects are _____, determining which members of an exposed group of individuals will develop cancer is not possible before the radiation dose is received.

14. When ionizing radiation damages reproductive cells, _____ may develop that could bring an injurious consequence in subsequent generations.

15. Stochastic responses to ionizing radiation may be determined with the use of both the _____ and _____ dose-response curves.

16. Revised concepts of radiation exposure and _____ have brought about recent changes in NCRP recommendations for limits on exposure to ionizing radiation.

17. The lifetime fatal risk in hazardous occupations such as logging and deep-sea fishing is many times _____ than the occupational risk associated with radiation exposure.

18. Epidemiologic studies of atomic bomb survivors exposed in utero have provided conclusive evidence of a dose-dependent increase in the incidence of severe intellectual disability for fetal doses greater than approximately _____ Sv.

19. Referring to the previous statement (number 18), the greatest risk for radiation-induced intellectual disability was found to occur when the embryo-fetus was exposed _____ to _____ weeks after conception.

20. The effective dose limiting system is an attempt to equate the various risks of _____ and _____ effects to the tissues or organs that were exposed to radiation.

21. The cumulative effective dose limit pertains to the _____ _____.

22. In addition to limits for occupationally exposed individuals, the NCRP also sets limits for _____ _____ exposed individuals who are not undergoing medical examinations. An example of such persons would be a spouse, parent, or guardian accompanying a patient to the radiology department.

23. For education and training purposes, the same dose limits should apply to students of radiography in general and to those individuals younger than 18 years of age. The dose limit is the _____ for kindergarten through twelfth-grade students attending science demonstrations involving ionizing radiation as it is for student radiologic technologists who begin their education before the age of 18 years.

24. The sum of both _____ and _____ whole-body exposures is considered when an effective dose limit is being established.

25. An annual occupational effective dose limit of _____ mSv (not including medical and natural background exposure) has been established for the whole body, with an added recommendation that the lifetime EfD in mSv should not exceed _____ times the occupationally exposed person's age in years.

Exercise 5: Labeling

Label the following tables.

A. Summary of radiation protection standards organizations.

Organization	Function
1. _____	Evaluates information on biologic effects of radiation and provides radiation protection guidance through general recommendations on occupational and public dose limits
2. _____	Reviews regulations formulated by the ICRP and decides ways to include those recommendations in U.S. radiation protection criteria
3. _____	Evaluates human and environmental ionizing radiation exposure and derives radiation risk assessments from epidemiologic data and research conclusions; provides information to organizations such as the ICRP for evaluation
4. _____	Reviews studies of biologic effects of ionizing radiation and risk assessment and provides the information to organizations such as the ICRP for evaluation

B. Summary of U.S. regulatory agencies.

Agency	Function
1. _____	Oversees the nuclear energy industry, enforces radiation protection standards, publishes its rules and regulations in Title 10 of the *U.S. Code of Federal Regulations,* and enters into written agreements with state governments that permit the state to license and regulate the use of radioisotopes and certain other material within that state
2. _____	Enforces radiation protection regulations through their respective health departments
3. _____	Facilitates the development and enforcement of regulations pertaining to the control of radiation in the environment
4. _____	Conducts an ongoing product radiation control program, regulating the design and manufacture of electronic products, including x-ray equipment
5. _____	Functions as a monitoring agency in places of employment, predominantly in industry

Chapter **10** Dose Limits for Exposure to Ionizing Radiation

C. Summary of National Council on Radiation Protection and Measurements (NCRP) recommendations*†
(NCRP Report No. 116).

A. Occupational exposures‡	
1. Effective dose limits	
a. Annual	1. __ mSv
b. umulative	2. __ mSv × age
2. Equivalent dose annual limits for tissues and organs	
a. Lens of eye	3. __ mSv
b. Localized areas of the skin, hands, and feet	4. __ mSv
B. Guidance for emergency occupational exposure‡ (see Section 14, NCRP Report No. 116)	
C. Public exposures (annual)	
1. Effective dose limit, continuous or frequent exposure‡	5. __ mSv
2. Effective dose limit, infrequent exposure‡	6. __ mSv
3. Equivalent dose limits for tissues and organs‡	
a. Lens of eye	7. __ mSv
b. Localized areas of the skin, hands, and feet	8. __ mSv
4. Remedial action for natural sources	
a. Effective dose (excluding radon)	9. >__ mSv
b. Exposure to radon and its decay products§	10. >__ J/(sm^{-3})‖
D. Education and training exposures (annual)‡	
1. Effective dose limit	11. __ mSv
2. Equivalent dose limit for tissues and organs	
a. Lens of eye	12. __ mSv
b. Localized areas of the skin, hands, and feet	13. __ mSv
E. Embryo-fetus exposures‡	
1. Equivalent dose limit	
a. Monthly	14. __ mSv
b. Entire gestation	15. __ mSv
F. Negligible individual dose (annual)‡	16. __ mSv

*Excluding medical exposures.
†See Tables 4.2 and 5.1 in NCRP Report No. 116 for recommendations on radiation weighting factors and tissue weighting factors, respectively.
‡Sum of external and internal exposures, excluding doses from natural sources.
§WLM stands for *working level month* and refers to a cumulative exposure for a working month (170 hours). As applied to radon and its daughter products, 1 WLM represents the cumulative exposure experienced in a 170-hour period resulting from a radon concentration of 100 pCi/L. The occupational limit for miners is 4 WLM per year, which results in a dose equivalent of approximately 0.15 Sv per year.
‖A measure of the rate of release of energy (joules per second) by radon and its decay products per unit volume of air (cubic meters).

Exercise 6: Short Answer
Answer the following questions by providing a short answer.

1. What have scientists developed to limit radiation exposure of the general public, patients, and radiation workers?

  _____

  _____

2. Why must medical imaging professionals be familiar with previous, existing, and new radiation safety guidelines?

  _____

  _____

  _____

3. Name four major organizations responsible for evaluating the relationship between radiation equivalent dose and induced biologic effects.

_____

_____

_____

_____

4. Name five U.S. regulatory agencies responsible for enforcing radiation protection standards for the protection of the general public, patients, and occupationally exposed personnel.

_____

_____

_____

_____

_____

5. Why should a health care facility have a radiation safety committee?

_____

_____

_____

_____

_____

6. What are the training and experience requirements for an RSO?

_____

_____

7. How do health care facilities define ALARA?

_____

_____

8. In practice, what does "keep occupational and nonoccupational dose limits ALARA" actually mean?

_____

_____

9. How is the occupational risk associated with radiation exposure equated?

_____

_____

10. Why have some U.S. states not complied with the Consumer-Patient Radiation Health and Safety Act of 1981?

_____

_____

Chapter **10** **Dose Limits for Exposure to Ionizing Radiation**

11. What term was adopted to replace the older terms *nonstochastic* and *deterministic*?

_____

12. What is the central principle for radiation protection underlying the ALARA concept?

_____

_____

13. What is the purpose of the Consumer-Patient Radiation Health and Safety Act of 1981?

_____

_____

14. The EPA was established for what purpose?

_____

_____

15. Define the term *exposure linearity.*

_____

_____

Exercise 7: General Discussion or Opinion Questions

The following questions are intended to allow students to express their knowledge and understanding of the subject matter or to present a personal opinion. The questions may be used to stimulate class discussion. Because answers to questions may vary, determination of the answer's acceptability is left to the discretion of the course instructor.

1. How does current radiation protection philosophy affect patient and personnel radiation exposure?

2. Using the concept of radiation hormesis and data from any available studies, explain how continuing exposure to small amounts of radiation could possibly have a beneficial aspect or result for groups of individuals.

3. What are some of the important provisions of the code of standards for diagnostic x-ray equipment that went into effect on August 1, 1974? How do these standards improve radiation safety?

4. What types of radiation exposures are not taken into consideration with the effective dose limiting system?

5. Since 2008, what changes have been made in the Nuclear Regulatory Commission's scope of responsibility?

Exercise 8: Calculation Problems

Solve the following problems.

A radiation worker's lifetime effective dose must be limited to his or her age in years times 10 mSv. This is called the *cumulative effective (CumEfD) limit,* which pertains to the whole body. Adherence to the limit ensures that the lifetime risk for these workers remains acceptable. The following problems demonstrate the application of the CumEfD limit.

1. Determine the CumEfD limit (in mSv) for the whole body of an occupationally exposed person who is 54 years old.

2. Determine the CumEfD limit (in mSv) for the whole body of an occupationally exposed person who is 46 years old.

3. Determine the CumEfD limit (in mSv) for the whole body of an occupationally exposed person who is 33 years old.

4. Determine the CumEfD limit (in mSv) for the whole body of an occupationally exposed person who is 25 years old.

5. Determine the CumEfD limit (in mSv) for the whole body of an occupationally exposed person who is 18 years old.

POST-TEST

The student should take this test after reading Chapter 10, finishing all accompanying textbook and workbook exercises, and completing any additional activities required by the course instructor. The student should complete the post-test with a score of 90% or higher before advancing to the next chapter. (Each of the following 20 questions is worth 5 points.)
Score = _____ %

1. To what may risk to a radiographer from radiation exposure be equated?

   _____

   _____

2. The NRC is a federal agency that has the authority to control the possession, use, and production of atomic energy in the interest of _____ _____.

3. What U.S. agency functions as a monitoring agency in places of employment, predominantly in industry?

   _____

4. In a health care facility, who is responsible for developing an appropriate radiation safety program to ensure that all people are adequately protected from radiation?

   _____

5. Determine the CumEfD limit (in mSv) for the whole body of an occupationally exposed person who is 39 years old.

6. What is the effective dose limit?

   _____

   _____

7. What system is the current method for assessing radiation exposure and the associated risk of biologic damage to radiation workers and the general public?

   _____

8. ALARA is the acronym for what term?

   _____

9. Biologic somatic effects of ionizing radiation that can be directly related to the dose received include:
   1. Early tissue reactions
   2. Stochastic effects
   3. Late tissue reactions
   A. 1 and 2 only
   B. 1 and 3 only
   C. 2 and 3 only
   D. 1, 2, and 3

10. Examples of stochastic effects include:
   1. Acute radiation syndrome
   2. Cancer
   3. Genetic alterations
   A. 1 and 2 only
   B. 1 and 3 only
   C. 2 and 3 only
   D. 1, 2, and 3

11. The NCRP now recommends a monthly EqD limit not exceeding _____ per month to the embryo-fetus of a pregnant radiation worker.

12. The current radiation protection philosophy is based on the assumption that a_____ _____ relationship exists between radiation dose and biologic response.

13. When does the greatest risk for radiation-induced intellectual disability occur during a pregnancy?

   _____

   _____

14. What essential concept underlies radiation protection?

   _____

   _____

15. What dose limit does the NCRP recommend as an equivalent dose limit for the embryo-fetus during the entire period of gestation?

_____

_____

16. What is the NCRP recommended annual occupational whole-body effective dose limit per year for radiation workers?

_____

17. What is the significance of tissue weighting factors?

_____

_____

18. Adherence to occupational and nonoccupational _____ dose limits helps prevent harmful biologic effects of radiation exposure.

19. What is radiation hormesis?

_____

_____

20. Why are internal action limits established by health care facilities?

_____

_____

Reference

1. National Council on Radiation Protection and Measurements (NCRP): Recommendations on limits for exposure to ionizing radiation, Report No. 9, Bethesda, MD, 1987, NCRP.

11 Equipment Design for Radiation Protection

Chapter 11 covers state-of-the-art diagnostic radiographic and fluoroscopic equipment that is designed with many devices that radiologists and technologists can use to optimize the quality of the image while at the same time reducing radiation exposure for patients. Multiple features have been built in to new x-ray–producing machines by the manufacturers to ensure radiation safety, and some characteristics have also been included to meet enhanced federal regulations. In addition, various accessories are available to further lower radiation dose. Lastly, in the newest systems, all dimensions for patient setups are now given in metric units. Table 11.1 in the textbook provides an overview of standard English system dimensions with their corresponding metric unit replacements. In summary, this chapter provides an overview of equipment components and accessories that imaging professionals can use to minimize radiation exposure of patients.

CHAPTER HIGHLIGHTS

- A diagnostic-type tube housing protects the patient and imaging personnel from off-focus, or leakage, radiation by restricting the emission of x-rays to the area of the useful, or primary, beam.
  - Leakage radiation from the tube housing measured at 1 m from the x-ray source must not exceed 1 Gy_a/hr (100 mR/hr) when the tube is operated at its highest voltage at the highest current that allows continuous operation.
- The control panel, or console, must be located behind a suitable protective barrier that has a radiation-absorbent window that permits observation of the patient during any procedure.
  - This panel must indicate the conditions of exposure and provide a positive indication when the x-ray tube is energized.[1]
- The radiographic examination tabletop must be of uniform thickness, and for under-table tubes as used in fluoroscopy, the patient support surface also should be as radiolucent as possible so that it will absorb only a minimal amount of radiation, thereby reducing the patient's radiation dose.
  - The tabletop is often made of a carbon fiber material.
- Radiographic equipment must have a source–to–image receptor distance (SID) indicator.
- X-ray beam limitation devices must be used to confine the useful beam before it enters the anatomic area of clinical interest.
  - The light-localizing variable-aperture rectangular collimator, cones, and extension cylinders are the beam limitation devices used.

- The patient's skin surface should always be at least 15 cm below the collimator to minimize exposure to the epidermis.
- Good coincidence between the x-ray beam and the light-localizing beam of the collimator is necessary; both alignment and length and width dimensions of the two beams must correspond to within 2% of the SID.
- States vary in their exact requirements for agreement of positive beam limitation (PBL) setting and radiation field, varying from 2% to 3% of SID.
- Exposure to the patient's skin may be reduced through proper filtration of the radiographic beam.
  - Inherent filtration amounting to 0.5-mm aluminum equivalent is always present in the x-ray beam reaching the collimator.
  - Together, the inherent filtration and added filtration comprise the total filtration. Stationary x-ray units operating at more than 70 kVp are required to have a total filtration on emerging x-rays of 2.5-mm aluminum equivalent.
  - The half-value layer (HVL) of the beam is measured to determine whether an x-ray beam is adequately filtered.
- Compensating filters are used in radiography to provide uniform imaging of body parts when considerable variation in thickness or tissue composition exists.
- Diagnostic x-ray units must have consistent exposure reproducibility, that is, the ability to duplicate certain radiographic exposures for any given combination of kVp, mA, and time.
- Exposure linearity is essential. When a change is made from one mA station to a neighboring mA station, the most linearity can vary is 10%.
- Radiographic grids increase patient dose in radiography. Their use for examination of thicker body parts is a fair compromise because they remove scattered radiation emanating from the patient that would otherwise degrade the recorded image.
  - Because of increased sensitivity of photostimulable phosphor to scatter radiation before and after exposure to a radiographic beam, a grid may be used more often during computed radiography (CR) imaging. The use of a grid does increase patient dose but significantly improves radiographic contrast and visibility of detail.
- To limit the effects of inverse square falloff of radiation intensity with distance during a mobile radiographic examination, an x-ray source–to–skin distance (SSD) of at least 30 cm (12 inches) must be used.
- With digital radiography, the latent image formed by x-ray photons on a radiation detector is actually an

electronic latent image. It is called a *digital image* because it is produced by computer representation of anatomic information. The image receptor is divided into small detector elements that make up the two-dimensional picture elements, or pixels, of the digital image.

- Radiographers must select correct technical exposure factors the first time to avoid overexposing patients when digital images are obtained.
- Computed radiography results when the invisible, or latent, image generated in conventional radiography is produced in a digital format using computer technology.
- The digital image can be displayed on a monitor for viewing, and it can be printed on a laser film when hard copy is needed.
- Fluoroscopic procedures produce the largest patient radiation exposure rate in diagnostic radiology.
  - □ Minimize patient exposure time whenever possible.
  - □ Limit the size of the fluoroscopic field to include only the area of anatomy that is of clinical interest.
  - □ Employ the practice of interrupted and pulsed fluoroscopy to reduce the overall length of exposure.
  - □ Select the correct technical exposure factors to help minimize the amount of radiation received by a patient.

  - □ Ensure that the SSD is no less than 38 cm (15 inches) for stationary (fixed) fluoroscopes and no less than 30 cm (12 inches) for mobile fluoroscopes.
- During C-arm fluoroscopic procedures, the patient–image intensifier distance should be as short as possible.
- Reduce patient dose by using intermittent activation of the fluoroscope to locate the catheter, limiting the time of the digital run, and using the last-image-hold feature to view the most recent image.
- During digital fluoroscopy (DF) the use of pulsed progressive systems lowers patient dose.
  - □ Use of the last-image-hold feature is another effective dose-reduction technique in DF.
- High-level-control fluoroscopy (HLCF) is used for interventional procedures and uses exposure rates that are substantially higher than those allowed for routine fluoroscopic procedures.
  - □ If skin dose is received in the range of 1 to 2 Gy_t, the U.S. Food and Drug Administration (FDA) requires that a notation be placed in the patient's record.
  - □ The radiographer generally has the responsibility for monitoring and documenting procedural fluoroscopic time when fluoroscopic equipment is used by nonradiologist physicians.

Exercise 1: Matching

Match the following terms with their definitions or associated phrases.

1. _____ Inherent filtration

2. _____ HVL

3. _____ Diagnostic-type protective tube housing

4. _____ Spacer bars

5. _____ Added filtration

6. _____ Control panel, or console

7. _____ Scattered radiation

8. _____ PBL

9. _____ Computed radiography (CR)

10. _____ Radiographic beam defining system

11. _____ High level control fluoroscopy (HLCF)

A. Equipment that should be used to perform radiographic procedures only on patients who cannot be transported to a fixed radiographic installation (an x-ray room)

B. Metal most widely selected as a filter material

C. Material used in a radiographic/fluoroscopic x-ray room tabletop that helps to reduce patient dose

D. Device that increases patient dose

E. Consists of two sets of adjustable lead shutters mounted within the collimator at different levels, a light source to illuminate the x-ray field and permit it to be centered over the area of clinical interest, and a mirror to deflect the light beam toward the patient to be radiographed

F. Feature of a radiographic collimator that, when activated, automatically adjusts the collimator so that the radiation field matches the size of the image receptor

G. Allows the fluoroscopist to see the most recent image without exposing the patient to another pulse of radiation

H. Brightness of a surface

I. Thickness of a designated absorber (customarily a metal such as aluminum) required to decrease the intensity (quantity or amount) of the primary beam by 50% of its initial value

J. Projects down from the x-ray tube housing of some collimators to prevent the collimator from moving closer than 15 cm away from the patient

K. Sheets of aluminum (or its equivalent) of appropriate thickness generally located outside the glass window of the x-ray tube housing above the collimator shutters

12. _____ Carbon fiber

13. _____ Nit

14. _____ Luminance

15. _____ Amorphous selenium

16. _____ Mobile (portable) x-ray unit

17. _____ Off-focus radiation

18. _____ Last image hold feature for dose reduction

19. _____ Digital radiography

20. _____ Source–to–image receptor distance (SID)

21. _____ Desquamation

22. _____ Radiographic grid

23. _____ Useful, or primary, x-ray beam

24. _____ Aluminum

25. _____ Digital image

L. Required to protect the patient and imaging personnel from off-focus, or leakage, radiation by restricting the emission of x-rays to the area of the useful, or primary, beam

M. The distance from the anode focal spot to the radiographic image receptor

N. The glass envelope encasing the x-ray tube, the insulating oil surrounding the tube, and the glass window in the tube housing

O. Where technical exposure factors such as mA and kVp are selected and seen on indicators by the operator

P. Process in which an image is captured on a removable digital storage cassette using storage phosphor technology. The cassette is then taken to a reader that interprets the stored signal and transfers it in a digital matrix to a picture archiving and communication system.

Q. An electronic latent image formed by x-ray photons on a radiation detector

R. Image produced by computer representation of anatomic information

S. A simple term for candelas per square meter

T. X-rays that can never be completely eliminated from an x-ray beam because the metal shutters cannot be placed immediately beneath the actual focal spot of the x-ray tube

U. An operating mode of fluoroscopic equipment in which exposure rates are substantially higher than those normally allowed in routine procedures. This higher exposure rate allows visualization of smaller and lower contrast objects that do not usually appear during standard fluoroscopy.

V. Sloughing off of skin cells

W. A photoconductor used to convert x-ray energy directly into electrical signals

X. X-rays emitted through the x-ray port tube window, or port

Y. All the radiation that arises from the interaction of an x-ray beam with the atoms of a patient or any other object in the path of the beam

Exercise 2: Multiple Choice

Select the answer that best completes the following questions or statements.

1. To meet radiation safety features, radiographic equipment must have a:
   1. Correctly functioning control panel
   2. Protective tube housing
   3. Radiographic examination table and other devices and accessories designed to reduce patient radiation dose
   A. 1 only
   B. 2 only
   C. 3 only
   D. 1, 2, and 3

2. There are various types of digital radiography image receptors. Some use a scintillator, such as amorphous silicon, to:
   A. Convert visible light into x-ray energy
   B. Convert x-ray energy into visible light
   C. Ensure adequate penetration of the anatomy to be imaged
   D. Reduce scattered radiation before it reaches the image receptor

3. The luminance of the collimator light source must be:
   A. Adequate to permit the localizing light beam to outline the margins of the radiographic beam adequately on the patient's anatomy
   B. Visible on the patient's anatomy only when all white light is turned off in the radiography room
   C. Less than 5 foot-candles
   D. At least 10 foot-candles

4. Which of the following results in an *increase* in the patient dose?
   A. Use of a radiographic grid
   B. Use of carbon fiber in the radiographic tabletop
   C. Use of filtration according to kVp selected
   D. Use of a variable rectangular collimator containing a spacer bar

5. The patient dose significantly *decreases* and the life of the fluoroscopic tube *increases* with which of the following?
   A. Restriction of the fluoroscopic field to include only the area of clinical interest
   B. Use of a conventional fluoroscope rather than image intensification, or the use of digital fluoroscopy equipment
   C. Pulsed, or intermittent, fluoroscopy
   D. Darkness adaptation

6. When fluoroscopic field size is limited to include only the area of clinical interest by adequately collimating the x-ray beam, patient area, or integral dose:
   A. Decreases substantially
   B. Increases substantially
   C. Remains the same as if the x-ray beam were not collimated
   D. Remains at zero

7. Digital radiography eliminates the need for almost all retakes resulting from improper technique selection because:
   A. The image contrast and overall brightness may be manipulated after image acquisition.
   B. The image contrast and overall brightness may not be manipulated after image acquisition.
   C. The image requires chemical processing to become visible.
   D. Pixel sizes can be altered after exposure to correct image contrast and overall brightness.

8. Computed radiography involves:
   1. Use of conventional radiographic equipment
   2. Selection and use of standard technical exposure factors
   3. Traditional patient positioning performed by a radiographer
   A. 1 only
   B. 2 only
   C. 3 only
   D. 1, 2, and 3

9. Which of the following is the *most* versatile for defining the size and shape of the radiographic beam?
   A. A square metal diaphragm shaped to a specific size
   B. Radiographic cone shaped as a flared metal tube
   C. Radiographic cone shaped as a straight cylinder
   D. Light-localizing variable-aperture rectangular collimator

10. The use of digital radiographic systems offers a number of advantages over CR systems. Some of these include:
    1. Immediate imaging results
    2. Lower dose
    3. Presence of a preinstalled grid
    A. 1 and 2 only
    B. 1 and 3 only
    C. 2 and 3 only
    D. 1, 2, and 3

11. In computed radiography imaging, when the use of a grid is necessary for radiographing anatomy sections more than 10 cm thick or for techniques that exceed 70 kVp, patient dose received is:
    A. About the same as with non-CR imaging because the same mAs is used
    B. Significantly higher than with non-CR imaging because the mAs required is significantly higher
    C. Significantly lower than with non-CR imaging because the mAs required is significantly lower
    D. Slightly lower than with non-CR imaging because the mAs required is slightly lower

12. Some fluoroscopically guided therapeutic interventional procedures have the potential for substantial patient exposure. In high-level control (HLC) mode, patient exposure rates have been estimated to range from:
    A. 50 to 99 mGy_a/min
    B. 100 to 500 mGy_a/min
    C. 200 to 1200 mGy_a/min
    D. 1300 to 2500 mGy_a/min

13. To protect the patient's skin from exposure to electrons produced by photon interaction with the collimator, the skin surface should be at least _____ *below* the collimator.
    A. 6 cm
    B. 12 cm
    C. 15 cm
    D. 20 cm

14. To reduce patient entrance dose during C-arm fluoroscopic procedures, the patient–image intensifier distance should be:
    A. As short as possible
    B. As long as possible
    C. Always set at a 100-cm (40-inch) SID
    D. Always set at a 180-cm (72-inch) SID

133

15. Which of the following may reduce patient exposure to off-focus radiation?
    A. Placing the second pair of shutters in the collimator below the level of the light source and mirror
    B. Placing the first pair of shutters in the collimator as close as possible to the x-ray tube window
    C. Transmitting an electric signal through the collimator's first and second pair of shutters
    D. Off-focus radiation in a collimator cannot be reduced.

16. When a digital fluoroscopic system is used, which of the following is an effective technique for reducing patient dose?
    A. Converting to non–image intensification fluoroscopy
    B. Increasing mAs significantly
    C. Using scotopic (rod) vision instead of photopic (cone) vision
    D. Using the last image hold feature

17. The ratio of the height of the lead strips in a grid to the distance between them defines:
    A. Grid ratio
    B. Grid alignment
    C. Grid types
    D. Grid weight

18. HLCF is an operating mode for state-of-the-art fluoroscopic equipment in which exposure rates are:
    A. Slightly higher than those normally allowed in routine procedures
    B. Substantially higher than those normally allowed in routine procedures
    C. Slightly lower than those normally used in routine procedures
    D. Substantially lower than those normally used in routine procedures

19. Monitoring and documentation of procedural fluoroscopic time are essential to good practice. The responsibility for monitoring and documentation generally belongs to:
    A. The nurse assisting the physician with the procedure
    B. The physician performing the fluoroscopic procedure
    C. The radiographer assisting with the procedure
    D. Radiology department secretarial personnel

20. HVL is expressed in:
    A. Centimeters of aluminum
    B. Centimeters of lead
    C. Millimeters of aluminum
    D. Millimeters of lead

21. Dose reduction and uniform imaging of body parts that vary considerably in thickness or tissue composition may be accomplished by use of:
    A. Compensating filters constructed of aluminum, lead-acrylic, or other suitable material
    B. Compensating filters constructed of lightweight plastic or wood
    C. Compensating filters made of carbon fibers
    D. Radiographic grids

22. Resolution of a digital image is sharper when pixels are:
    A. Larger
    B. Smaller
    C. Variable in size
    D. Variable in thickness

23. A primary protective barrier of _____ is required for a fluoroscopic unit.
    A. 2-mm aluminum equivalent
    B. 2-mm lead equivalent
    C. 4-mm aluminum equivalent
    D. 4-mm lead equivalent

24. Compared with the resolution of an optimal quality image produced with a screen-film radiographic system, the resolution of a digital image is:
    A. Actually somewhat less
    B. Comparable to the quality of the image produced with a screen-film radiographic system
    C. Actually somewhat greater
    D. Significantly greater

25. Some of the causes for high exposures to personnel during interventional procedures include:
    1. Operating the fluoroscopic tube for longer periods in continuous mode in place of pulsed mode
    2. Failure to use the protective curtain or floating shields on the stationary fluoroscopic equipment's image intensifier as a means of protection
    3. Lack of familiarity with the x-ray equipment leading to longer fluoroscopic time for completion of a procedure
    A. 1 and 2 only
    B. 1 and 3 only
    C. 2 and 3 only
    D. 1, 2, and 3

Exercise 3: True or False

Circle *T* if the statement is true; circle *F* if the statement is false.

1. (T) F — State-of-the-art diagnostic radiographic and fluoroscopic equipment is designed with many devices that radiologists and technologists can use to optimize the quality of the image while at the same time reducing radiation exposure for patients undergoing various imaging procedures.

2. T (F) — During routine radiographic examinations, it is acceptable for the radiographer to adjust the collimator so that the radiographic beam is ~~slightly~~ larger than the size of the image receptor. *no larger*

3. T (F) — Radiographic cones are earlier x-ray beam filtration devices.

4. (T) F — When PBL is activated, the collimators are automatically adjusted so that the radiation field matches the size of the image receptor.

5. T (F) — Inherent filtration in an x-ray tube used for routine radiography amounts to approximately 2.5-mm aluminum equivalent. *.5mm*

6. (T) F — Because HVL is a measure of beam quality, or effective energy of the x-ray beam, a certain minimal HVL is required at a given peak kilovoltage.

7. T (F) — Radiographic tubes do ~~not~~ need a device in place to ensure accurate x-ray beam alignment.

8. T (F) — Because filtration absorbs some of the photons in a radiographic beam, it ~~increases~~ the overall intensity of the incident radiation. *decreases*

9. (T) F — When operating a mobile radiographic unit, the radiographer must use an SID of at least 30 cm (12 inches) to limit the effects of the inverse square falloff of radiation intensity with distance.

10. (T) F — In digital radiography the size of the pixels determines the sharpness of the image.

11. T (F) — Barium ~~platinocyanide~~ is the most commonly used photostimulable phosphor used in computed radiography imaging plates. *Fluorohalide*

12. (T) F — Technical exposure factors for fluoroscopic procedures for children necessitate a decrease in kVp by as much as 25%.

13. T (F) — In standard image intensification fluoroscopy an x-ray beam HVL of ~~7- to 9.5-mm~~ aluminum is considered acceptable when kVp ranges from 80 to 100. *3 - 4.5*

14. T (F) — Patient dose ~~decreases~~ as the grid ratio increases. *increases*

15. T (F) — When a radiographic procedure is performed with a CR system, it is acceptable practice to overexpose a patient initially because the image obtained can be technically adjusted to an acceptable quality, thereby avoiding the possibility of repeat exposure for the patient. *not acceptable*

16. T (F) — In CR imaging, the routine practice of overexposing patients to possibly avoid repeat radiographic exposures is ethical and acceptable. *not*

17. (T) F — For dose-reduction purposes it is preferable to position a C-arm so that the x-ray tube is under the patient.

18. (T) F — In the newest x-ray imaging systems all dimensions for patient setup are now given in metric units.

19. (T) F — For the computer to form a CR image correctly, the body area or part being radiographed must be positioned in or near the center of the CR image receptor.

20. T (F) — The coincidence requirements between the radiographic beam and the localizing light beam are known as *linearity* and *luminance*. *alignment and congruence*

21. (T) F — Added filtration is generally located outside the glass window of the x-ray tube housing above the collimator shutters.

22. T (F) — The effective metric equivalent of 40 inches is 180 cm. *100cm*

23. T (F) — A primary protective barrier of 2-mm ~~aluminum~~ equivalent is required for a fluoroscopic unit. *lead*

Chapter **11** Equipment Design for Radiation Protection

24.  T F   The use of C-arm fluoroscopy, in procedures such as a surgical pinning of a fractured hip, carries the potential for a relatively large patient radiation dose. C-arm fluoroscope operators, if standing close to the patient, could also receive a significant increase in occupational exposure from patient scatter radiation during such cases.

25. T F   Ongoing education and training in the safe use of fluoroscopic equipment should be mandatory for nonradiologist physicians and equipment operators.

Exercise 4: Fill in the Blank

Using the following Word Bank, fill in the blanks with the word or words that best complete the statements.

brightness	exit	mAs
center	federal	mispositioning
collimator	filtration	multifield
dead-man	fluoroscopy	quality
decreases	image matrix	resolution
distance	incapacitated	same
dose reduction	latitude	technique
electronic	less	under
energized	limitation	wedge
entrance	manufacturers	

1. Multiple features have been built into new x-ray–producing machines by the _____ to ensure radiation safety, and some extra characteristics have also been included to meet enhanced _____ regulations.

2. Patient exposure can be substantially reduced by using appropriate beam _____ devices.

3. For dose reduction purposes, it is preferable to position the C-arm so that the x-ray tube is _____ the patient.

4. The fluoroscopic exposure control switch (e.g., the foot pedal) must be of the _____ type so that the exposure automatically terminates if the person operating the switch becomes_____ or for any reason removes his or her foot from the pedal.

5. Filtration _____ the overall intensity of the radiation.

6. Many quality assurance teams are now realizing that CR, because of its higher exposure _____, makes grid use on the pediatric population _____ necessary than was previously believed.

7. For the computer to form a CR image correctly, the body area or part being radiographed must be positioned in or near the _____ of the CR image receptor.

8. _____ charts indicating optimal kVp values for all CR projections must be available in the x-ray room near the operating console for the radiographer.

9. When a dorsoplantar projection of a foot is being obtained, a _____ filter may be used to provide uniform density of the anatomic structures.

10. With digital radiography, the latent image formed by x-ray photons on a radiation detector is actually an _____ latent image.[1]

11. DR images can be accessed at several workstations at the _____ time, thus making image viewing very convenient for physicians providing patient care.

12. To limit the effects of inverse fall-off of radiation intensity with _____ during a mobile radiographic examination, an SSD of at least 30 cm (12 inches) must be used.

13. The numeric values of the digital image are aligned in a fixed number of rows and columns (an array) that form many individual miniature square boxes, each of which corresponds to a particular place in the image. These individual boxes collectively constitute the _____ _____.

14. When using a radiographic grid, because some fraction of the image receptor is covered with lead, _____ must be increased to compensate for the use of this device.

Chapter **11 Equipment Design for Radiation Protection**

15. Overall _____ of the radiographic image is improved when scattered photons do not reach the image receptor.

16. The _____ is the most versatile device for defining the size and shape of the radiographic beam.

17. Low-energy photons should be removed from the radiographic beam through _____.

18. _____ is sharper when pixels are smaller.

19. In digital radiography, _____ is defined as the amount of luminance (light emission) of a display monitor.

20. _____ procedures produce the largest patient exposure rate in diagnostic radiology.

21. Even though DR eliminates the need for almost all retakes required because of improper technique selection, repeat rates for reasons of _____ are not lowered.

22. Because an image intensification system greatly increases brightness, image intensification fluoroscopy requires less milliamperage than the discontinued non–image intensifier fluoroscopic systems. The consequent decrease in exposure rate can result in a sizable _____ _____ for the patient.

23. Depending on their manufacturer and geographic location, _____ image intensification tubes vary in size, but the 30/25/20-cm (12/10/8-inch) diameter trifield model is typical for general-purpose fluoroscopic units.

24. When the SSD is small (e.g., for mobile radiographic examinations), patient _____ exposure is significantly greater than _____ exposure. By increasing the SSD, the radiographer maintains a more uniform distribution of exposure throughout the patient.

25. When the enclosed phosphor of a CR cassette is exposed to x-rays, it becomes _____.

Exercise 5: Labeling

Label the following illustrations and table.

A. X-ray tube, collimator, and image receptor.

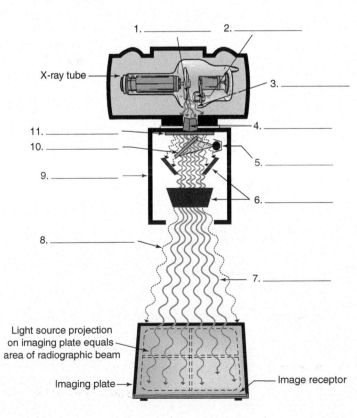

B. Image intensification fluoroscopic unit.

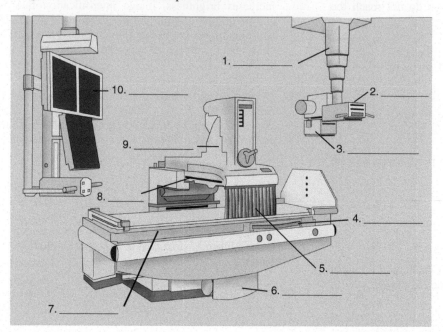

From Bushong SC: *Radiologic science for technologists: physics, biology and protection,* ed 10, St. Louis, 2013, Elsevier.

C. HVL required by the Radiation Control for Health and Safety Act of 1968 and detailed by the Bureau of Radiological Health* in 1980.

Peak Kilovoltage	Minimum Required HVL in Millimeters of Aluminum
30	1. _____
40	2. _____
50	3. _____
60	4. _____
70	5. _____
80	6. _____
90	7. _____
100	8. _____
110	9. _____
120	10. _____

*The Bureau of Radiological Health changed its name to the Center for Devices and Radiological Health in 1982.

Exercise 6: Short Answer

Answer the following questions by providing a short answer.

1. If adequate filtration of the radiographic beam were not present, how would the patient's radiation dose and the image process be affected?

_____

_____

2. Why is it impossible to eliminate all off-focus radiation coming from the primary beam and exiting at various angles from the x-ray tube window?

_____

_____

3. Why is aluminum the metal most widely selected for filter material in general diagnostic radiology?

_____

_____

4. Why is a certain minimal HVL required at a given kVp?

_____

_____

5. What should be done in DR imaging to hold technologists accountable for retakes necessitated by mispositioning?

_____

_____

6. What is the purpose of a protective x-ray tube housing?

_____

_____

7. What does inherent filtration include?

_____

_____

8. What are two causes of high radiation exposure to personnel during an interventional procedure that is performed by a nonradiologist physician?

_____

_____

_____

9. According to FDA recommendation, at what range of skin dose received from a fluoroscopic procedure should a notation be placed in a patient's record?

_____

_____

10. What is the advantage of using a pulsed progressive system for digital fluoroscopy?

_____

_____

11. How does filtration reduce the overall intensity of radiation in a radiographic beam? How does this affect the remaining photons in the beam?

_____

_____

139

12. With regard to the diagnostic x-ray tube, where is added filtration located?

_____

_____

13. What are the requirements for the construction of the x-ray tube housing?

_____

_____

_____

14. Where must the control panel or console in a fixed radiographic room be located?

_____

_____

15. What requirement must be met by the thickness of a radiographic examination tabletop?

_____

_____

16. What is a synonymous term for a bilateral wedge filter?

_____

17. List 11 procedures involving extended fluoroscopic time.

_____

_____

_____

_____

_____

_____

18. Why is a cumulative timing device needed on fluoroscopic equipment?

_____

_____

_____

19. For dose reduction purposes, why is it best to position the C-arm of a C-arm fluoroscopic unit so that the x-ray tube is under the patient whenever possible?

_____

_____

20. What is scattered radiation?

_____

_____

Exercise 7: General Discussion or Opinion Questions

The following questions are intended to allow students to express their knowledge and understanding of the subject matter or to present a personal opinion. The questions may be used to stimulate class discussion. Because answers to questions may vary, determination of the answer's acceptability is left to the discretion of the course instructor.

1. What radiation safety features that will reduce patient radiation exposure can be found on state-of-the-art diagnostic radiographic and fluoroscopic equipment?

2. During interventional fluoroscopic procedures, what strategies can be used to manage radiation dose to patients, x-ray equipment operators, and other staff?

3. What are the responsibilities of a radiographer who is working with a nonradiologist physician, using a C-arm or stationary fluoroscope with HLC mode, while performing an interventional procedure?

4. What radiation safety features may be found on state-of-the-art radiographic and fluoroscopic equipment that will reduce radiation exposure for the equipment operator?

5. What are the benefits and the consequences of using a radiographic grid when the anatomy to be radiographed is greater than 10 cm?

POST-TEST

The student should take this test after reading Chapter 11, finishing all accompanying textbook and workbook exercises, and completing any additional activities required by the course instructor. The student should complete the post-test with a score of 90% or higher before advancing to the next chapter. (Each of the following 20 questions is worth 5 points.)
Score = _____ %

1. Define the term *half-value layer.*

   _____

2. What type of material is commonly used in the tabletop of a radiographic examination table?

   _____

3. Every diagnostic imaging system must have a _____ tube housing and a correctly functioning _____ panel, or console.

4. What is the most versatile x-ray beam limitation device currently in use?

   _____

5. Define *scattered radiation.*

   _____

   _____

6. How does the use of a radiographic grid affect the patient dose?

   _____

   _____

7. The numeric values of the _____ image are aligned in a fixed number of rows and columns (an array) that form many individual miniature square boxes, each of which corresponds to a particular place in the image. These individual boxes collectively constitute the _____ _____.

8. Which of the following reduces patient exposure?
    1. Carbon fiber material in a radiographic tabletop
    2. Use of appropriate beam limitation devices
    3. Use of automatic collimation
   A. 1 and 2 only
   B. 1 and 3 only
   C. 2 and 3 only
   D. 1, 2, and 3

9. Filtration that includes the glass envelope encasing the x-ray tube, the insulating oil surrounding the tube, and the glass window in the tube housing is called:
   A. Added filtration
   B. Inherent filtration
   C. Total filtration
   D. HVL

10. When fluoroscopic field size is limited to include only the area of clinical interest by adequately collimating the x-ray beam, patient area, or _____ _____, decreases substantially.

11. When _____ _____ _____ is activated, the collimators are automatically adjusted so that the radiation field matches the _____ of the image receptor.

12. For what type of procedures is high-level-control fluoroscopy used?

   _____

13. By increasing _____, the radiographer maintains a more uniform distribution of _____ throughout the patient.

14. What fluoroscopic practice should a radiologist use to reduce the overall length of the exposure for a given procedure?

   _____

   _____

15. To protect the patient's skin from exposure to electrons produced by photon interaction with the collimator, the skin surface should be at least _____ cm below the collimator.
   A. 3
   B. 5
   C. 10
   D. 15

16. During C-arm fluoroscopic procedures, what should the patient–image intensifier distance be?

   _____

17. In digital radiography the size of the _____ determines the sharpness of the image.

18. What must radiographic imaging equipment have so that the radiographer can determine how far the image receptor is from the anode focal spot?

   _____

19. Placing the first pair of shutters in the collimator as close as possible to the x-ray tube window may:
    A. Eliminate the need for a second pair of shutters
    B. Eliminate the need for added filtration
    C. Reduce patient exposure from the primary beam
    D. Reduce patient exposure from off-focus radiation

20. In CR imaging, the routine practice of overexposing patients to possibly avoid repeat radiographic exposures is _____ and _____.

Reference

1. Bushong SC: *Radiologic science for technologists: physics, biology and protection,* ed 8, p. 589, St. Louis, 2013, Mosby Elsevier

12 Management of Patient Radiation Dose During Diagnostic X-Ray Procedures

Chapter 12 covers management of patient radiation dose during diagnostic x-ray procedures. During such procedures, a holistic approach to patient care is essential. This means treating the whole person rather than just the area of concern. Holistic patient care must begin with effective communication between the radiographer and the patient. This type of dialogue alleviates the patient's uneasiness and increases the likelihood for cooperation and successful completion of the procedure. To take care of all patients appropriately, the radiographer should develop easily understandable communication skills.

Radiographers must limit the patient's exposure to ionizing radiation by employing appropriate radiation reduction techniques and by using protective devices that minimize radiation exposure. Patient exposure can be substantially reduced by using proper body or part immobilization, motion reduction techniques, appropriate beam limitation devices, adequate filtration of the x-ray beam, and gonadal or other specific area shielding. Selection of suitable technical exposure factors used in conjunction with computer-generated digital images, use of appropriate digital image processing, and the elimination of repeat radiographic exposures can also contribute significantly to limiting patient exposure. This chapter provides an overview of methods and techniques that radiographers can use to minimize the patient's exposure to radiation during radiologic examinations.

CHAPTER HIGHLIGHTS

- Effective communication with the patient is the first step in holistic patient care.
  - Imaging procedures should be explained in simple terms.
  - Patients must have an opportunity to ask questions and receive truthful and clear answers within ethical limits.
- Adequate immobilization of the patient is necessary to eliminate voluntary motion.
  - Restraining devices are available to immobilize either the whole body or the individual body part to be radiographed.
  - Involuntary motion can be compensated for by shortening exposure time with an appropriate increase in mA and by using very-high-speed image receptors.
- Protective shielding may be used to reduce or eliminate radiation exposure of radiosensitive body organs and tissues.
  - The reproductive organs should be protected from exposure to the useful beam when they are inside or within approximately 5 cm of a properly collimated

beam, unless this would compromise the diagnostic value of the study.
  - Correctly placed, appropriate gonadal shielding can greatly reduce the exposure received by patients of both sexes (50% reduction for female patients, 90% to 95% reduction for male patients).
- The clear lead shadow shield and a posteroanterior (PA) projection can significantly reduce the dose to the breast of a young patient undergoing a scoliosis examination.
- Appropriate technical exposure factors for each examination that ensure a diagnostic image of optimal quality with minimal patient dose must be selected.
  - Standardized technique charts must be available for each x-ray unit to help provide a uniform selection of technical exposure factors. High kVp and lower mAs should be chosen whenever possible to reduce the amount of radiation received by the patient.
- When digital images are acquired, correct postprocessing is essential to produce a high-quality diagnostic image.
  - Imaging departments should establish a quality control program that ensures standardization in the postprocessing of digital images.
- An air gap technique can be used as an alternative to the use of a grid.
- Repeat radiographic exposures must be minimized to prevent the patient's skin and gonads from receiving a double dose of radiation.
- Radiographic examinations are to be performed only when patients will benefit from useful information gained from the procedure. Nonessential radiologic examinations should not be performed.
- The amount of radiation received by a patient from diagnostic imaging procedures may be specified as entrance skin exposure (ESE) (including skin and glandular), gonadal dose, or bone marrow dose.
  - ESE is the easiest quantity to obtain and the most widely used.
  - The estimated genetically significant dose (GSD) for the population of the United States is approximately 0.20 mSv.
- Fluoroscopically guided positioning is an unethical and unacceptable practice that leads to increased patient radiation dose.
- Abdominal radiologic examinations that have been requested after full consideration of the clinical status of a patient, including the possibility of pregnancy, need not be postponed or selectively scheduled.[1]
  - The NCRP recommendation for elective abdominal examinations of women of childbearing years states that such examinations should be performed during

144

the first few days after the onset of menses to minimize the possibility of irradiating an embryo.[2,3]

- ☐ A radiographer must carefully question female patients of childbearing age regarding any possibility of pregnancy before they undergo an x-ray examination.
- ☐ If irradiation of an unknown pregnancy occurs, a calculated estimate of the approximate equivalent dose to the embryo-fetus as a result of the examination should be obtained. A radiologic physicist determines the fetal dose.

■ Children are much more vulnerable to late effects of radiation than are adults.

- ☐ Use a PA projection to protect the breasts of female patients.
- ☐ In small girls, shielding of the ovaries requires protection of the iliac wings as well as the sacral area when shielding is needed.
- ☐ Adequate collimation of the radiographic beam to include only the area of clinical interest is essential, and effective immobilization techniques should be used when necessary. The use of a high-mA station and a short exposure time also helps to minimize patient motion.

■ A developing embryo-fetus is especially sensitive to exposure from ionizing radiation.

- ☐ Use the smallest technical exposure factors that will generate a diagnostically useful radiographic image, carefully collimate the beam to include only the anatomic area of interest, and cover the lower abdomen and pelvic regions with a suitable contact shield if they do not need to be included in the examination.
- ☐ The goal of the Image Gently Campaign is to change practice by increasing awareness about methods to lower radiation dose during pediatric medical imaging examinations (Alliance for Radiation Safety in Pediatric Imaging, 2016).[4]
- ☐ Radiographers and imaging facilities can pledge to Image Gently.
- ☐ Radiographers can pledge to Image Wisely.

Exercise 1: Matching

Match the following terms with their definitions or associated phrases.

1. _____ Body language

2. _____ External anatomic landmarks

3. _____ Air gap technique

4. _____ Flat contact shields

5. _____ Referring physician

6. _____ Gonadal shielding

7. _____ Nonessential radiologic examinations
8. _____ Epidermis

9. _____ Double dose

10. _____ Shaped contact shield

11. _____ Bone marrow

A. Standardization in the processing of digital images, which includes regular monitoring and maintenance of all processing and image display equipment in a facility

B. Suspended from above the radiographic beam-defining system, this device hangs over the area of clinical interest to cast a shadow in the primary beam over the patient's reproductive organs

C. These are made of transparent lead-acrylic material impregnated with approximately 30% lead by weight

D. Something that a radiographer should ask a female patient of childbearing age about before the patient undergoes an x-ray examination

E. Cup-shaped radiopaque device that encloses the scrotum and penis to protect the male reproductive organs from exposure to ionizing radiation

F. Campaign to promote lowering the amount of radiation used in medically necessary imaging procedures and eliminating unnecessary procedures in adult medical imaging

G. The recorded detail in the radiographic image

H. "An interaction that produces a satisfying result through an exchange of information"[5]

I. A campaign to change long-established practice by raising awareness about methods for lowering radiation dose during pediatric medical imaging examinations

J. Areas on the patient that can be used to guide placement of a testicular or ovarian shield

K. Its primary function is to protect underlying tissues and structures

145

12. _____ Possibility of pregnancy

13. _____ Gonadal dose

14. _____ Effective communication

15. _____ Spatial resolution

16. _____ Quality control program

17. _____ Quantum noise, or mottle

18. _____ Clear lead shields

19. _____ Entrance skin exposure (ESE)

20. _____ Image Wisely

21. _____ Genetically significant dose (GSD)

22. _____ Elective x-ray examinations

23. _____ Image Gently

24. _____ Shadow shield

25. _____ Fluoroscopically guided positioning (FGP)

L. Alternative procedure to the use of a radiographic grid for reducing scattered radiation during certain examinations

M. Individual responsible for ordering a radiologic examination

N. Unconscious actions, or nonverbal messages, that if understood as intended will promote effective communication between the radiographer and patient

O. Devices used on patients during diagnostic x-ray procedures to protect the reproductive organs from exposure to the useful beam when these organs are in or within approximately 5 cm of a properly collimated beam

P. What the patient's skin and possibly the gonads receive whenever a repeat examination occurs

Q. Most commonly reported and simplest way to specify the amount of radiation received by a patient from a diagnostic imaging procedure

R. Nonurgent x-ray procedures that can be booked at an appropriate time to meet patient needs and safety

S. Radiation exposure received by the male and female reproductive organs

T. The practice of using fluoroscopy to determine the exact location of the central ray before taking a radiographic exposure[6]

U. A blotchy radiographic image that results when an insufficient quantity of x-ray photons reaches the image receptor

V. The equivalent dose to the reproductive organs that, if received by every human, would be expected to bring about an identical gross genetic injury to the total population, as does the sum of the actual doses received by exposed individual members of the population

W. Some traditional radiographic examinations performed in the absence of definite medical indications

X. Of great importance because it contains large numbers of stem, or precursor, blood cells that could be either depleted or, worse, even eliminated by substantial exposure to ionizing radiation

Y. Not suited for nonrecumbent positions or projections other than anteroposterior (AP) or posteroanterior (PA)

Exercise 2: Multiple Choice

Select the answer that *best* completes the following questions or statements.

1. Effective communication between the radiographer and the patient does which of the following?
   1. Alleviates the patient's uneasiness
   2. Increases the patient's likelihood for cooperation during the procedure
   3. Makes possible successful completion of the procedure
   A. 1 only
   B. 2 only
   C. 3 only
   D. 1, 2, and 3

2. According to the National Council of Radiation Protection and Measurements, the chance of malformations from fetal radiation exposure is significantly increased above control levels only at doses:
   A. Greater than 25 cGy
   B. Greater than 15 cGy
   C. Less than 10 cGy
   D. Less than 5 cGy

3. During a fluoroscopic examination, because no localizing light field exists and the field of view is usually moved about:
   A. A flat contact shield is not suitable for use.
   B. A shadow shield is not suitable for use.
   C. A shaped contact shield is not suitable for use.
   D. A shield that provides any type of gonadal protection is not suitable for use.

4. Which of the following results in an *increase* in the patient dose?
   A. Use of the lowest possible kVp with the highest possible mAs for each examination
   B. Use of gonadal or specific area shielding
   C. Use of standardized technique charts, when automatic exposure control is not used
   D. Use of the highest practicable kVp with the lowest possible mAs for each examination

5. Flat contact shields are made of:
   A. Aluminum strips or aluminum-impregnated materials 1 mm thick
   B. Tin strips or tin-impregnated materials 2 mm thick
   C. Lead strips or lead-impregnated materials 1 mm thick
   D. Wood strips or wood-impregnated materials 2 mm thick

6. Using appropriate technical exposure factors and an 8:1 ratio grid, an optimal quality cross-table lateral projection of the cervical spine was obtained. If another radiograph is obtained, using an air gap technique and technical exposure factors that are comparable to those used with the 8:1 ratio grid, the patient dose will be:
   A. About the same
   B. Significantly higher
   C. Significantly lower
   D. Not a concern because an air gap technique cannot be used in place of a grid for a lateral projection of the cervical spine

7. The skin and gonads of the patient receive a "double dose" of x-radiation whenever:
   A. Specific area shielding is used.
   B. An air gap technique is used.
   C. Gonadal shielding is used.
   D. A repeat radiograph is necessary, as a consequence of human or mechanical error.

8. When an effective repeat analysis program is implemented and maintained in an imaging department, improving the overall importance of that department includes:
   1. Increased awareness among staff and student radiographers of the need to produce optimal quality images from the start
   2. Radiographers becoming more careful in producing radiographic images because they are aware that images are being reviewed
   3. Designing and providing in-service education programs for imaging personnel covering problems or concerns on specific topics that have been identified
   A. 1 only
   B. 2 only
   C. 3 only
   D. 1, 2, and 3

9. Exposure of the fetus to radiation arising from diagnostic procedures:
   A. Is not of concern because radiation from diagnostic procedures cannot cause any harm to an unborn fetus
   B. Will result in the immediate need for the patient to have a therapeutic abortion because of fetal demise as a consequence of a diagnostic radiation exposure
   C. Would definitely be a cause in all instances, by itself, for terminating a pregnancy
   D. Would rarely be cause, by itself, for terminating a pregnancy

10. When an individual of childbearing age undergoes a diagnostic x-ray procedure, gonadal shielding should be used to protect the reproductive organs from exposure to the useful beam:
    1. When these organs are in or within approximately 5 cm of a properly collimated x-ray beam
    2. Unless shielding will compromise the diagnostic value of the examination
    3. When the radiographer chooses to substitute gonadal shielding for adequate collimation of the x-ray beam
    A. 1 and 2 only
    B. 1 and 3 only
    C. 2 and 3 only
    D. 1, 2, and 3

11. Which of the following are *most often* used to assess skin doses?
    A. Compensating filters
    B. Filtration equivalent to 4-mm aluminum placed in the path of the x-ray beam
    C. Radiographic grids
    D. Thermoluminescent dosimeters

12. Areas of the body that should be shielded from the useful beam whenever possible are the:
    1. Lens of the eye
    2. Breasts
    3. Thyroid gland
    4. Reproductive organs
    A. 1 and 4 only
    B. 2 and 3 only
    C. 3 and 4 only
    D. 1, 2, 3, and 4

13. Some clinical manifestations that can cause involuntary motion during a radiographic procedure include:
    1. Chills
    2. Tremors
    3. Muscle spasms
    4. Pain
    A. 1 and 2 only
    B. 2 and 3 only
    C. 3 and 4 only
    D. 1, 2, 3, and 4

14. If in the course of performing a specific radiographic procedure 75% of the active bone marrow were in the useful beam and received an average absorbed dose of 0.4 mGy_t, the mean marrow dose would be which of the following?
    A. 0.3 mGy_t
    B. 0.6 mGy_t
    C. 0.9 mGy_t
    D. 1 mGy_t

15. Exposure of patients to medical x-ray examinations is commanding increasing attention in our society because:
    1. An increasing risk of early tissue reactions from diagnostic x-ray has caused alarm in the general public.
    2. The frequency of x-ray examinations, including many repetitive studies in short periods, among all age groups is expanding annually, which indicates that physicians are relying more and more on radiographic examinations to assist them in patient care and diagnosis.
    3. Concern among public health officials is growing regarding the risk of late effects associated with these multiple medical x-ray exposures.[7]
    A. 1 and 2 only
    B. 1 and 3 only
    C. 2 and 3 only
    D. 1, 2, and 3

16. Before the start of a diagnostic radiographic procedure, the radiographer should thoroughly explain the procedure to the patient in simple terms that the patient can understand. If a patient has questions, how should the radiographer respond?
    A. The radiographer must listen attentively to these questions and then find a way to avoid answering the patient's questions to save time.
    B. The radiographer must listen attentively to these questions and answer them truthfully in an appropriate tone of voice and in accordance with ethical guidelines.
    C. The radiographer must listen attentively to these questions and then tell the patient that he or she is not permitted to answer his or her questions because it is not legally acceptable to do so.
    D. The radiographer must listen attentively to these questions but refuse to answer the questions so as not to incriminate himself or herself.

17. To ensure a diagnostic image with minimal patient dose, the selection of scientifically correct technical exposure factors chosen for each examination, whether digital or non-digital, must ensure:
    1. A high quality image that has sufficient brightness or density to display anatomic structures
    2. An appropriate level of subject contrast to differentiate amount the anatomic structures
    3. The maximum amount of spatial resolution and a minimum amount of distortion
    A. 1 only
    B. 2 only
    C. 3 only
    D. 1, 2, and 3

18. If a radiographic procedure will cause pain, discomfort, or any strange sensations, the patient:
    A. Must be informed before the procedure begins, but the radiographer should not overemphasize this aspect of the examination
    B. Must be informed before the procedure begins, and the radiographer should really stress this aspect of the examination
    C. Should not be informed before the procedure begins because he or she may decide not to have the procedure
    D. Should not be informed before the procedure begins so that he or she will not worry about this part of the examination

19. If a flat contact shield is used during a typical fluoroscopic examination, to protect the patient, it must be placed:
    A. To the side of the patient away from the fluoroscopist to absorb scattered radiation
    B. On top of the patient to reduce the scattered radiation emanating from the patient
    C. Underneath the patient because the x-ray tube is located beneath the radiographic table
    D. To the side of the patient near the fluoroscopist to absorb scattered radiation

20. When automatic exposure control (AEC) is not used, neglecting to use standardized technique charts necessitates estimating the technical exposure factors, which may result in:
    1. Poor-quality images
    2. Repeat examinations
    3. Additional and unnecessary exposure for the patient
    A. 1 only
    B. 2 only
    C. 3 only
    D. 1, 2, and 3

21. Entrance skin exposure may be converted to patient _____ by using well-documented multiplicative factors.
    A. Gonadal dose
    B. Skin dose
    C. Bone marrow dose
    D. Genetically significant dose

22. Unwanted densities in the image that are not part of the patient's anatomy and may negatively affect the ability of a radiologist to interpret the image correctly are called:
    A. Artifacts
    B. Blobs
    C. Grids
    D. Irregularities

23. Shadow shields are made of:
    A. Aluminum
    B. Copper
    C. Radiopaque material
    D. Rubber

24. If a pregnant patient is inadvertently irradiated, which of the following medical professionals should determine fetal dose?
    A. Attending physician
    B. Administrator of the health care facility
    C. Radiologic physicist
    D. Radiology resident

25. Which of the following radiographic procedures are considered unnecessary?
    1. Chest x-ray examination as part of a preemployment physical
    2. Chest x-ray examination for mass screening for tuberculosis
    3. Whole-body multislice spiral computed tomography (CT) screening
    A. 1 and 2 only
    B. 1 and 3 only
    C. 2 and 3 only
    D. 1, 2, and 3

Exercise 3: True or False

Circle *T* if the statement is true; circle *F* if the statement is false.

1. T F Patient exposure can be substantially reduced by using proper body or part immobilization and motion reduction techniques.

2. T F Patients do not need to be given the opportunity to ask questions about their examination when they are having a routine x-ray procedure.

3. T F Shadow shields are suspended from the ceiling of the radiographic room.

4. T F Shaped contact shields are not recommended for PA projections because the shield covers the anterior and lateral surfaces of the male reproductive organs and because the x-ray beam enters the posterior surface in a PA projection; the shield does not protect the reproductive organs.

5. T F An air gap technique removes scatter radiation by using a decreased object–to–image receptor distance.

6. T F With computed radiography (CR) or digital radiography (DR), it is necessary to develop a policy whereby the digital files that correspond to retaken images can be recovered for analysis because this would not happen automatically.

7. T F During a diagnostic radiographic examination, the lens of the eye, breasts, thyroid gland, and reproductive organs need not be selectively shielded from the primary beam.

8. T F Primary beam exposure for male patients may be reduced by only 25% when the gonads are covered with a contact shield containing 1 mm of lead.

149

9. T F For safeguarding the ovaries of a female patient, the shield should be placed approximately 2.5 cm (1 inch) medial to each palpable anterior superior iliac spine.

10. T F External anatomic landmarks on the patient can be used to guide placement of a testicular or ovarian shield.

11. T F Use of a lower peak kilovoltage (kVp) and a higher milliamperage and exposure time in seconds (mAs) reduces the patient dose.

12. T F Skin dose is used in radiation safety terminology to refer to the dose to the epidermis, the most superficial layer of the skin.

13. T F Collimation should be a secondary protective measure, not a substitute for adequate gonadal shielding.

14. T F The ESE dose levels set in regulations can be exceeded.

15. T F When a radiographic procedure is performed with a CR system, it is an acceptable practice to overexpose a patient initially because the image obtained can be technically adjusted to an acceptable quality, thereby avoiding the possibility of repeat exposure for the patient.

16. T F Shielding of particularly sensitive breast tissue during a scoliosis examination may be accomplished using a clear lead shadow shield. The radiation dose to the breast of a young patient may be further reduced by performing the scoliosis examination with the x-ray beam entering the anterior surface of the patient's body instead of the posterior surface.

17. T F Problems that occur in digital imaging (either CR or DR) tend to be systematic, which can affect the quality of every image and the degree of radiation exposure of every patient until the problems are identified and corrected.

18. T F Words and actions of medical imaging personnel must demonstrate understanding and respect for human dignity and individuality.

19. T F Inadequate or misinterpreted instructions may prevent the patient from being able to cooperate.

20. T F During a routine diagnostic examination, body or body part immobilization is of no value and therefore unnecessary.

21. T F Patient protection during a diagnostic x-ray procedure should begin with clear, concise instructions.

22. T F Motion controlled by a patient's will is classified as involuntary motion.

23. T F Imaging departments do not need to establish a written shielding protocol for each of their radiologic procedures.

24. T F Because much evidence suggests that the developing embryo-fetus is very radiation sensitive, special care is taken in radiography to prevent unnecessary exposure of the abdominal area of pregnant women.

25. T F The GSD is the average annual gonadal equivalent dose (EqD) to members of the population who are of childbearing age.

Exercise 4: Fill in the Blank

Using the following Word Bank, fill in the blanks with the word or words that best complete the statements.

0.20	less	primary
50	leukemia	protective
additional	male	protocol
beam-defining	mean marrow	reduces
benefits	menstrual period	reduction
clinical interest	milliampere-seconds	remote
cooperate	minimal	reproductive
compromised	minimize	risks
effective	over	smaller
female	poor	symphysis pubis
holistic	pregnancy	

Chapter 12 Management of Patient Radiation Dose During Diagnostic X-Ray Procedures

1. Radiographers must limit the patient's exposure to ionizing radiation by employing appropriate radiation _____ techniques and by using _____ devices that _____ radiation exposure.

2. _____ patient care must begin with _____ communication between the radiographer and the patient.

3. When patients understand the procedure and their responsibilities, they can more fully _____ .

4. Repeat radiographic exposures sometimes can be attributed to _____ communication between the radiographer and the patient.

5. If gonadal shields are not placed correctly, the _____ organs will not be protected.

6. As a consequence of their anatomic location, the _____ reproductive organs receive about three times more exposure during a given radiographic procedure involving the pelvic region than do the _____ reproductive organs.

7. Specific area shielding for selective body areas other than the gonads significantly _____ radiation exposure to those areas and should be used whenever possible.

8. When a male patient is in the supine position, the _____ _____ can be used to guide shield placement over the testes.

9. Some fluoroscopic tubes are located above the patient and are referred to as _____ rooms because personnel set up the patient for the examination and then leave the room before activating the x-ray tube. In these rooms the shield should be placed _____ the patient.

10. The _____ light must be accurately positioned to ensure correct placement of the shadow shield.

11. When estimating approximate equivalent dose to the embryo-fetus, radiation output can be specified in milligray in air per _____.

12. Patients with the potential to reproduce should be gonadally protected during x-ray procedures whenever the diagnostic value of the examination is not _____.

13. Standardizing exposure techniques does not mean that radiographers use the same _____ for all patients in all situations.

14. Adequate collimation of the radiographic beam to include only the area of _____ _____ is essential.

15. According to the U.S. Public Health Service, the estimated GSD for the population of the United States is about _____ mSv.

16. In general, _____ doses of ionizing radiation are sufficient to obtain useful images in pediatric imaging procedures than are necessary for adult imaging procedures.

17. Suspended from above the radiographic beam–defining system, shadow shields hang over the area of clinical interest to cast a shadow in the _____ beam over the patient's reproductive organs.

18. Selection of appropriate technical exposure factors for each x-ray examination is essential to ensure a diagnostic image with _____ patient dose.

19. For female patients a flat contact shield containing 1 mm of lead placed over the reproductive organs reduces exposure by about _____ %.

20. Occasionally it is permissible to obtain an _____ image, when recommended by the radiologist for the purpose of obtaining additional diagnostic information.

21. In simple terms the GSD concept suggests that the genetic consequences of substantial absorbed doses of gonadal radiation become significantly _____ when averaged over an entire population rather than applied to just a few of its members.

22. Bone marrow dose may also be referred to as the _____ _____ dose.

23. In humans, radiation dose to bone marrow is of great importance because it may induce _____.

24. No diagnostic procedure using ionizing radiation should be conducted unless its _____ outweigh its _____.

25. Whenever a female patient of childbearing age is to undergo an x-ray examination, it is essential that the radiographer carefully question the patient about the possibility of _____. Part of this questioning involves asking the patient for the date of her last _____ _____.

151

Exercise 5: Labeling

Label the following illustration and complete the lists.

A. Technical exposure factor considerations.

1. _____

2. _____

3. _____

4. _____

5. _____

6. _____

7. _____

B. Lead filter with breast and gonad shielding device.

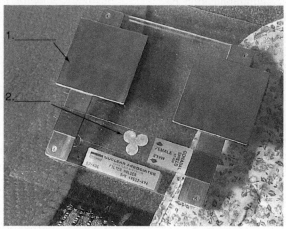

Courtesy Fluke Biomedical. Everett, WA.

1. _____

2. _____

C. Reasons for unacceptable images.

1. _____

2. _____

3. _____

4. _____

5. _____

6. _____

Exercise 6: Short Answer

Answer the following questions by providing a short answer.

1. How must radiographers limit the patient's exposure to ionizing radiation during a diagnostic x-ray procedure?

_____

_____

2. Why must the radiographer achieve a balance in technical radiographic exposure factors?

_____

_____

3. List four basic types of gonadal shielding devices that can be used during a diagnostic x-ray procedure.

_____

_____

4. When performing a routine diagnostic x-ray procedure on a pediatric patient, how can a radiographer minimize or possibly eliminate patient motion?

_____

_____

5. What is protective shielding?

_____

_____

6. How is an air gap technique performed? How does use of this technique for certain examinations help reduce scattered x-rays? How does the patient dose received from an air gap technique compare with the dose received from use of a midratio grid?

_____

_____

_____

_____

7. What decision regarding the patient must the referring physician make before ordering a radiologic examination?

_____

_____

8. Why can an accurate determination of a patient's skin, or surface, dose be made with a thermoluminescent dosimeter (TLD)?

_____

_____

_____

9. List three ways to specify the amount of radiation a patient receives from a diagnostic imaging procedure.

_____

_____

10. What does the selection of scientifically correct technical exposure factors for each examination ensure for patients?

_____

_____

11. What members of a population would be excluded from genetically significant dose considerations?

_____

_____

12. If a patient is to receive substantial pelvic irradiation and there is some doubt about her pregnancy status but no overriding medical concerns, what would be recommended before the pelvis is irradiated?

_____

_____

13. List the four basic types of gonadal shielding devices that can be used during routine diagnostic x-ray procedures.

_____

_____

14. When a radiographer listens attentively to a patient's questions and answers them truthfully in an appropriate tone of voice and in accordance with ethical guidelines, what benefit is derived?

_____

_____

15. List six x-ray procedures that are now considered nonessential.

_____

_____

16. Approximately what percent lead by weight does a clear lead shield contain?

_____

17. What type of shield for the lens of the eye is always used and positioned directly on a patient?

_____

18. Why is protection of the reproductive organs of particular concern in diagnostic radiology?

_____

_____

19. If in the course of performing a specific radiographic procedure 50% of the active bone marrow were in the useful beam and received an average absorbed dose of 0.6 mGy_t, what would the mean marrow dose received be?

_____

20. How are TLDs used to measure skin dose directly?

_____

_____

Exercise 7: General Discussion or Opinion Questions

The following questions are intended to allow students to express their knowledge and understanding of the subject matter or to present a personal opinion. The questions may be used to stimulate class discussion. Because answers to questions may vary, determination of the answer's acceptability is left to the discretion of the course instructor.

1. If a pregnant patient is irradiated inadvertently, what procedure should be followed?

2. Give examples of poor radiographer-patient communication, and explain in each situation how the radiographer could improve communication with the patient.

3. What are the benefits of the Image Gently and Image Wisely campaigns?

4. How do adults and children differ in terms of vulnerability to radiation exposure?

5. Describe various patient clinical situations and explain how effective communication can be used in each situation to improve the chance for successful completion of the diagnostic x-ray imaging procedure.

6. Explain why fluoroscopically guided positioning is not an ethical or acceptable practice when performing radiographic procedures.

7. Describe various methods that can be applied in a clinical situation to reduce patient exposure.

POST-TEST

The student should take this test after reading Chapter 12, finishing all accompanying textbook and workbook exercises, and completing any additional activities required by the course instructor. The student should complete the post-test with a score of 90% or higher before advancing to the next chapter. (Each of the following 20 questions is worth 5 points.)
Score = _____ %

1. What can radiographers and imaging facilities do to Image Gently?

2. What is the current position of the American College of Radiology (ACR) regarding abdominal radiologic examinations that have been requested by a physician after full consideration of the clinical status of a patient, including the possibility of pregnancy?

3. Whenever a repeat radiograph must be taken as a consequence of human or mechanical error, the skin and gonads of the patient receive a _____ _____ of x-radiation.

4. What patients should have gonadal protection during x-ray procedures whenever the diagnostic value of the examination is not compromised?

5. Define the term *genetically significant dose.*

6. To safeguard the ovaries of a female patient, where on the anatomy should an ovarian shield be placed?

7. How is the practice of fluoroscopically guided positioning viewed by the American Society of Radiologic Technologists (ASRT)?

Chapter **12** **Management of Patient Radiation Dose During Diagnostic X-Ray Procedures**

8. Which of the following substantially reduce patient exposure?
     1. Use of proper body or part immobilization
     2. Use of appropriate technical exposure factors
     3. Use of gonadal or other specific area shielding
   A. 1 and 2 only
   B. 1 and 3 only
   C. 2 and 3 only
   D. 1, 2, and 3

9. Which of the following x-ray procedures are considered unnecessary?
     1. Chest x-ray examination as part of a preemployment physical
     2. Chest x-ray examination for mass screening for tuberculosis
     3. Whole-body CT screening
   A. 1 and 2 only
   B. 1 and 3 only
   C. 2 and 3 only
   D. 1, 2, and 3

10. Gonadal shielding should be a secondary protective measure, not a substitute for an adequately _____ beam.

11. Shielding of particularly sensitive breast tissue during a scoliosis examination may be accomplished using a clear lead shadow shield. The radiation dose to the breast of a young patient may be further reduced by performing the scoliosis examination with the x-ray beam entering the _____ surface of the patient's body instead of the _____ surface.

12. Who is responsible for ordering a diagnostic x-ray procedure?

   _____

13. Correctly placed, appropriate gonadal shielding can greatly reduce the exposure received by patients of both genders (____ % for female patients, 90% to 95% for male patients).

14. According to the U.S. Public Health Service, what is the estimated GSD for the population of the United States?

   _____

15. Which of the following is a type of sensing device that is most often used to measure skin dose directly?
   A. Personnel digital ionization dosimeter
   B. Optically stimulated luminescence (OSL) dosimeter
   C. Pocket ionization chamber
   D. Thermoluminescent dosimeter

16. If irradiation of an unknown pregnancy occurs, what should be obtained?

   _____

   _____

17. Because of their anatomic location, the female reproductive organs receive about _____ times more exposure during a radiographic procedure involving the pelvic region than do the male reproductive organs.

18. When a male patient is in the supine position, what external anatomic landmark can a radiographer use for placement of a testicular shield?

   _____

   _____

19. Selection of appropriate technical exposure factors for each x-ray examination is essential to ensure a diagnostic image with:
    A. Maximal patient dose
    B. Minimal patient dose
    C. No patient dose
    D. Selective organ dose only

20. What must always be the first step for the radiographer to provide gonadal protection for patients?

_____

References

1. Reynold FB: Prepared remarks for the October 20, 1976, American College of Radiology press conference.

2. National Council on Radiation Protection and Measurements (NCRP): Medical x-ray, electron beam and gamma ray protection up to 50 MeV (equipment design, performance and use), Report No. 102, Bethesda, Md, 1989, NCRP.

3. National Council on Radiation Protection and Measurements (NCRP): Medical exposure of pregnant and potentially pregnant women, Report No. 54, Washington, DC, 1977, NCRP.

4. Alliance for Radiation Safety in Pediatric Imaging, 2016. www.imagegently.org/About us/TheAlliance

5. Torres LS: *Basic Medical Techniques and Patient Care for Radiologic Technologists,* ed 5, Philadelphia, 1997, Lippincott Williams & Williams.

6. Haynes K, Curtis T: Fluoroscopic vs. blind positioning: comparing entrance skin exposure. *Radiol Technol,* 81:1, 2009.

7. Bushong SC: *Radiologic Science for Technologists: Physics, Biology, and Protection,* ed 10, St. Louis, 2013, Mosby.

13 Special Considerations on Safety in Computed Tomography and Mammography

Some types of radiographic examinations require special consideration for radiation safety. Chapter 13 addresses these concerns for computed tomography and for mammography.

CHAPTER HIGHLIGHTS

- Computed tomography (CT) is a commonly employed diagnostic x-ray imaging modality that is considered to be a relatively high radiation exposure examination.
  - With higher radiation exposure to the patient, there is potentially an increased associated cancer risk.
  - Skin dose and dose distribution are two concerns related to patient dose in CT scanning.
  - CT examinations generally expose a smaller mass of tissue than that exposed during an ordinary x-ray series.
- The entrance exposure from a computed tomography examination may be compared with the entrance exposure received during a routine fluoroscopic examination.
  - When a series of adjacent slices is obtained, some radiation scatters from the slice being made into the adjacent slices. This is called interslice scatter.
  - Direct patient shielding is not typically used in CT.
  - When the spiral scan pitch ratio is approximately 1, the spiral CT patient dose is comparable to that produced by conventional or axial CT.
  - Tube current modulation in CT scanning can help to reduce patient dose.
- Recent advances in computer technology allow scan data to be reconstructed, modified, reconstructed again, modified, and so on, until an image having the lowest noise possible is obtained. Such a repeat process is referred to as *iteration* and is used in iterative reconstruction in CT.
  - In CT, all other factors being equal, increasing kVp tends to increase patient dose.
  - A miscentering of 2 cm can produce as much as a 25% increase in patient dose.[1]

- CT dose index volume ($CTDI_{VOL}$) and dose length product (DLP) are required dose markers.
- Effective DLP (EfDLP) is expressed in millisieverts per milligray-centimeter (mSv/mGy-cm).
- For routine head and body CT examinations, effective doses fall in the 1 to 10 mSv effective dose range.
- From a radiation protection point of view, the goal of all CT imaging should be to obtain the best possible anatomic scan while delivering an acceptable level of ionizing radiation to the patient.
- Nonpalpable breast cancer may be detected through mammography.
  - Federal regulations state that the mean dose to the glandular tissue of a 4.5-cm compressed breast using a screen-film or digital mammography system should not exceed 3 mGy_t per view.
  - Studies have found that well-calibrated mammographic systems are capable of providing excellent imaging performance with an average glandular dose of not more than 2 Gy_t.[2]
  - Digital mammography units with the ability to enhance contrast with image gray-level manipulation offer substantial visualization improvement for patients with dense breasts.
  - Dose reduction in standard mammography can be achieved by limiting the number of projections taken.
  - Axillary projections in mammography should only be done at the request of the radiologist.
  - Metallic elements such as molybdenum (Z = 42) and rhodium (Z = 45) are commonly employed as filters in mammography. However, molybdenum x-ray tube targets with molybdenum or rhodium filtration are being replaced in newer digital systems by tungsten targets with rhodium or silver filtration.
  - Beryllium (Z = 4) takes the place of glass in the window of the low-kVp mammographic x-ray tube.

Exercise 1: Matching

Match the following terms with their definitions or associated phrases.

1. _____ Computed tomography (CT)

2. _____ Helical (spiral) CT

3. _____ Dose distribution

4. _____ Dose parameters

5. _____ CTDI$_W$
6. _____ CTDI$_{VOL}$

7. _____ Interslice scatter

8. _____ Iterative reconstruction

9. _____ Pitch

10. _____ Tube current modulation

11. _____ Filtered back projection

12. _____ Sharpening filter

13. _____ Angular tube current modulation

14. _____ Patient centering in CT

15. _____ Dose length product (DLP)

16. _____ Radiation risk estimates less than 50 mSv

17. _____ Scan length

18. _____ Mammography

19. _____ Screening mammography

20. _____ 3 mGy

21. _____ Effective dose in CT

22. _____ Molybdenum
23. _____ Silver

24. _____ Craniocaudal and mediolateral

25. _____ Beryllium

A. Tube current is altered during a CT scan to adjust for different patient thicknesses and densities

B. The "window" or exit port for x-rays in a mammographic x-ray tube is composed of this element

C. Changes in the x-ray tube output during a rotation of the tube. Primarily used to reduce dose to structures on one side of the patient

D. Two centimeters of misalignment of the center of the patient with the center of the gantry can produce as much as a 25% unnecessary increase in patient dose

E. CTDI$_{VOL}$ × scan length

F. Scanning technique in which the x-ray tube rotates around the patient while the patient couch moves through the gantry

G. The relationship between the movement or advance of the patient couch, also known as table increment (I), and the x-ray beam collimator dimension (Z)

H. A dose level below which, according to the American Association of Physicists in Medicine, risks are too low to be detectable and may be nonexistent

I. A radiographic technique used to detect breast cancer that may not be palpable by physical examination

J. The product of dose length product (DLP) and a body region–specific conversion factor

K. The superior-inferior extent of the patient's irradiation during CT

L. An element used for a filter in mammography when a molybdenum target is used

M. A process in which repeated reconstructions are used to improve on a single mathematical reconstruction in CT

N. Food and Drug Administration (FDA) maximum breast dose for screening mammography

O. CT-specific dose markers or quantities needed to determine patient dose

P. Breast radiography used to detect disease in the general asymptomatic population

Q. The standard method for reconstruction of CT images from CT scan data in a single mathematical operation

R. The two projections recommended for routine screening mammography

S. Variation of radiation dose to the patient throughout the region imaged in a CT slice or slices

T. A weighted average of two measured CTDI values, one that is obtained with the pencil chamber placed in the center of the acrylic phantom and the other derived from the average of four peripheral measurements

U. The process of creating a cross-sectional tomographic plane of any part of the body

V. Radiation scattered from one slice to another

W. A mathematical modification to back projection that may be used to enhance the appearance of abrupt edges or small features within the image

X. An element used for filters with a tungsten target in mammography for thicker than average breasts

Y. CTDI$_W$/pitch

159

Exercise 2: Multiple Choice

Select the answer that *best* completes the following questions or statements.

1. Patient dose in CT is a topic of special interest because:
   A. Visible radiation damage is always produced.
   B. It has no detectable radiation exposure.
   C. It is used often and produces doses higher than those in general radiography.
   D. It has been associated with increased cancer incidence, particularly in the middle-aged population.

2. Which of the following describes the dose distribution within a slice of the patient for CT?
   A. It is more uniform than for radiography.
   B. It has a higher exit dose than entrance dose.
   C. There is an exponential decrease in dose with depth in the patient.
   D. Dose in the center of the patient is much higher than the dose at the periphery.

3. Which of the following *best* describes the use of direct patient shielding (such as contact shields or drapes) in CT?
   A. It is always used.
   B. It is used infrequently.
   C. It is used for all women of childbearing age.
   D. It is only used for imaging of the lumbar spine.

4. If I = table increment, L = overall length of the patient, Z = x-ray beam collimation thickness, and D = number of detectors, what is the definition of pitch?
   A. I/L
   B. D/I
   C. Z/L
   D. I/Z

5. What is the meaning of pitch = 1?
   A. The spiral scan dose is comparable to that of a single slice dose.
   B. The effective dose equals the skin exposure.
   C. The CT dose is 1 Gy.
   D. The dose distribution is uniform.

6. What is the relationship between patient dose and pitch in CT?
   A. They are unrelated.
   B. Half of the pitch equals the dose.
   C. Twice the pitch equals the dose.
   D. Greater pitch means lower dose.

7. How does tube current modulation affect patient dose in CT?
   A. It changes the reconstruction diameter during a scan.
   B. It changes tube current according to attenuation of the patient.
   C. It modifies collimator settings according to patient density.
   D. It sets a cumulative exposure timer.

8. What is the purpose of angular dose modulation in CT?
   A. To reduce patient dose in the center
   B. To increase pitch effect
   C. To reduce exposure of objects on one side of the patient
   D. To modify x-ray tube output along the long axis of the patient

9. A mathematical filter is applied during CT back projection to:
   A. Reduce patient dose
   B. Increase image noise
   C. Compare successive reconstructions with the "ideal" reconstruction
   D. Remove blur that would appear as a result of simple back projection

10. Different types of mathematical filters are used in back projection to change the amount of _____ in the CT image.
    A. Sharpness
    B. Collimation
    C. Surface exposure
    D. Dose overlap

11. If all other scan parameters are kept constant and the tube voltage is increased in CT, the patient dose will:
    A. Increase
    B. Decrease
    C. Stay the same
    D. Be unaffected

12. Miscentering of the patient in the CT scanner will most likely affect:
    A. Noise
    B. Resolution
    C. Patient dose
    D. Slice thickness

13. Which of the following parameters are the two CT-specific dose indicators or markers?
    A. Tube current and mAs
    B. $CTDI_{VOL,}$ DLP
    C. Filter function, exposure time
    D. CTDI, $CTDI_{VOL}$

14. What is the typical shape of an ionization chamber used to measure CTDI?
    A. Rectangular
    B. Spherical
    C. Cylindrical
    D. Trapezoidal

15. An acrylic phantom used to measure CT dose indices could be the approximate size of:
    A. A small room
    B. A human cell
    C. An adult head
    D. A fetal extremity

16. A CT scan consisting of 50 1-mm slices with a pitch of 2 has a scan length of _____ cm.
    A. 100
    B. 51
    C. 50
    D. 12

17. The dose length product equals:
    A. Scan length/$CTDI_{VOL}$
    B. $CTDI^2$
    C. Off axis centering $\times$ scan length
    D. $CTDI_{VOL} \times$ scan length

18. Effective dose is calculated from scan region–specific factors (CF) and other CT dose parameters as follows:
    A. $CF \times E_f DLP$
    B. CTDI/CF
    C. $CTDI_{VOL} \times$ scan length $\times$ CF
    D. $CF/CTDI_{VOL}$

19. During mammography, FDA regulations state that the mean dose to the glandular tissue of a 4.5 cm compressed breast should not exceed:
    A. 0.3 mGy per view
    B. 3 mGy per view
    C. 0.3 mGy total for three views
    D. 3 mGy total for three views

20. The imaging technique in which multiple views of the breast are reconstructed by a computer after being acquired by a mammography tube that rotates over a small range of angles is called:
    A. Digital breast dispersion
    B. Digital angular mammography
    C. Digital tomography
    D. Digital scintigraphy

21. The American College of Radiology (ACR), American Cancer Society (ACS), and American Medical Association (AMA) recommend mammography screening of the general population of women:
    A. Older than age 20
    B. Older than age 30
    C. Ages 30 to 60
    D. Ages 40 to 49

22. To limit the dose to the patient from screening mammography, it is generally recommended that screening examinations consist of the following projections:
    A. Craniocaudal, mediolateral, and axillary
    B. Craniocaudal and mediolateral
    C. Mediolateral and axillary
    D. Axillary only

23. Filters are used in mammography x-ray tubes to:
    A. Increase the milliamperage
    B. Decrease the energy spectra
    C. Remove photons that are not in the useful energy range
    D. Shape the voltage waveform of the x-ray generator

24. Which of the following materials are commonly used as x-ray tube targets?
    A. Molybdenum, rhodium, tungsten
    B. Beryllium, molybdenum, rhodium
    C. Silver, tungsten, molybdenum
    D. Molybdenum, silver

25. Which of the following materials are commonly used as filters in mammography systems?
    A. Rhodium, silver
    B. Molybdenum, tungsten
    C. Tungsten, silver, rhodium
    D. Molybdenum, rhodium, silver

Exercise 3: True or False

Circle *T* if the statement is true; circle *F* if the statement is false.

1. T F Computed tomography has been referred to as CAT scanning. The *A* stands for *acquisition.*

2. T F Patient dose in CT tends to be higher than dose from radiography of the same regions.

3. T F Dose at the center of a slice is generally 5 to 10 times higher than the dose at the periphery.

4. T F Interslice scatter tends to increase the overall patient dose when multiple slices are imaged.

5. T F Direct or contact shields are mandatory for use in CT to reduce dose to the anterior of the patient.

6. T F When the spiral scan pitch ratio is approximately 1, the spiral CT patient dose is comparable to that produced by conventional or axial CT.

161

7. T F Pitch is defined as $CTDI_{VOL}$ divided by the dose length product.

8. T F Tube current modulation cannot be used to lower patient dose on the anterior versus the posterior side of the patient.

9. T F Breast shields made of aluminum are mandatory for CT scanning in women younger than 49 years.

10. T F Iterative reconstruction techniques, however, can be used to reduce dose to levels less than those of filtered back projection while maintaining acceptable noise levels.

11. T F A highpass filter enhances the appearance of sharp edges in the CT image.

12. T F In CT, increasing kVp tends to increase patient dose.

13. T F Patient centering in the gantry has no effect on CT dose.

14. T F All the CTDI dose parameters are based on dose to an acrylic cylindrical phantom.

15. T F Effective dose in CT does not depend on the body part that is in the field of view.

16. T F Dose length product is equal to the product of $CTDI_{VOL}$ and scan length.

17. T F $CTDI_{VOL}$ is equal to $CTDI_W$ multiplied by the pitch.

18. T F According to the American Association of Physicists in Medicine (AAPM),[3] "Risks of medical imaging at effective doses below 50 mSv for single procedures or 100 mSv for multiple procedures over short time periods are too low to be detectable and may be nonexistent."

19. T F Yearly screening mammograms are generally recommended for women older than age 50.

20. T F Although doses for screening mammography must be less than 3 mGy to meet FDA requirements, most screening is associated with doses of no more than 2 mGy.

21. T F Mammographic image quality is easier to maintain in women with denser breast tissue.

22. T F Digital tomosynthesis only allows one view but requires a much smaller radiation dose than full-field digital mammography.

23. T F X-ray tube targets for mammography must emit photons of only 17 and 19 keV to meet FDA guidelines.

24. T F Cellophane takes the place of glass in the window of the low kVp mammographic unit.

25. T F Axillary projections in mammography should only be done on request of the radiologist.

Exercise 4: Fill in the Blank

Using the following Word Bank, fill in the blanks with the word or words that best complete the statements.

16	dose	molybdenum
32	dose length product	overlap of margins
40	effective	pitch
49	false-positive	rhodium (can be used twice)
acrylic	filtered	"scout view" or "radiographic
an acceptable	greater than	mode"
automatic exposure control	internal	silver
best	interslice scatter	spiral, or helical
collimated	iterative	tube current modulation
craniocaudal	low	tungsten
dense	mediolateral	yearly

1. Multislice, _____, CT scanners acquire images by rotating the x-ray tube around the patient as he or she is moved through the gantry.

2. The skin dose for a succession of adjacent scans is _____ _____ the skin dose from a single scan.

3. Scatter dose is reduced in CT compared with radiography because the CT beam is _____.

4. There are two reasons why multislice CT dose is slightly higher than the sum of the doses from individual slices. These are _____ _____ and _____ _____.

5. Dose outside of the field of view in CT is caused primarily by _____ scatter.

6. The distance that the couch travels during a scan divided by the beam thickness is the _____ ratio.

7. CT manufacturers utilize information from the initial _____ _____ or _____ _____ image to modulate or change the current as the tube moves along the longitudinal axis of the patient.

8. Angula-based _____ _____ _____ can be used to reduce dose to tissues on one side of the patient.

9. Tube current modulation is also referred to as _____ _____ _____ for CT.

10. Before CT scan data are back projected, they are _____ to remove blur.

11. Repeated reconstruction of CT images until constraints such as noise are minimized is referred to as _____ reconstruction.

12. When the patient is miscentered in the gantry, the patient _____ usually increases when AEC is used.

13. If $CTDI_{VOL}$ and DLP are known, then _____ dose (EfD) to the patient may be determined.

14. CTDI is determined with an ionization chamber in a cylindrical _____ phantom.

15. Phantoms used for CT dose measurement are cylindrical with diameters of _____ cm for the head and _____ cm for the abdomen.

16. _____ _____ _____ is equal to $CTDI_{VOL}$ × scan length.

17. According to the American Association of Physicists in Medicine, "Risks of medical imaging at effective doses below 50 mSv for single procedures or 100 mSv for multiple procedures over short time periods are too _____ to be detectable."[3]

18. The goal of CT imaging should be to obtain the _____ possible image while delivering _____ _____ level of ionizing radiation to the patient.

19. Experts agree that _____ mammographic screening of women 50 years of age and older leads to earlier detection of breast cancer.

20. Digital tomosynthesis lowers the percentage of _____ readings caused by increased density and consequently permits a more effective screening of younger women.

21. Younger women generally have breast tissue that is more radiographically _____ than older women.

22. The American Cancer Society currently recommends mammographic screening for women between the ages of _____ and _____.

23. For mammography screening examinations in asymptomatic women with no significant risk factors it is generally recommended that only _____ and _____ projections be taken.

24. Three x-ray tube target materials used for mammography x-ray tubes are: _____, _____, and _____.

25. Two filters that are used with tungsten targets in mammography systems are _____ and _____.

Exercise 5: Labeling

Complete the list and table.

A. List four dose reduction methods that lead to optimization of patient dose in CT.

1. _____

2. _____

3. _____

4. _____

B. Fill in the typical effective dose values for the CT examinations listed in the following table.

Examination	Effective dose (mSv)
Head	
Chest	
Abdomen	
Pelvis	
Coronary artery calcification	
Coronary angiography	

Exercise 6: Short Answer

Answer the following questions by providing a short answer.

1. What are the two concerns related to patient dose in CT scanning?

_____

_____

2. Why is the skin dose usually smaller for a CT scan than for a radiographic or fluoroscopic image of the same region of the body?

_____

_____

3. What factors increase the dose of multislice examinations compared with a single-slice examination in CT?

_____

_____

4. Why is direct (contact, surface) shielding not usually recommended for patients undergoing CT examinations?

_____

_____

5. What is the relationship between pitch and patient dose in CT?

_____

_____

6. What feature of a CT scanner adjusts output according to the density of various parts of the patient?

_____

_____

_____

_____

7. Name two methods for image reconstruction in CT.

_____

_____

8. What is the effect of patient miscentering on patient dose in CT if the patient is placed closer to the x-ray tube during the scout (radiographic) view?

_____

_____

_____

9. List four CT dose parameters.

_____

_____

10. By what factor is DLP multiplied to calculate effective dose?

_____

_____

11. What is the maximum allowed dose for FDA-approved screening mammography?

_____

_____

12. What technique allows the radiologist to get three-dimensional views of the breast?

_____

13. To maintain acceptably low radiation dose, typical screening mammograms are limited to what projections?

_____

14. Why are target materials other than tungsten sometimes used in mammography?

_____

_____

15. What materials are used as filters when tungsten targets are used for digital mammography?

_____

_____

Exercise 7: General Discussion or Opinion Questions

The following questions are intended to allow students to express their knowledge and understanding of the subject matter or to present a personal opinion. The questions may be used to stimulate class discussion. Because answers to questions may vary, determination of the answer's acceptability is left to the discretion of the course instructor.

1. Why are the higher doses associated with CT considered acceptable compared with lower doses from radiographic studies or zero doses from ultrasound?

2. Why are breast shields generally not used in CT?

3. How is radiation dose in CT tailored to the varying thicknesses and densities of parts of different patients?

4. What dose parameters are most relevant to a general question from a referring physician or a patient, such as, What is the dose from this CT scan?

5. What are the issues of concern with regard to dose to pediatric patients in CT, and how are they addressed?

6. Why is there some disagreement among various organizations about the age at which women should undergo screening mammograms?

7. What are the relevant advantages and disadvantages to the use of digital tomosynthesis in screening mammography? What is its role in a diagnostic workup previously diagnosed as suspicious findings?

POST-TEST

The student should take this test after reading Chapter 12, finishing all accompanying textbook and workbook exercises, and completing any additional activities required by the course instructor. The student should complete the post-test with a score of 90% or higher before advancing to the next chapter. (Each of the following 20 questions is worth 5 points.)
Score = _____ %

1. The dose distribution within a CT slice is _____ (more/less) uniform than it is for general radiography.

2. Multislice CT scans produce higher radiation doses than single-slice scans to the area within individual slices because of:
   A. Beam hardening
   B. Filtration
   C. Interslice scatter
   D. Tomographic recentering

3. Direct patient shielding such as aprons or other contact shields are not generally used within the irradiated field of view of CT because:
   A. Tube rotation and AEC would attempt to compensate
   B. Lead is of the wrong k edge for attenuation of CT photons
   C. Interslice scatter
   D. Sharpening filter disruption

4. The amount of movement of the patient couch as the x-ray tube rotates completely around the patient is referred to as the _____ _____.

5. A pitch of 1.5 means that:
   A. The patient dose exceeds FDA guidelines.
   B. The couch increments exceed the beam width.
   C. The filter is a sharpening filter.
   D. The kVp exceeds the mAs.

Chapter **13** Special Considerations on Safety in
Computed Tomography and Mammography

6. Which of the following are methods to optimize patient dose in CT?
    A. Tube current modulation
    B. Iterative reconstruction
    C. Correct patient centering
    D. All of the above

7. The main method of automatic exposure control in CT is: _____ _____ _____.

8. _____ _____ tube current modulation reduces tube current while the x-ray tube is on the anterior side of the patient and maintains or increases dose as it rotates on the posterior side. This method has been found to underdose the superficial anterior organs without adversely affecting image quality.

9. In the past, CT images were usually produced by _____ back projection. Newer scanners provide the option to use _____ reconstruction.

10. When scan time is fixed in CT, if kVp is increased, the output of the x-ray tube increases during a scan and the patient exposure actually_____ (increases/decreases).

11. If the patient is mispositioned toward the x-ray tube in the scout (radiographic) view, then the AEC system may produce a _____ (greater/lower) exposure to compensate for the magnified size of the patient.

12. $CTDI_{VOL}$ is the:
    A. Average absorbed dose within the scanned volume of a phantom
    B. Effective dose to the patient within the scanned volume
    C. Ionization chamber reading at the center of the cylindrical phantom
    D. Ionization chamber reading outside of a phantom, between contiguous slices

13. Scan direction collimation is equal to the product of the number of _____ _____ used during one axial acquisition (N) and the nominal slice width of one axial image (T).

14. If the $CTDI_{VOL}$ is multiplied by the scan length, the _____ _____ _____ is obtained.

15. A helical scan that is composed of 80 5-mm slices with a pitch of 1.25 has a scan length of _____ cm.

16. A scan region–specific conversion factor is multiplied by _____ _____ _____ to calculate effective dose in CT.

17. Federal regulations for FDA certification of screening mammography facilities state that the mean dose to the glandular tissue of a_____-cm compressed breast using a screen-film or digital mammography system should not exceed 3 mGy_t per view.

18. Before the onset of menopause, a _____ is also highly recommended for comparison with mammograms taken at a later age.
    A. Diagnostic ultrasound
    B. Screening CT
    C. Complete blood cell count
    D. Baseline mammogram

19. Digital tomosynthesis mammography x-ray tubes often use the same tube target material as is used for general purpose radiography, which is _____.

20. If a tungsten target is used for mammography, what materials are commonly used as filters?
    A. Silver and aluminum
    B. Rhodium and silver
    C. Rhodium and molybdenum
    D. Molybdenum and aluminum

References

1. Mayo-Smith WW et al: How I do it: managing radiation dose in CT, *Radiology* 273(3):657-672, 2014.

2. Yaffe M, Mawdslwy GE: Equipment requirements and quality control for mammography, in specification, acceptance testing and quality control of diagnostic x-ray imaging equipment. In Siebert JA, Barnes GT, Gould RG, eds: *American Association of Physicists in Medicine medical physics monograph,* No. 20, College Park, Md, 1994, American Association of Physicists in Medicine.

3. American Association of Physicists in Medicine, AAPM website. AAPM position statement on radiation risk from medical imaging procedures, policy no. pp. 25 A.

14 Management of Imaging Personnel Radiation Dose During Diagnostic X-Ray Procedures

Some x-ray procedures increase the radiographer's risk of exposure to scatter radiation. Chapter 14 presents an overview of methods that can be used to reduce exposure for imaging professionals during diagnostic x-ray procedures. In addition, a brief explanation of diagnostic x-ray suite radiation protection design is presented.

CHAPTER HIGHLIGHTS

- An annual occupational effective dose of 50 mSv for whole-body exposure during routine operations and an annual effective dose of 1 mSv for individuals in the general population have been established.
- A cumulative effective dose (CumEfD) limits a radiation worker's whole-body lifetime effective dose to his or her age in years times 10 mSv.
- Radiation workers can receive a larger equivalent dose than the general public without altering the genetically significant dose (GSD).
- Occupational exposure must be kept as low as reasonably achievable (ALARA).
- The following methods of reducing scatter radiation also reduce the occupational hazard for the radiographer:
  - ☐ Use of beam-limitation devices, higher-kVp and lower-mA techniques, appropriate beam filtration, and adequate protective shielding
  - ☐ Proper use of protective apparel (lead aprons, gloves, thyroid shields)
  - ☐ Reduction of repeat images
- The basic principles of time, distance, and shielding are to be employed to minimize occupational radiation exposure.
- Pregnant radiographers can wear an additional monitoring device at waist level to ensure that their monthly equivalent dose does not exceed 0.5 mSv.
- Primary and secondary protective barriers must be designed so that annual effective dose limits are not exceeded.
- A lead-lined, metal, diagnostic-type protective tube housing protects the radiographer and the patient from leakage radiation.
- The following practices are important in protecting the radiographer during routine fluoroscopy:
  - ☐ The radiographer, in addition to wearing appropriate protective apparel, should stand as far away from the patient as is practical and move closer to the patient only when assistance is required.
  - ☐ A protective curtain and Bucky slot shielding device must be used.
  - ☐ The x-ray beam must be adequately collimated, and a cumulative timing device should be used.
- The following are required to protect the radiographer during mobile radiographic examinations:
  - ☐ The radiographer must wear protective garments.
  - ☐ The radiographer should stand at least 2 m from the patient, x-ray tube, and useful beam.
  - ☐ If possible, the radiographer should also stand at a right angle to the x-ray beam–scattering object (the patient) line.
- Limited exposure time and dose-reduction features are required to protect the radiographer during high-level-control fluoroscopy.
- Distance is the most effective means of protection from ionizing radiation.
- If the peak energy of the x-ray beam is 100 kVp, a lead apron of at least 0.25-mm lead equivalent thickness should be worn if the radiographer cannot remain behind a protective barrier. A lead apron of 0.5- or 1-mm lead equivalent thickness affords much greater protection.
- Lead gloves, a thyroid shield, and protective glasses are sometimes required.
- Radiographers should never stand in the primary beam to hold a patient during a radiographic exposure.
- When designing diagnostic x-ray suites, equivalent dose to radiation workers, nonoccupationally exposed personnel, and the general public must be taken into consideration.
  - ☐ Facilities must be equipped with radiation-absorbent barriers.
  - ☐ Occupancy factor, workload, and use factor must be considered when thickness requirements for a protective barrier are being determined. Whether an area beyond a structure is designated as a controlled or uncontrolled area is significant in determining the amount of radiation shielding to be added to that structure.
- Radiation warning signs are an important component of safety in a radiology department.

Exercise 1: Matching

Match the following terms with their definitions or associated phrases.

1. _____ 50 mSv

2. _____ Control booth barrier

3. _____ 0.5 mSv

4. _____ ALARA concept

5. _____ Lead and concrete

6. _____ Secondary radiation

7. _____ Workload (W)

8. _____ Protective curtain

9. _____ CumEfD limit

10. _____ Occupancy factor (T)

11. _____ Bucky slot shielding device

12. _____ GSD

13. _____ Inverse square law (ISL)

14. _____ Use factor (U)

15. _____ Scatter radiation

16. _____ Protective eyeglasses

17. _____ Secondary protective barrier

18. _____ High-level-control

19. _____ Protective apparel

20. _____ Remote control fluoroscopic system

A. "The intensity of radiation is inversely proportional to the square of the distance from the source"

B. Protects against leakage and scatter radiation

C. Annual occupational effective dose in metric units for whole-body exposure during routine operations

D. Restricts the dimensions of the radiographic beam so that its margins do not extend beyond the image receptor

E. Prevents direct, or unscattered, radiation from reaching personnel or members of the general public on the other side of the barrier

F. Monthly allowable equivalent dose to the embryo-fetus in metric units from occupational exposure of a pregnant technologist

G. Beam direction factor

H. Annual effective dose (EfD) limit set for members of the general public

I. Specified either in units of milliampere-seconds (mAs) per week or milliampere-minutes (mA-min) per week

J. During a standard fluoroscopic examination, when the Bucky tray is positioned at the foot end of the table, this device automatically covers the Bucky slot opening in the side of the x-ray table. It protects the radiologist and radiographer at the gonadal level

K. Most common materials used for structural protective barriers

L. This is used to modify the shielding requirement for a particular barrier by taking into account the fraction of the work week during which the space beyond the barrier is occupied

M. Permits the radiologist and assisting radiographer to remain outside the fluoroscopic room at a control console behind a protective barrier until needed

N. Mode of operation in which the exposure rate may significantly exceed the rate used in routine fluoroscopy

O. During a fluoroscopic examination, this device should be positioned between the fluoroscopist and the patient to intercept scattered radiation above the tabletop

P. A permanent protective barrier for the radiographer that is located in an x-ray room housing stationary radiographic equipment

Q. A radiation worker's whole-body lifetime effective dose in mSv should not exceed 10 times the person's age in years

R. All the radiation that arises from interactions of an x-ray beam with the atoms of an object in the path of the beam

S. Principle that holds that occupational exposure of the radiographer and other occupationally exposed persons should be kept as low as reasonably achievable

T. The average annual gonadal equivalent dose to members of the population who are of childbearing age

21. _____ Primary protective barrier

22. _____ C-arm fluoroscope

23. _____ 1 mSv

24. _____ Positive beam limitation (PBL)

25. _____ Mechanical restraining devices

U. Consists of radiation that has been deflected from the primary beam. This radiation is made up of leakage radiation from the tube housing and scatter primarily from the patient

V. Glasses with optically clear lenses that contain a minimal lead equivalent protection level of 0.35 mm

W. Should be used to immobilize patients during radiographic exposures, whenever possible, instead of people

X. Special garments (e.g., aprons, gloves, and thyroid shields) that conventionally are made of lead-impregnated vinyl and are worn during fluoroscopic and certain radiographic procedures

Y. A portable device for producing real-time (motion) images of a patient. This device holds an x-ray tube at one end and an image intensifier at the other end; exposure of personnel is caused by scattered radiation from the patient

Exercise 2: Multiple Choice

Select the answer that *best* completes the following questions or statements.

1. Because the workforce in radiation-related jobs is small compared with the population as a whole, the amount of radiation received by this workforce can be larger than the amount received by the general public without altering the:
   A. Genetically significant dose (GSD)
   B. Lethal dose (LD) 50/30
   C. Mean marrow dose (MMD)
   D. Tumor induction risk ratio (TIRR)

2. Which of the following is a tenet of the ALARA concept?
   A. The radiographer's occupational exposure should not exceed the annual EfD limit allowed for individual members of the general population.
   B. The radiographer's occupational exposure should be as high as necessary to allow for holding of patients during diagnostic x-ray procedures.
   C. The radiographer's occupational exposure for the whole body should limit that individual's lifetime EfD to his or her age times 50 mSv.
   D. The radiographer's exposure should be kept as low as reasonably achievable.

3. A facility that employs a pregnant diagnostic imaging staff member should provide that individual with an additional monitor to be worn at waist level during *all* radiation procedures. The purpose of this additional monitor is to ensure that the monthly equivalent dose (EqD) to the embryo-fetus does not exceed _____ in metric units.
   A. 50 mSv
   B. 10 mSv
   C. 5 mSv
   D. 0.5 mSv

4. Which of the following are radiation sources that can be generated in a diagnostic x-ray room?
   1. Primary radiation
   2. Scatter radiation
   3. Leakage radiation
   A. 1 only
   B. 2 only
   C. 3 only
   D. 1, 2, and 3

5. During C-arm fluoroscopy, the exposure rate caused by scatter near the entrance surface of the patient (the x-ray tube side) _____ the exposure rate caused by scatter near the exit surface of the patient (the image intensifier side).
   A. Equals
   B. Exceeds
   C. Is slightly less than
   D. Is considerably less than

6. For high-level-control interventional procedures, the radiographer should verify that which of the following dose reduction features are available and in good working order?
   1. High-quality, low-dose fluoroscopy mode and pulsed beam operation
   2. Manual collimation, correct beam filtration, and removable grids
   3. Roadmapping, time-interval differences, and last-image-hold mode
   A. 1 only
   B. 2 only
   C. 3 only
   D. 1, 2, and 3

171

7. In diagnostic radiology, which of the following radiation sources poses the *greatest* occupational hazard for the radiographer?
   A. Image-formation radiation
   B. Leakage radiation
   C. Primary radiation
   D. Scattered radiation

8. During a fluoroscopic examination, which of the following methods and devices reduce(s) the radiographer's exposure?
   1. Adequate x-ray beam collimation
   2. Control of technical exposure factors
   3. Use of a cumulative timing device
   A. 1 only
   B. 2 only
   C. 3 only
   D. 1, 2, and 3

9. If the peak energy of the diagnostic x-ray beam is 120 kVp, the primary protective barrier in a typical installation consists of at least _____ and extends _____ upward from the floor of the x-ray room, when the tube is 1.5 to 2.1 m from the wall in question.
   A. 1.6 mm lead, 2.1 m
   B. 1.6 mm lead, 6.3 m
   C. 0.8 mm lead, 2.1 m
   D. 0.8 mm lead, 6.3 m

10. Of the following radiation sources, which is the control booth barrier *not* intended to intercept in a diagnostic x-ray room?
    1. Leakage radiation
    2. Primary radiation
    3. Scattered radiation
    A. 1 only
    B. 2 only
    C. 3 only
    D. 1 and 3 only

11. A radiographic x-ray suite is in operation 5 days per week. The average number of patients per day is 25, and the average number of images per patient is 3. The average technical exposure factors are 70 kVp, 300 mA, and 0.2 sec. Find the weekly workload.
    A. 125 mA-min/wk
    B. 250 mA-min/wk
    C. 375 mA-min/wk
    D. 450 mA-min/wk

12. Which of the following statements is *true*?
    A. When wearing a protective apron, a radiographer may stand in the useful beam to restrain a patient during a difficult radiologic procedure.
    B. When wearing protective aprons, nurses, orderlies, relatives, or friends may stand in the useful beam to restrain a patient during a difficult radiologic procedure.
    C. When wearing protective aprons, pregnant radiographers or other nonoccupationally exposed pregnant women may stand in the useful beam to restrain a patient during a difficult radiologic procedure.
    D. Radiographers and nonoccupationally exposed individuals should never stand in the useful beam to restrain a patient during a radiographic procedure.

13. Of the devices listed here, which eliminates nonuseful low-energy photons from the primary beam?
    1. Collimator light source
    2. Electronic sensors
    3. Aluminum filtration
    A. 1 only
    B. 2 only
    C. 3 only
    D. 1, 2, and 3

14. Which of the following is the *most effective* means of protection from ionizing radiation normally available to the radiographer?
    A. Reducing the amount of time spent near a source of radiation
    B. Placing as much distance as possible between oneself and the source of radiation
    C. Remaining behind a mobile protective shield during an exposure
    D. Using protective shielding garments

15. The lead glass window of the control booth barrier in a stationary (fixed) radiographic installation typically consists of which of the following?
    A. 0.25-mm lead equivalent
    B. 0.5-mm lead equivalent
    C. 1-mm lead equivalent
    D. 1.5-mm lead equivalent

16. The beam direction factor is also known as the:
    A. Occupancy factor
    B. ISL
    C. Workload
    D. Use factor

17. If the intensity of the x-ray is inversely proportional to the square of the distance from the source, how does the intensity of the x-ray beam change when the distance from the source of radiation and a measurement point is quadrupled?
    A. It increases by a factor of 4 at the new distance.
    B. It increases by a factor of 16 at the new distance.
    C. It decreases by a factor of 16 at the new distance.
    D. It decreases by a factor of 4 at the new distance.

18. Leakage radiation and scatter radiation are forms of:
    A. Cosmic radiation
    B. Natural background radiation
    C. Nonionizing radiation
    D. Secondary radiation

19. Diagnostic x-ray installations must be equipped with:
    A. Barriers made of aluminum
    B. Barriers made of Sheetrock
    C. Radiation-absorbent barriers
    D. Radiation-nonabsorbent barriers

20. Which of the following principles can be used to minimize occupational radiation exposure?
        1. Time
        2. Distance
        3. Shielding
    A. 1 and 2 only
    B. 1 and 3 only
    C. 2 and 3 only
    D. 1, 2, and 3

21. Pregnant radiographers can wear an additional monitoring device at waist level to ensure that the monthly EqD does not exceed:
    A. 0.1 mSv
    B. 0.2 mSv
    C. 0.3 mSv
    D. 0.5 mSv

22. During fluoroscopy, which of the following will provide radiation protection for the radiographer and the radiologist?
        1. Using appropriate source-to-skin distance
        2. Having a diagnostic-type x-ray tube housing
        3. Using a remote control fluoroscopic system
    A. 1 and 2 only
    B. 1 and 3 only
    C. 2 and 3 only
    D. 1, 2, and 3

23. Floors of radiation rooms except dental installations, doors, walls, and ceilings of radiation rooms exposed routinely to the primary beam are given a use factor of:
    A. 1
    B. $^1/_2$
    C. $^1/_4$
    D. $^1/_{16}$

24. If a radiographer stands 1 m away from an x-ray tube and receives an exposure rate dose of 4.0 mGy$_a$ /hr, what will the exposure rate dose be if the same radiographer moves to stand at a position located 2 m from the x-ray tube?
    A. 1 mGy$_a$/hr
    B. 2 mGy$_a$/hr
    C. 8 mGy$_a$/hr
    D. 16 mGy$_a$/hr

25. If a radiographer moves closer to a source of radiation, the radiation exposure to the radiographer:
    A. Decreases slightly
    B. Decreases significantly
    C. Increases slightly
    D. Increases significantly

Exercise 3: True or False

Circle *T* if the statement listed below is true; circle *F* if the statement is false.

1. T   F   Compared with routine radiographic procedures, general fluoroscopic procedures increase the radiographer's risk of exposure to ionizing radiation.

2. T   F   A radiographer's annual occupational EfD includes personal medical and natural background radiation exposure.

3. T   F   The ALARA concept takes economic and social factors into consideration.

4. T   F   Protective lead aprons and shielded barriers function as gonadal shields for diagnostic imaging personnel.

5. T   F   The intensity of radiation is directly proportional to the square of the distance from the source.

6. T   F   Radiographic and fluoroscopic exposures can be made when room doors are open.

7. T   F   If the peak energy of an x-ray beam is 100 kVp, a protective lead (Pb) apron must be equivalent to at least a 2.5-mm thickness of lead.

173

8. T   F   During a routine fluoroscopic examination, if the radiographer's immediate presence is not required near the x-ray table to assist the radiologist, the radiographer may either stand behind the radiologist, who is also wearing protective apparel, or stand behind the control-booth barrier until his or her services are required.

9. T   F   The protective curtain on a fluoroscopic unit protects the radiologist and radiographer at the gonadal level.

10. T   F   For C-arm devices with similar fields of view, the dose rate for personnel located within a meter of the patient is comparable to that in routine fluoroscopy—approximately several milligray in air (mGy_a) per hour.

11. T   F   The physical configuration of a C-arm fluoroscopic unit allows the operator many methods of achieving protection from scattered radiation.

12. T   F   From the perspective of increased radiation safety, it is best to reverse the C-arm to place the x-ray tube under the table and the image intensifier over the table.

13. T   F   A radiographer may hold a patient during a radiographic exposure as long as the radiographer stands in the useful beam.

14. T   F   The primary radiation intensity for a selected kVp at the barrier location for an x-ray suite may be determined by making air kerma measurements on the suite's x-ray unit at a reference distance (e.g., 100 cm) from the x-ray tube target with the aid of a calibrated ionization chamber.

15. T   F   Because scatter and leakage radiation emerge in all directions in the x-ray room, every wall, door, viewing window, and other surface are always struck by some quantity of radiation.

16. T   F   Filtration primarily benefits the radiographer.

17. T   F   During a diagnostic x-ray procedure, the patient becomes a source of scattered radiation as a consequence of the coherent scattering process.

18. T   F   At a 90-degree angle to the primary x-ray beam, at a distance of 1 m, the scattered x-ray intensity is generally approximately $\frac{1}{1000}$ of the intensity of the primary x-ray beam.

19. T   F   Methods and techniques that reduce patient exposure also reduce exposure for the radiographer.

20. T   F   Pregnant diagnostic imaging department staff members must immediately stop performing their respective duties and discontinue employment as a consequence of pregnancy.

21. T   F   The amount of radiation a worker receives at a particular location is inversely proportional to the length of time the individual is exposed to ionizing radiation.

22. T   F   If a declared pregnant radiographer is reassigned to a lower radiation exposure risk area, then the other remaining radiographers in the higher risk area, who must fill in, can be subject to increased risk. Therefore the declared-pregnant radiographer does not necessarily need to be reassigned to a lower radiation exposure area as a direct consequence of the declared pregnancy.

23. T   F   In accordance with ALARA guidelines, work schedules are designed to distribute radiation exposure risk evenly to all employees.

24. T   F   In a typical x-ray room, a secondary barrier should overlap the primary barrier by about 1.27 cm.

25. T   F   During a fluoroscopic examination, a radiographer need not wear a protective apron when he or she is in the x-ray room during a procedure.

Exercise 4: Fill in the Blank

Using the following Word Bank, fill in the blanks with the word or words that best complete the statements.

2.1 meters	Compton scatter (may be used more than once)	perpendicular
0.25 mm lead		right angles
0.5 mm lead (may be used more than once)	direct	routine
	distance (may be used more than once)	safety (may be used more than once)
0.8 mm lead	embryo-fetus	
1.0 mm lead	equivalent dose	scattered (may be used more than once)
1.6 mm lead	four	
0.5 mSv	gloves	shielding (may be used more than once)
4	high-tension	
5.0 mSv	housing	shortening
90	least	thyroid shields
aprons	magnify	time
assistance	patient	wraparound

1. Although the radiographer and other diagnostic imaging personnel are allowed to absorb more radiation than the general public, the _____ _____ received must be minimized whenever possible.

2. _____ radiation poses the greatest occupational hazard in diagnostic radiology.

3. Radiation warning signs are an important component of _____ in a radiology department.

4. After receiving radiation safety counseling, a pregnant radiologic technologist must read and sign a form acknowledging that she has received counseling and understands the practices to be followed to ensure the _____ of the _____.

5. Primary radiation is also known as _____ radiation.

6. _____ the length of time spent in a room where x-radiation is produced reduces occupational exposure.

7. The most effective means of protection from ionizing radiation is _____.

8. Structural barriers such as walls and doors in an x-ray room provide protective _____ for both imaging department personnel and the general public.

9. Accessory protective shielding includes _____, _____, and _____ _____ made of lead-impregnated vinyl.

10. No one should touch the tube _____ or _____ cables while a radiographic exposure is in progress.

11. When high-speed image receptor systems are used, smaller radiographic exposure (less milliamperage) is required, which results in fewer x-ray photons being available to produce _____ _____. Because of this reduction in _____ _____, personnel exposure is decreased.

12. It is imperative that the EqD to the embryo-fetus from occupational exposure of the mother not exceed the National Council on Radiation Protection and Measurements (NCRP)–recommended monthly EqD limit of _____ _____ or a limit of _____ _____ during the entire pregnancy.

13. Maternity protective aprons consist of _____ _____ _____ equivalent over their entire length and width and also have an extra _____ _____ _____ equivalent protective panel that runs transversely across the width of the apron to provide added safety for the embryo-fetus.

14. Shortening the length of _____ spent in a room where x-radiation is produced, standing at the greatest _____ possible from an energized x-ray beam, and interposing a radiation-absorbent _____ material between the radiation worker and the source of radiation all reduce occupational exposure.

15. When the distance from the x-ray target, a point source of radiation, is doubled, the radiation at the new location spans an area _____ times larger than the original area. However, because the same amount of radiation exists to cover this larger area, the intensity at the new distance decreases by a factor of _____.

175

16. Primary protective barriers are located _____ to the undeflected line of travel of the x-ray beam.

17. If the peak energy of the x-ray beam is 120 kVp, the primary protective barrier in a typical installation consists of approximately _____ _____ _____ and extends _____ _____ upward from the floor of the x-ray room when the x-ray tube is 1.5 to 2.1 meters from the wall in question.

18. In a typical diagnostic x-ray installation, the secondary barrier consists of _____ _____ _____.

19. During general fluoroscopy and x-ray special procedures, a neck and thyroid shield can guard the thyroid area of occupationally exposed people. It should be _____ _____ _____ equivalent.

20. To ensure protection from _____ radiation emanating from the patient during a fluoroscopic examination, the radiographer should stand as far from the _____ as is practical and should move closer to the patient only when _____ is required.

21. Protective lead gloves of at least _____ _____ _____ equivalent should be worn whenever the hands must be placed near the fluoroscopic field.

22. For better visualization of small body parts, C-arm fluoroscopes have the capability to _____ the image.

23. During a fluoroscopic examination, a_____ protective apron is recommended to protect personnel who must move around the x-ray room.

24. The radiographer should attempt to stand at _____ _____ (_____ degrees) to the x-ray beam-scattering object (the patient) line; when the protective factors of distance and shielding have been accounted for, this is the place where the _____ amount of scattered radiation is received.

25. In _____ imaging, because the image contrast and overall brightness can be manipulated after image acquisition, the need for almost all retakes resulting from improper technique selection is eliminated.

Exercise 5: Labeling

Label the following illustrations and solve the following problems.

A. Relationship between distance and intensity.

More distance = Less intensity (quantity of radiation)

1. $2 \times d =$ _____

2. $3 \times d =$ _____

3. $4 \times d =$ _____

B. Protective barriers.

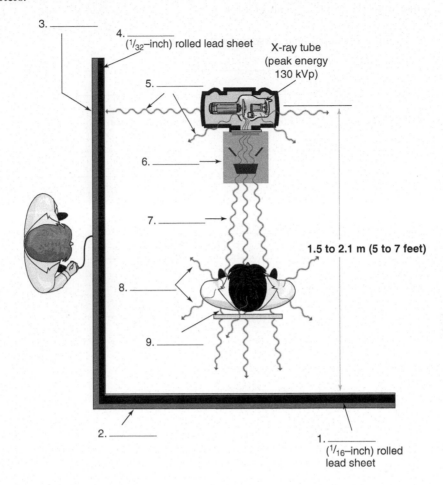

3. _____

4. _____
($^1/_{32}$–inch) rolled lead sheet

X-ray tube
(peak energy
130 kVp)

5. _____

6. _____

7. _____

1.5 to 2.1 m (5 to 7 feet)

8. _____

9. _____

2. _____

1. _____
($^1/_{16}$–inch) rolled
lead sheet

C. Standing at right angles to the scattering object.

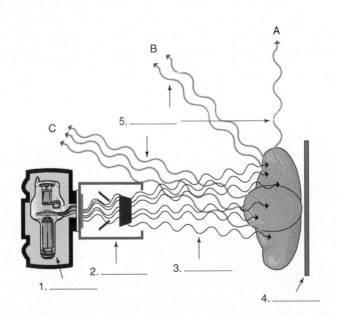

A

B

C

5. _____

1. _____

2. _____

3. _____

4. _____

Exercise 6: Short Answer

Answer the following questions by providing a short answer.

1. What does the annual limit for occupational personnel *not* include?

   _____

   _____

2. From what types of x-radiation are lead aprons designed to provide protection?

   _____

   _____

3. What colors are radiation warning signs required to be?

   _____

   _____

4. Why should a pregnant radiographer "declare" a pregnancy?

   _____

   _____

5. List the three basic principles of radiation protection.

   _____

   _____

6. Who should determine the exact requirements for protective structural shielding for a particular imaging facility?

   _____

   _____

7. Of what material are protective aprons, gloves, and thyroid shields made?

   _____

   _____

8. How can scattered radiation to the lens of the eyes of diagnostic imaging personnel be substantially reduced?

   _____

   _____

9. How does a lead-lined, metal, diagnostic-type protective tube housing protect the radiographer and the patient from off-focus, or leakage, radiation?

   _____

   _____

10. How does the use of a remote control fluoroscopic unit increase the safety of imaging personnel?

   _____

   _____

11. From the perspective of increased radiation safety, why is it best to place the x-ray tube end of the C-arm under the table and the image intensifier over the table whenever possible?

_____

_____

12. During operating room procedures in which cross-table exposures are obtained with a mobile C-arm fluoroscope, where is the potential for scatter dose lower in relation to the patient?

_____

_____

13. How can the radiologist or other interventional physician reduce radiation exposure during a high-level-control interventional procedure?

_____

_____

14. Why should physicians performing interventional procedures wear extremity monitors? What is the annual EqD limit in metric units for localized areas of the skin and hands? What can physicians use to protect their hands during an interventional procedure?

_____

_____

15. List eight radiation-absorbent barrier-design considerations.

_____

_____

Exercise 7: Discussion or Opinion Questions

The following questions are intended to allow students to express their knowledge and understanding of the subject matter or to present a personal opinion. The questions may be used to stimulate class discussion. Because answers to these questions may vary, determination of the answer's acceptability is left to the discretion of the course instructor.

1. Of what importance is protective structural shielding in an imaging facility? What factors must be considered in planning structural shielding? Who is responsible for the planning of this shielding?

2. What are some of the requirements for posting caution signs to alert others of the presence of radioactive materials or radiation areas? What do these signs look like?

3. What types of protective apparel are usually available for personnel in most health care facilities? Give examples of appropriate use of each of these items in a clinical setting.

4. When performing a mobile radiographic examination, what radiation protection problems can a radiographer encounter? How can each problem be safely resolved?

5. When operating a mobile C-arm fluoroscope in the operating room during a surgical procedure, what radiation protection problems may a radiographer encounter? How can each problem be safely resolved?

Exercise 8: Calculation Problems

Solve the following problems.

The inverse square law (ISL) expresses the relationship between distance and intensity (quantity) of radiation and is significant as a tool to be used in governing the dose received by personnel. The law is stated as "The intensity of radiation is inversely proportional to the square of the distance from the source." To be more explicit, as the separation between the radiation source and a measurement point increases, the quantity of radiation measured at the more distant position decreases by the square of the ratio of the original distance from the source to the new distance from the source.

This lowering of radiation concentration physically occurs because the area, which the same flux of x-rays at the original location now covers at the new location, has increased by the square of the relative distance change. For example, as demonstrated in the sample problem that follows, when the distance from the x-ray target, a point source of radiation, is doubled, the radiation at the new location spans an area four times larger than the original area. However, because the same amount of radiation exists to cover this larger area, the intensity at the new distance consequently decreases by a factor of four.

The ISL may be stated as a formula, shown in the following equation. A mathematical example is also provided.

$$\frac{I_1}{I_2} = \frac{(d_2)^2}{(d_1)^2}$$

I_1 expresses the exposure (intensity) at the original distance; I_2 expresses the exposure (intensity) at the new distance; d_1 expresses the original distance from the source of radiation; and d_2 expresses the new distance from the source of radiation.

Example: If a radiographer stands 2 m away from an x-ray tube and receives an exposure rate dose of 6.0 mGy$_a$/hr, what will the exposure rate dose be if the same radiographer moves to stand at a position located 4 m from the x-ray tube?

Answer:

$$\frac{I_1}{I_2} = \frac{(d_2)^2}{(d_1)^2}$$

$$\frac{6}{I_2} = \frac{(4)^2}{(2)^2}$$

$$\frac{6}{I_2} = \frac{16}{4}(\text{cross-multiply})$$

$$16I_2 = 24$$

$$I_2 = 1.5 \text{ mGy}_a/\text{hr}$$

1. If a radiographer stands 3 m *away* from an x-ray tube and receives an exposure rate dose of 9.0 mGy$_a$/hr, what will the exposure rate dose be if the same radiographer moves to stand at a position located 6 m from the x-ray tube?

2. If a radiographer stands 2 m away from an x-ray tube and receives an exposure rate dose of 5.0 mGy$_a$/hr, what will the exposure rate dose be if the same radiographer moves to stand at a position located 4 m from the x-ray tube?

3. If a radiographer stands 5 m away from an x-ray tube and receives an exposure rate dose of 4.0 mGy$_a$/hr, what will the exposure rate dose be if the same radiographer moves to stand at a position located 10 m from the x-ray tube?

4. If a radiographer stands 1 m away from an x-ray tube and receives an exposure rate dose of of 7.0 mGy$_a$/hr, what will the exposure rate dose be if the same radiographer moves to a position located 2 m from the x-ray tube?

5. If a radiographer stands 6 m away from an x-ray tube and receives an exposure rate dose of 6.0 mGy$_a$/hr, what will the exposure rate dose be if the same radiographer moves to a position located 12 m from the x-ray tube?

6. If a radiographer stands 2 m away from an x-ray tube and receives an exposure rate dose of 6.0 mGy$_a$/hr, what will the exposure rate dose be if the same radiographer moves to a position located 6 m from the x-ray tube?

The ISL also implies that if a radiographer moves closer to a source of radiation, radiation exposure to the radiographer dramatically increases.

Example: If a radiographer stands 2 m away from an x-ray source instead of 6 m away, the radiographer's exposure increases by a factor of $(6/2)^2 = 9$.

$$6 \div 2 = 3$$
$$3 \times 3 = 9$$

7. If a radiographer stands 5 m away from an x-ray source instead of 10 m away, the radiographer's exposure increases by a factor of _____.

8. If a radiographer stands 4 m away from an x-ray source instead of 12 m away, the radiographer's exposure increases by a factor of _____ .

9. If a radiographer stands 1 m away from an x-ray source instead of 4 m away, the radiographer's radiation exposure increases by a factor of _____.

10. If a radiographer stands 2 m from an x-ray source instead of 8 m, the radiographer's radiation exposure increases by a factor of _____.

POST-TEST

The student should take this test after reading Chapter 14, finishing all accompanying textbook and workbook exercises, and completing any additional activities required by the course instructor. The student should complete the post-test with a score of 90% or higher before advancing to the next chapter. (Each of the following 20 questions is worth 5 points.)
Score = _____ %

1. What is the most effective means of protection from ionizing radiation?

   _____

2. Most health care facilities have policies for protecting pregnant personnel from radiation. Under these policies an imaging professional who becomes pregnant first informs her supervisor. After this voluntary _____ has been made, the health care facility officially recognizes the pregnancy.

3. According to ALARA guidelines, how should work schedules for radiographers be designed?

   _____

   _____

4. What poses the greatest occupational hazard for the radiographer in diagnostic radiology?

   _____

5. Protective lead aprons and shielded barriers function as _____ shields for diagnostic imaging personnel.

6. State the inverse square law (ISL).

   _____

   _____

181

7. During a radiographic exposure, radiographers and nonoccupationally exposed individuals should never stand in the useful beam to _____ a patient.

8. What are the three basic principles of radiation protection?

   _____

9. Primary protective barriers are located:
   A. At a 45-degree angle to the undeflected line of travel of the x-ray beam
   B. At a 60-degree angle to the undeflected line of travel of the x-ray beam
   C. Parallel to the undeflected line of travel of the x-ray beam
   D. Perpendicular to the undeflected line of travel of the x-ray beam

10. During general fluoroscopic and x-ray special procedures, a neck and thyroid shield can guard the thyroid area of occupationally exposed persons. This protective device should be:
    A. 1-mm lead equivalent
    B. 0.5-mm lead equivalent
    C. 0.25-mm lead equivalent
    D. 0.1-mm lead equivalent

11. For most mobile radiographic units that are not remote controlled, the cord leading to the exposure switch must be long enough to permit the radiographer to stand at least _____ from the patient, the x-ray tube, and the useful beam.
    A. 1 m
    B. 2 m
    C. 4 m
    D. 6 m

12. During high-level-control fluoroscopic interventional procedures, _____ should be kept so that the cumulative fluoroscopic exposure time may be determined.

13. When determining _____ requirements for a protective barrier, occupancy factor, workload, and use factor must be considered.

14. A protective curtain consisting of a minimum thickness of 0.25-mm lead equivalent normally should be positioned between the fluoroscopist and the patient to intercept _____ radiation above the tabletop.

15. If a radiographer stands 3 m away from an x-ray tube and receives an exposure rate dose of 10 mGy_a/hr, what will the exposure rate dose be if the same radiographer moves to a position located 6 m from the x-ray tube?

16. What type of protective barrier is needed to protect personnel against scatter and leakage radiation?

    _____

17. If the image intensifier of a mobile C-arm fluoroscope is positioned as close to the _____ as possible, the required fluoroscopic x-ray beam intensity is minimized.

18. In metric units, what does the NCRP currently recommend as an annual EqD limit to localized skin and hands?

    _____

19. Methods and techniques that reduce patient exposure also reduce exposure for the _____.

20. It is imperative that the EqD to the embryo-fetus from occupational exposure of the mother not exceed the NCRP-recommended monthly EqD limit of _____ mSv or a limit of _____ mSv during the entire pregnancy.

15 Radioisotopes and Radiation Protection

Chapter 15 provides a brief description of the use of radioisotopes in both diagnostic and therapeutic medical procedures and discusses some relevant radiation safety issues. The use of radiation as a terrorist weapon is also considered, and the chapter includes some fundamental principles for dealing with radioactive contamination in a health care setting. To assist the learner, both English and metric units are used in this chapter.

CHAPTER HIGHLIGHTS

- Isotopes are atoms that have the same number of protons within the nucleus but have different numbers of neutrons.
  - Some nuclei of isotopes have too many neutrons or too many protons for stability.
  - Radioactive isotopes spontaneously undergo changes or transformations to rectify their unstable arrangement.
- Rapidly dividing cells that are well oxygenated are very radiosensitive.
  - When cells are radiosensitive, cancerous growths or tumors can be either eliminated or at least controlled by irradiation of the area containing the growth.
- Therapeutic isotopes generally have relatively long half-lives compared with diagnostically employed isotopes.
- Fast electrons are beta radiation.
- Gamma rays and x-ray photons differ only in their point of origin.
- Iodine-125 decays with a half-life of 59.4 days by a process called *electron capture*.
- The most practical radiation protection to follow for patients having therapeutic prostate seed implants is use of the concepts of distance and time.
- When iodine-131 is being administered to treat a hospitalized patient for thyroid cancer, a large, up to 2.5-cm- or 1-inch-thick, rolling lead shield can be positioned between the patient and any attending personnel for protection.
- Residual unused nonreturned radioisotopes as well as radioactively contaminated items must be held in a secure, shielded, and posted storage area for a period of 10 half-lives of the isotope before being able to be discarded in ordinary trash. Proper record-keeping of storage and disposal is to be maintained.
- Diagnostic techniques in nuclear medicine typically make use of short-lived radioisotopes as radioactive tracers.
  - Technetium-99m is the most common radioisotope used in nuclear medicine.
- Positron emission tomography (PET) makes use of annihilation radiation events.
  - When matter-antimatter annihilation occurs, a positron and an electron interact destructively and disappear. Their respective masses are converted into energy that will be carried off by two photons emerging from the annihilation site in opposite directions, each with a kinetic energy of 511 keV.
  - A neutrino is a particle that has almost negligible mass and no electric charge but carries away any excess energy from the nucleus of the atom in processes such as beta and positron decay.
  - Fluorine-18 is the most important isotope used for PET scanning.
  - PET is an important imaging modality because it can examine metabolic processes within the body.
  - Fluorodeoxyglucose (FDG) is a radioactive tracer that is taken up or metabolized by cancerous cells and that reveals their location through positron emission decay and subsequent generation of oppositely traveling annihilation photons.
  - A PET/computed tomography (CT) scanner can detect the presence of regions of abnormally high glucose metabolism, thus providing evidence of cancer metastasis to other body areas, and at the same time can obtain detailed information about the location and size of these lesions or growths.
  - Positron emitters result in the production of high-energy radiation, and for this reason, the design of a PET/CT imaging suite involves significant radiation safety concerns.
- Most hospitals have radiation emergency plans for handling emergency situations involving radioactive contamination.
- A radioactive dispersal device, or "dirty bomb," is a radioactive source mixed with conventional explosives, the actual long-term health effects of which will most likely be minimal.
  - If radioactive material from a dirty bomb remains in a small area, only a few people may be seriously affected.
  - Conversely, if enough explosives are used to spread the radioactive material over a broad area, radioactivity will be diluted and may not be much higher than background levels.
  - If a dirty bomb were to explode with the same force as the explosion at Chernobyl, the actual number of radiation injuries could be quite small.

- The United States currently has emergency responders who are prepared and equipped to monitor and assess personnel exposure on-site in an emergency situation.
  - After an explosion of a dirty bomb, externally contaminated individuals can be decontaminated by removal of contaminated clothing and immersion in a shower.
  - Geiger-Müller (GM) detectors may be used by trained emergency personnel to monitor contamination levels.
  - During an emergency situation, individuals engaged in non-lifesaving activities are to work under a dose limit of 50 mSv per event, whereas those persons performing lifesaving activities have a dose limit of 250 mSv.
  - If surface contamination is suspected, emergency personnel should protect themselves by wearing gowns, masks, and gloves while working with the patient.
  - Handling of patients with internal contamination varies depending on the clinical and radiologic form of contamination. Strategies may include dilution and blocking absorption in the gastrointestinal tract. Potassium iodide can be administered to block further uptake of radioactive iodine in the thyroid gland.

Exercise 1: Matching

Match the following terms with their definitions or associated phrases.

1. _____ PET/CT scanner

2. _____ Radiation emergency plan

3. _____ Beta decay

4. _____ Decontamination

5. _____ Environmental Protection Agency (EPA)

6. _____ Half-value layer (HVL)

7. _____ Radioisotopes

8. _____ Radioactive contamination

9. _____ ^{18}F

10. _____ Surface contamination

11. _____ Neutrino

12. _____ Annihilation radiation

13. _____ Proton

A. A particle that has no electric charge and almost negligible mass but its energy of motion balances the energy of the reaction

B. Dirty bomb

C. Process wherein an inner-shell electron is captured by one of the nuclear protons, followed directly by the two combining to produce a neutron

D. Atoms that have the same number of protons within the nucleus but have different numbers of neutrons

E. By-product of the pair production interaction

F. A radioactive tracer that is very similar in chemical behavior to ordinary glucose and so is readily taken up or metabolized by cancerous cells. As such it reveals the locations of these cells through its positron emission decay and subsequent generation of oppositely traveling annihilation photons

G. Modality that uses ionizing radiation for the treatment of disease—namely, cancer

H. Isotopes of a particular element that are unstable because of their neutron-proton configuration

I. Modality that produces axial images by making use of annihilation radiation initiated by the radioactive decay of the nucleus of an unstable isotope

J. Removal of radioactive material from an area or from clothing or a person

K. Process wherein a nucleus relieves instability by one of its neutrons transforming itself into a combination of a proton and an energetic electron (called a *beta particle*). There is also the emission of another particle called a *neutrino*

L. Branch of medicine that employs radioisotopes to study organ function in a patient, to detect the spread of cancer into bone, and to treat certain types of diseases

M. U.S. government agency that facilitates the development and enforcement of regulations controlling radiation in the environment. It sets limits for radioactive contamination that assume that a 1 in 10,000 risk of causing a fatal cancer is unacceptable

14. _____ Nuclear medicine

15. _____ Isotopes

16. _____ FDG

17. _____ Electron capture

18. _____ Neutron

19. _____ Computed tomography (CT) scanner

20. _____ Positron

21. _____ Geiger-Müller (GM) detector

22. _____ Kinetic energy

23. _____ Radiation therapy

24. _____ PET

25. _____ Radioactive dispersal device

N. Radioactive isotope used for PET scanning

O. Radioactive material that is attached to or associated with dust particles or is in liquid form on various surfaces

P. Imaging unit that can be mechanically joined in a tandem configuration with a PET scanner

Q. Energy of motion

R. A device that detects individual radioactive particles or photons and that also serves as the primary radiation survey instrument for area monitoring in nuclear medicine facilities

S. A unit that is mechanically joined in a tandem configuration with a CT scanner to produce a single-joint imaging device. Using FDG ^{18}F, it can detect the presence of abnormally high regions of glucose metabolism, yielding evidence of cancer spread (metastasis) in other body areas. It also provides detailed information about the anatomic location and extent of these lesions or growths

T. The thickness of a designated absorber required to reduce the intensity of the primary beam by 50% of its initial value

U. A positively charged electron, which is a form of antimatter

V. A plan hospitals can implement for handling emergency situations involving radioactive contamination

W. External contamination of the skin or clothing with radioactive material

X. An electrically neutral particle found in the nucleus of the atom; one of the fundamental constituents of the atom

Y. One of the three main constituents of an atom, it carries a positive electrical charge

Exercise 2: Multiple Choice

Select the answer that *best* completes the following questions or statements.

1. Isotopes are atoms that have the *same* number of _____ within the nucleus but have *different* numbers of _____.
   A. Electrons, protons
   B. Neutrons, electrons
   C. Protons, neutrons
   D. Protons, neutrinos

2. Which two terms are synonymous?
   A. X-rays and gamma rays
   B. Alpha rays and beta rays
   C. Fast electrons and beta rays
   D. Neutrons and neutrinos

3. Which of the following radioisotopes is produced from the radioactive decay of molybdenum-99?
   A. ^{125}I
   B. ^{125}Te
   C. ^{131}I
   D. ^{99m}Tc

4. A particle that has no electric charge and almost negligible mass but carries away any excess energy from the nucleus of the atom is a(n):
   A. Electron
   B. Neutron
   C. Neutrino
   D. Proton

5. The branch of medicine that uses radioisotopes to study organ function in a patient, to detect the spread of cancer into bone, and to treat certain types of diseases is:
   A. Chemotherapy
   B. Computed radiography
   C. Nuclear medicine
   D. Ultrasonography

6. The radioisotope *most often* used in nuclear medicine diagnostic studies is:
   A. ^{123}I
   B. ^{125}I
   C. ^{131}I
   D. ^{99m}Tc

7. PET makes use of what radiation event?
   A. Annihilation radiation
   B. Compton scattering
   C. Photodisintegration
   D. Photoelectric interaction

8. During the process of annihilation, the positron and the electron annihilate each other, and their rest masses are converted into energy, which appears in the form of two 511-keV photons, each moving:
   A. At exactly a 45-degree angle to the other
   B. In the same direction
   C. In opposite directions
   D. Toward the nucleus of the original atom

9. The isotope *most often* used in PET scanning is:
   A. ^{60}Co
   B. ^{18}F
   C. ^{131}I
   D. ^{125}I

10. Positron emitters result in the production of:
    A. High-energy radiation
    B. Intermediate-energy radiation
    C. Low-energy radiation
    D. No radiation

11. Most hospitals have _____ _____ for handling emergency situations involving radioactive contamination.
    A. No radiation emergency plans
    B. No trained personnel
    C. Radiation emergency plans and trained personnel
    D. A and B only

12. A 1 in 10,000 probability of causing a fatal cancer corresponds to an effective dose of approximately:
    A. 1 mSv
    B. 2 mSv
    C. 3 mSv
    D. 5 mSv

13. For exposures localized to specific regions of the body, medical management involves:
    1. Prevention of infection
    2. Control of pain
    3. Possibly skin grafts
    A. 1 and 2 only
    B. 1 and 3 only
    C. 2 and 3 only
    D. 1, 2, and 3

14. The physical half-life of ^{18}F is:
    A. 10 minutes
    B. 110 minutes
    C. 10 years
    D. 110 years

15. ^{125}I is an unstable isotope of the element iodine with:
    A. 73 protons and 102 neutrons
    B. 102 protons and 73 neutrons
    C. 53 protons and 72 neutrons
    D. 72 protons and 53 neutrons

16. The design of a PET/CT imaging suite involves:
    A. No radiation safety concerns
    B. Minimal radiation safety concerns
    C. Moderate radiation safety concerns
    D. Significant radiation safety concerns

17. Each _____ nuclear transformation by positron decay yields two highly penetrating 511-keV photons.
    A. ^{18}Cl
    B. ^{18}F
    C. ^{18}I
    D. ^{18}Sr

18. In beta decay a neutron transforms itself into a combination of:
    A. A positron and an alpha particle
    B. A positron and a negatron
    C. A proton and an energetic electron
    D. A proton and an alpha particle

19. High energy photons (particles of electromagnetic radiation) that are emitted by the nucleus as a result of an unstable situation are known as:
    A. Alpha rays
    B. Beta rays
    C. X-rays
    D. Gamma rays

20. Fast electrons are:
    A. Alpha radiation
    B. Beta radiation
    C. Gamma radiation
    D. X-radiation

21. A neutrino is a particle that has _____ electric charge and almost _____ mass but carries away any excess energy from the nucleus of the atom.
    A. Positive, significant
    B. Negative, significant
    C. No, negligible
    D. Positive, negligible

22. Gamma rays and x-ray photons only differ in their:
    A. Wavelength
    B. Position on the electromagnetic spectrum
    C. Point of origin
    D. Energy and frequency

23. If a dirty bomb were to explode with the same force as the explosion at the Chernobyl nuclear power station in 1986, the actual number of injuries attributed to radiation exposure could be:
    A. Catastrophic
    B. Enormous
    C. Quite small
    D. Nonexistent

24. Potassium iodide may be administered to block further uptake of radioactive iodine in the:
    A. Gallbladder
    B. Liver
    C. Kidneys
    D. Thyroid gland

25. The thickness of a designated absorber required to reduce the intensity of the primary beam by 50% of its initial value defines:
    A. Radioisotope shielding barrier equivalent
    B. Lead apron thickness requirement
    C. HVL
    D. Positron emission

Exercise 3: True or False

Circle *T* if the statement is true; circle *F* if the statement is false.

1. T   F ^{125}I is a stable isotope.

2. T   F   Distance and time are the best radiation safety practices for therapeutic implants such as the ^{125}I seed implant for the prostate gland.

3. T   F   Hospital rooms for ^{131}I-treated patients usually are isolated and carefully prepared with absorbent cloths to substantially minimize radiation exposure to personnel and visitors either from emitted gamma radiation from the patient or from contaminated surfaces.

4. T   F   In a PET device, annihilation radiation is initiated by the radioactive decay of the nucleus of a stable atom.

5. T   F   The nucleus of ^{18}F has 18 neutrons.

6. T   F   The possible use of radiation as a terrorist weapon is of no concern to the general population.

7. T   F   If radioactive material from a dirty bomb remains in a small area, few people may be affected.

8. T   F   Because it may be difficult to monitor all workers involved in a radiation emergency, a dose rate criterion is often used.

9. T   F   The same procedures that control infection are not useful for preventing the spread of radioactive contamination.

10. T   F   Diagnostic techniques in nuclear medicine typically make use of long-lived radioisotopes as radioactive tracers.

11. T   F ^{131}I is the radioisotope most often used in nuclear medicine.

12. T   F   With the aid of computerized treatment planning and real-time ultrasound imaging, ^{125}I seeds are permanently inserted into the prostate gland in a calculated prescribed arrangement.

13. T   F   Neutrinos almost never interact in matter and are therefore nearly impossible to detect.

14. T   F   In the United States, emergency responders are equipped to monitor and assess personnel exposure on-site in an emergency situation.

15. T   F   Most hospitals stock cutie pies to monitor radiation contamination levels during an emergency.

16. T   F   Radiation therapy uses ionizing radiation for the radiologic diagnosis of disease.

17. T   F   Radioactive contamination may consist of surface, internal (inhaled or ingested), internal wound, or external wound contamination.

18. T   F   A positron is a normal form of matter.

19. T   F ^{123}I undergoes radioactive decay by the process of electron capture and has an average half-life of 13.3 hours.

Chapter **15** **Radioisotopes and Radiation Protection**

20. T F ^{99m}Tc is an extremely versatile radioisotope because it can be incorporated into a wide variety of different compounds or biologically active substances, each with a specificity for different tissues or organs of the body.

21. T F Each ^{18}F nuclear transformation by positron decay yields two highly penetrating 511-keV photons, which can be shielded by an ordinary lead apron.

22. T F ^{18}F has a physical half-life of 110 minutes; therefore the patient's degree of radioactivity will diminish naturally throughout the preparation time, losing approximately 25% to 30% by the time of scanning.

23. T F The only cases of acute radiation syndrome at Chernobyl were among emergency workers, primarily firefighters who worked very near the reactor.

24. T F A dirty bomb is unlikely to cause contamination with so much radioactive material that a victim could not receive medical attention.

25. T F Removal of surface radioactive contamination involves removal of the patient's contaminated clothing and immersion in a shower to cleanse the skin.

Exercise 4: Fill in the Blank

Using the following Word Bank, fill in the blanks with the word or words that best complete the statements.

6 (may be used more than once)	full	positron
90	Geiger	pregnant
adjacent	isolated	prep
annihilation	metabolic	radiation
beta	minimize	radiosensitive
cancer spread	monitoring	radiotracer
decay	nine	residual
dirty bomb	nucleus	sparing
electron capture	patient	unstable
	plastic container	vary

1. For ^{125}I seed implants, the goal is to deliver 145 Gy to at least _____% of the prostate's volume while limiting the radiation dose as much as possible to _____ structures such as the urethra, bladder, and anterior rectal wall.

2. ^{99m}Tc concentrates in bone and permits evaluation of potential _____ _____ to bony areas.

3. ^{99m}Tc has a half-life of _____ hours and decays primarily by emission from its _____ of a gamma ray photon with energy of 140 keV.

4. _____ emitters produce high-energy radiation.

5. Every patient who is to have a PET/CT scan requires _____ time.

6. After the attack on the World Trade Center by hijacked airplanes on September 11, 2001, the use of other possible terrorist weapons, such as _____, became a public health concern.

7. A radioactive source mixed with conventional explosives describes a radioactive dispersal device, or _____ _____.

8. Rapidly dividing cells that are well oxygenated are very _____.

9. Fast-moving electrons are called _____ radiation.

10. ^{125}I decays with a 59.4 half-life process called _____ _____.

11. During administration of iodine-131 to treat a hospitalized patient for thyroid cancer, a large, up to 1-inch-thick, rolling lead shield can be positioned between the _____ and any attending personnel for protection.

12. Radioactive isotopes spontaneously undergo changes or transformations to rectify their _____ arrangement.

13. PET makes use of _____ radiation events.

14. PET is an important imaging modality because it can examine _____ processes in the body.

15. _____ counters can be used by trained emergency personnel to monitor radioactive contamination levels.

16. Handling of patients with internal contamination will _____, depending on the clinical and radiologic form of contamination.

17. Clothing that has been contaminated with radioactive material should be placed in a _____ _____ and set aside for later evaluation.

18. ^{125}I-treated patients should significantly limit the duration of close contact (less than 30 cm or 1 foot) with small children and _____ women for a period of _____ months after the implant procedure.

19. In the case of PET scanning, annihilation radiation is initiated by the radioactive _____ of the nucleus of an unstable isotope.

20. For a patient who has thyroid cancer, it is desirable to strongly irradiate any _____ thyroid tissue not removed by surgery while significantly _____ surrounding tissue and other organs.

21. Hospital rooms for ^{131}I-treated patients usually are _____ and carefully prepared with absorbent cloths to substantially _____ radiation exposure to both personnel and visitors from gamma radiation emitted from the patient or from contaminated surfaces.

22. ^{123}I is a _____ compound.

23. The nucleus of ^{18}F has _____ neutrons.

24. A well-designed PET/CT facility is arranged so that no areas of _____ occupancy are adjacent to a high-energy radiation source.

25. _____ of all radiation workers involved in a radiation emergency may be difficult.

Exercise 5: Labeling
Label the following table.

A. Dose-effect relationship after acute whole-body radiation from gamma rays or x-rays.

Whole-Body Absorbed Dose	Effect
0.05 Gy_t	No symptoms
1.	No symptoms, but possible chromosomal aberrations in cultured peripheral blood lymphocytes
2.	No symptoms (minor decreases in white blood cell and platelet counts in a few persons)
3.	Nausea and vomiting in approximately 10% of persons within 48 hr after exposure
4.	Nausea and vomiting in approximately 50% of persons within 24 hr, with marked decreases in white blood cell and platelet counts
5.	Nausea and vomiting in 90% of persons within 12 hr, and diarrhea in 10% within 8 hr; 50% mortality in the absence of medical treatment
6.	100% mortality within 30 days because of bone marrow failure in the absence of medical treatment
7.	Approximate dose that is survivable with the best medical therapy available
8.	Nausea and vomiting in all persons in less than 5 min; severe gastrointestinal damage; death likely in 2-3 wk in the absence of treatment
9.	Cardiovascular collapse and central nervous system damage, with death in 24-72 hr

From Gusev I, Guskova AK, Mettler FA Jr, eds: *Medical management of radiation accidents*, ed 2, Boca Raton, Fla, 2001, CRC Press.

Chapter **15 Radioisotopes and Radiation Protection**

Exercise 6: Short Answer

Answer the following questions by providing a short answer.

1. How are therapeutic isotopes characterized?

   _____

   _____

2. How does electron capture occur?

   _____

   _____

3. How does beta decay occur?

   _____

   _____

4. What types of radioisotopes are typically used in nuclear medicine as radioactive tracers? How do these radionuclides work?

   _____

   _____

5. Why is PET an important imaging modality?

   _____

   _____

6. What benefit does the radioactive tracer FDG provide in PET imaging?

   _____

   _____

7. What benefit is obtained by combining PET and CT into one imaging device, called a *PET/CT scanner*?

   _____

   _____

8. What event led to the possibility of radiation being used as a terrorist weapon?

   _____

   _____

9. Why does the EPA set limits for radioactive contamination?

   _____

   _____

10. If a patient has surface radioactive contamination, what protective apparel should personnel wear?

   _____

   _____

11. Besides trained emergency personnel, who would be available to assess radioactive contamination in a health care facility during a radiation emergency?

_____

_____

12. How do personnel adhere to normal badge limits during a radiation emergency?

_____

_____

13. Describe the medical management of a patient during the first 48 hours of treatment for acute radiation syndrome.

_____

_____

14. What is annihilation radiation?

_____

_____

15. What is a radioactive dispersal device?

_____

_____

Exercise 7: General Discussion or Opinion Questions

The following questions are intended to allow students to express their knowledge and understanding of the subject matter or to present a personal opinion. The questions may be used to stimulate class discussion. Because answers to these questions may vary, determination of the answer's acceptability is left to the discretion of the course instructor.

1. How is PET/CT scanning accomplished? What value does this modality have in diagnosing the spread of cancer in the human body?

2. What are some of the problems that may be encountered in designing shielding for a PET/CT department?

3. During a radiation emergency situation, what role does a radiologic technologist in a health care facility fulfill?

4. When medical care is being provided to a patient contaminated with radiation either externally or internally, what protective measures should be taken by physicians and staff members coming in contact with the patient?

5. Describe a scenario that involves a radioactive dispersal device (dirty bomb). Include possible health and community consequences and the emergency response to the situation, with emphasis on radiation safety.

POST-TEST

The student should take this test after reading Chapter 14, finishing all accompanying textbook and workbook exercises, and completing any additional activities required by the course instructor. The student should complete the post-test with a score of 90% or higher before advancing to the next chapter. (Each of the following 20 questions is worth 5 points.) Score = _____ %

1. What U.S. government agency facilitates the development and enforcement of regulations controlling radiation in the environment and sets limits for radioactive contamination that assume that a 1 in 10,000 risk of causing a fatal cancer is unacceptable?

_____

Chapter **15 Radioisotopes and Radiation Protection**

2. Define *radioactive dispersal device.*

_____

_____

3. How are therapeutic radioisotopes characterized?

_____

_____

4. ^{18}F has a physical half-life of:
   A. 110 seconds
   B. 110 minutes
   C. 110 hours
   D. 110 years

5. Isotopes are atoms that have the same number of protons in the nucleus but have different numbers of _____.

6. _____ dividing cells that are well oxygenated are very radiosensitive.

7. What is a neutrino?

_____

_____

8. After a dirty bomb explosion, how can externally contaminated individuals be decontaminated?

_____

_____

9. Of what radiation events does PET make use?

_____

10. A 1-in-10,000 probability of causing a fatal cancer corresponds to an effective dose of approximately _____ mSv.

11. A radioactive tracer that is readily taken up or metabolized by cancerous cells and as such reveals the locations of these cells through its positron emission decay and subsequent generation of oppositely traveling annihilation photons is _____.

12. Diagnostic techniques in nuclear medicine typically make use of _____ radioisotopes as radioactive tracers.

13. During an emergency, under what dose limit are individuals performing lifesaving activities allowed to work?

_____

14. Define the term *electron capture.*

_____

_____

15. In what do positron emitters result?

_____

_____

16. What radiation survey instrument is used by emergency personnel to monitor radioactive contamination?

_____

17. What radioisotope is most often used in nuclear medicine diagnostic studies?

_____

18. What do most hospitals have for handling emergency situations involving radioactive contamination?

_____

19. A well-designed PET/CT facility is arranged so that no areas of full occupancy are adjacent to a _____ radiation source.

20. Fast-moving electrons are _____ radiation.

Answer Key

Chapter 1

Exercise 1: Matching

1. P	6. A	11. I	16. J	21. L
2. X	7. H	12. E	17. O	22. S
3. F	8. Y	13. T	18. R	23. M
4. C	9. G	14. D	19. N	24. Q
5. K	10. B	15. W	20. U	25. V

Exercise 2: Multiple Choice

1. C	6. D	11. D	16. A	21. B
2. B	7. D	12. D	17. B	22. C
3. A	8. B	13. D	18. D	23. D
4. A	9. D	14. D	19. C	24. B
5. A	10. D	15. B	20. A	25. C

Exercise 3: True or False

1. F (X-rays are a form of ionizing radiation.)
2. T
3. F (Since the early 1900s they have been known to cause injury.)
4. F (No threshold exists for radiation-induced malignant disease.)
5. F (3 mSv/yr)
6. T
7. T
8. F (The danger is the same.)
9. F (Humans are continuously exposed.)
10. T
11. T
12. T
13. F (It is the employer's responsibility.)
14. T
15. T
16. F (BERT does not imply risk from radiation exposure; it is simply a means of comparison.)
17. T
18. T
19. F (Production of low-energy x-ray photons is a consequence of ionization in human cells.)
20. T
21. T
22. F (Repeated with an increase in radiation dose)
23. F (Natural radiation in their own body)
24. F (Diagnostic efficacy is an important part.)
25. T

Exercise 4: Fill in the Blank

1. innate
2. lowest
3. Exposure
4. benefits, far outweigh, chance
5. energy, biologic effects
6. maximized
7. ALARA
8. justified
9. time
10. follow-up
11. unsafe
12. ALARA
13. ALARA
14. BERT
15. first
16. protective
17. audit
18. more
19. subunit
20. ionizing, protective
21. education
22. beneficial, destructive
23. smallest
24. unstable
25. occupational

Exercise 5: Labeling

Label the following illustration and table.

A. **X-ray tube.**

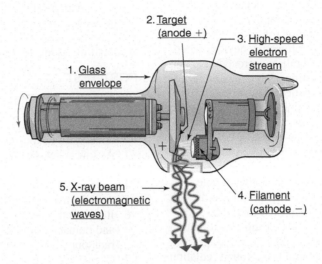

2. Target (anode +)

3. High-speed electron stream

1. Glass envelope

5. X-ray beam (electromagnetic waves)

4. Filament (cathode −)

B. **Typical Adult Patient Effective Dose (EfD) and Background Equivalent Radiation Time (BERT) Values.**

Radiologic Procedure	EfD mSv	BERT (Amount of Time to Receive the Same EfD from Natural)
1. Dental, intraoral	0.06	1 wk
2. Chest radiograph	0.08	10 days
3. Lumbar spine	3.0	1 yr
4. Abdomen	0.7	4 mo
5. CT chest	8.0	3.6 yr
6. CT abdomen/pelvis	10.0	4.5 yr

Sources: Adapted from Wall BF: *Patient dosimetry techniques in diagnostic radiology,* York, UK, 1988, Institute of Physics and Engineering in Medicine, pp 53 and 117; Cameron JR: *Med Phys World,* 15:20, 1999; and Stabin MG: *Radiation protection and dosimetry: an introduction to health physics,* New York, 2008, Springer.
CT, Computed tomography; *mSv,* millisievert.

Exercise 6: Short Answer

1. Humans can safely control the use of radiant energy by using the knowledge of radiation-induced hazards that has been gained over many years and by employing effective methods to limit or eliminate those hazards.

2. Radiologic technologists and radiologists can reduce radiation exposure to patients and to themselves by using protective devices whenever possible, by following established procedures, and by selecting x-ray machine settings that significantly reduce radiation exposure to patients and themselves.

3. When passing through normal matter, ionizing radiation produces positively and negatively charged particles (ions) along its path. The production of these ions, as well as the electrons ejected in the process, are the events that may cause injury in normal biologic tissue.

4. The three cardinal principles of radiation protection are time, distance, and shielding.

5. Occupational radiation exposure of imaging personnel can be minimized by the use of these cardinal principles: (1) shortening the length of time spent in a room where x-radiation is produced, (2) standing at the greatest distance possible from an energized x-ray beam, and (3) interposing a radiation-absorbent shielding material between the radiographer and the source of the radiation.

6. The ALARA principle provides a method for comparing the amount of radiation used in various health care facilities in a particular area for specific imaging procedures.

7. The goals of modern radiation protection programs are twofold: to protect persons from both short term and long term effects of radiation.

8. In a hospital setting, the radiation safety officer (RSO) is expressly charged by the administration to be directly responsible for the execution, enforcement, and maintenance of the ALARA program.

9. When ionizing radiation is used for the welfare of the patient, the realized benefits of this exposure to radiant energy must far outweigh any slight chance of inducing a radiogenic malignancy or any genetic defects.
10. Radiologic technologists and radiologists (1) are educated in the safe operation of x-ray producing imaging equipment, (2) use protective devices whenever possible, (3) follow established procedures, and (4) select x-ray machine settings that significantly reduce radiation exposure to patients and to themselves.
11. Six consequences of ionization in human cells are (1) creation of unstable atoms, (2) production of free electrons, (3) production of low-energy x-ray photons, (4) creation of highly reactive free molecules (called *radicals*) capable of producing substances poisonous to the cell, (5) creation of new biologic molecules detrimental to the living cell, and (6) injury to the cell that may manifest itself as abnormal function.
12. The radiographer can respond by using an estimation based on the comparison of radiation received from the x-ray examination to natural background radiation received, for example, over a certain number of days. Thus the radiographer can say, "The radiation received from having a chest x-ray examination is equivalent to what would be received while spending approximately 10 days in your natural surroundings."
13. Reference values for patient dose are usually based on large scale surveys of actual measurement of x-ray machines in hospitals.
14. For all medical imaging procedures, the selection of exposure factors should always follow the ALARA concept or principle.
15. Using the background equivalent radiation time (BERT) method to compare the amount of radiation received with natural background radiation received over a given period has three advantages: (1) BERT does not imply radiation risk, it is simply a means for comparison; (2) BERT emphasizes that radiation is an innate part of our environment; and (3) BERT provides an answer that is easy for the patient to comprehend.
16. Radiation workers' responsibilities to maintain an effective radiation safety program are to (1) be aware of rules governing the workplace and (2) perform duties consistent with ALARA.
17. Two objectives of the Image Wisely campaign are (1) lowering the amount of radiation used in medically necessary imaging studies and (2) eliminating unnecessary procedures.
18. Adverse biologic effects are damage to living tissue of animals and humans exposed to ionizing radiation.
19. X-rays travel in straight lines and at the speed of light (300 million meters per second) until they interact with atoms.
20. The responsibility of the radiologic technologist is to make sure that the radiologist and/or medical physicist has the information needed to carry out the dose estimate.

Exercise 7: General Discussion or Opinion Questions

The questions in this exercise are intended to allow students to express their knowledge and understanding of the subject matter covered in this chapter. Because the answers may vary, determination of an answer's acceptability is left to the discretion of the instructor.

POST-TEST

1. *Radiation protection* may be defined as effective measures employed by radiation workers to safeguard patients, personnel, and the general public from unnecessary exposure to ionizing radiation.
2. As low as reasonably achievable (ALARA)
3. The referring physician
4. chance or risk
5. An effective radiation safety program in place
6. It is based on evidence that living tissue of animals and humans can be damaged by exposure to ionizing radiation.
7. C
8. The milligray (mGy) is the subunit of measure for absorbed dose.
9. C
10. D
11. The goals of modern radiation programs are twofold: to protect persons from both short term and long term effects of radiation.
12. High-quality mammography
13. Image Gently campaign
14. Background equivalent radiation time (BERT)
15. A
16. D
17. The radiation safety officer
18. smallest, repeat
19. comparison
20. F (The level of danger is the same.)

Chapter 2
Exercise 1: Matching

1. K	6. B	11. I	16. D	21. J
2. X	7. H	12. E	17. O	22. S
3. F	8. Y	13. T	18. R	23. M
4. L	9. G	14. C	19. N	24. Q
5. A	10. P	15. W	20. U	25. V

Exercise 2: Multiple Choice

1. C	6. C	11. C	16. B	21. D
2. D	7. D	12. D	17. C	22. C
3. C	8. B	13. A	18. C	23. C
4. B	9. C	14. D	19. C	24. A
5. D	10. C	15. A	20. A	25. C

Exercise 3: True or False

1. T
2. F (About 6.3 mSv)
3. T
4. T
5. F (Sunspots indicate regions of increased electromagnetic field activity.)

6. T
7. F (Particulate radiations vary in their ability to penetrate matters.)
8. F (EqD enables the calculation of EfD.)
9. T
10. T
11. F (Atmospheric nuclear testing has not escalated since 1980.)
12. F (They produce negligible radiation exposure.)
13. F (Steel vault)
14. T
15. F (Alpha particles can be absorbed; they are very damaging to radiosensitive epithelial tissue.)
16. T
17. T
18. T
19. F (A neutron has approximately the same mass as a proton.)
20. F (Changes in white blood cell count are a classic example of organic damage.)
21. T
22. F (Smokers exposed to high radon levels face a higher risk of lung cancer than do nonsmokers.)
23. F (The solar contribution to the cosmic ray background increases.)
24. T
25. T

Exercise 4: Fill in the Blank

1. radiation dose, dose rates
2. unplanned
3. ETHOS Project
4. fetal dose
5. electromagnetic spectrum
6. terrestrial
7. Cosmic
8. radionuclides
9. equivalent dose
10. x-ray machines, radiopharmaceuticals
11. constant
12. solar flare
13. 0.08 mGy
14. millisievert (mSv)
15. radon
16. Radionuclides
17. greatest, lowest
18. alpha particles
19. atmosphere, magnetic field
20. Thyroid
21. 4
22. radium
23. 40, molten
24. higher
25. noble

Exercise 5: Labeling

Label the following illustration and tables.

A. **Percentage contribution of each natural and manmade radiation source to the total collective effective dose for the population of the United States, 2006.**

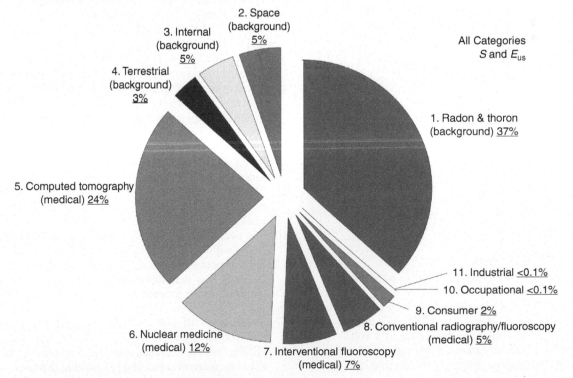

From National Council on Radiation Protection and Measurements (NCRP): *Ionizing radiation exposure of the population of the United States,* Report No. 160, Bethesda, Md, 2009, NCRP.

B. Radiation equivalent dose (EqD) and subsequent biologic effects resulting from acute whole-body exposures.[*]

Radiation EqD	Subsequent Biologic Effects
0.25 Sv	Blood changes (e.g., measurable hematologic depression, substantially decreases within a few days in the number of lymphocytes that are the body's primary defense against disease
1.5 Sv	Nausea, diarrhea
2.0 Sv	Erythema (diffuse redness over an area of skin after irradiation)
2.5 Sv	If dose is to gonads, temporary sterility
3.0 Sv	50% chance of death; lethal dose (LD) for 50% of population over 30 days (LD 50/30)
6.0 Sv	Death

Adapted from *Radiologic health,* unit 4, slide 17, Denver, Multi-Media Publishing (slide program).

C. Average annual radiation equivalent dose (EqD) for estimated levels of radiation exposure for humans.

Category	Type of Radiation	mSv
Natural	Radon	2.0
	Cosmic	0.3
	Terrestrial and internally deposited radionuclides	0.7
	Total	3.0
Medical imaging	CT scanning	1.5
	Radiography	0.6
	Nuclear medicine	0.7
	Interventional procedures	0.4
	Total	3.2
Other manmade		0.1
	Total annual EqD from all sources	6.3

Exercise 6: Short Answer

1. Energy is the ability to do work—that is, to move an object against resistance.
2. An electron volt (eV) is a unit of energy equal to the quantity of kinetic energy an electron acquires as it moves through a potential difference of 1 volt.
3. While penetrating body tissue, ionizing radiation produces biologic damage primarily by ejecting electrons from the atoms comprising the tissues.

4. The amount of energy absorbed by human tissue from ionizing radiation is an important determinant of the extent of biologic harm that may occur.
5. If excessive cellular damage occurs as a consequence of radiation exposure, the living organism will have a significant possibility of exhibiting genetic or somatic changes.
6. Cosmic rays are of extraterrestrial origin and result from nuclear interactions that have taken place in the sun and other stars.
7. Potassium-40 (^{40}K), carbon-14 (^{14}C), hydrogen-3 (^{3}H), tritium, and strontium-90 (^{90}Sr).
8. An accurate estimate of the total annual equivalent dose from fallout cannot be made because actual radiation measurements do not exist. The dose commitment that may ultimately be delivered from a given intake of radionuclide may be estimated by using a series of approximations and simplistic models that are subject to considerable speculation.
9. It is necessary to control artificial sources of radiation because humans are unable to control natural background radiation. Also, if artificial sources of radiation that can be controlled are limited, the general public can be protected from further biologic damage.
10. For radiation protection purposes the electromagnetic spectrum can be divided into ionizing radiation and nonionizing radiation.
11. Radiations such as visible light and radio waves are considered to be nonionizing because they do not have sufficient kinetic energy to eject electrons from the atom.
12. Mesons are short-lived (only a few hundredths of a microsecond) subatomic particles, smaller than a proton, and are generated as by-products from very-high energy collisions between protons or between protons and neutrons. They can carry an electric charge of the same value as that of an electron or be neutral.
13. A millisievert (mSv) is equal to $^{1}/_{1000}$ of a sievert.
14. Seven sources of manmade (artificial) ionizing radiation are (1) consumer products containing radioactive material, (2) air travel, (3) nuclear fuel for generation of power, (4) atmospheric fallout from nuclear weapons testing, (5) nuclear power plant accidents, (6) nuclear power plant accidents as a consequence of natural disasters, and (7) medical radiation.
15. Thyroid cancer continues to be the main adverse health effect of the 1986 accident at the Chernobyl nuclear power plant.
16. The average dose received by the exposed population living within a 50-mile radius of the Three Mile Island nuclear power plant during the accident that occurred in 1979 was determined to be 0.08 mSv, which is well below the average annual background radiation level.
17. Three ways of indicating the amount of radiation received by a patient are (1) entrance skin exposure (ESE), which includes skin and glandular dose; (2) bone marrow dose; and (3) gonadal dose.
18. The radiation quantity equivalent dose enables the calculation of the effective dose.

19. In the electromagnetic spectrum, higher frequencies are associated with shorter wavelengths and higher energies.
20. In terms of ability to penetrate biologic matter, alpha particles are less penetrating than beta particles. Because alpha particles interact readily and lose their kinetic energy quite rapidly as they travel a short distance through biologic matter (e.g., into the superficial layers of the skin), they are considered virtually harmless as an external source of radiation. However, if an alpha emitter is inhaled or ingested, there is a significant risk to the live cells it will encounter in the respiratory or digestive tract.

Exercise 7: General Discussion or Opinion Questions

The questions in this exercise are intended to allow students to express their knowledge and understanding of the subject matter covered in this chapter. These questions may be used to stimulate class discussion. Because the answers may vary, determination of an answer's acceptability is left to the discretion of the instructor.

POST-TEST

1. *Radiation* refers to kinetic energy that passes from one location to another.
2. Three electromagnetic radiations that are classified as ionizing radiations are (1) x-rays, (2) gamma rays, and (3) ultraviolet radiation with energy above 10 eV.
3. The process that is the foundation of the interactions of x-rays with human tissue is ionization.
4. False. As an external source of radiation, beta particles are more penetrating than are alpha particles.
5. Both occupational and nonoccupational dose limits are expressed as effective dose (EfD) and are stated in millisievert (mSv).
6. Electrically charged particles
7. lung cancer
8. Millisievert (mSv)
9. B
10. D
11. the amount of radiation received by a patient
12. The electromagnetic spectrum
13. Natural sources of ionizing radiation
14. organic or somatic
15. C
16. D
17. As an internal source of radiation
18. Because it is extremely difficult to measure the amount of radiation people received
19. Thyroid cancer
20. Genetic damage

Chapter 3
Exercise 1: Matching

1. G	6. M	11. N	16. F	21. E
2. O	7. J	12. I	17. S	22. V
3. K	8. C	13. A	18. B	23. Y
4. P	9. Q	14. R	19. T	24. X
5. D	10. L	15. H	20. U	25. W

Exercise 2: Multiple Choice

1. D	6. B	11. D	16. C	21. D
2. D	7. D	12. C	17. D	22. D
3. B	8. B	13. B	18. C	23. A
4. A	9. B	14. D	19. C	24. C
5. C	10. B	15. A	20. C	25. C

Exercise 3: True or False

1. T
2. F (When only direct transmission photons reach the image receptor)
3. T
4. F (An x-ray photon interacts with an outer-shell electron.)
5. T
6. F (Absorption properties of different body structures must be different.)
7. T
8. F (It is not. The effective atomic number [Z_{eff}] of air is 7.6.)
9. T
10. F (The use of positive contrast media leads to an increase in absorbed dose.)
11. T
12. F (A Compton scattered electron is also known as a secondary, or recoil, electron.)
13. T
14. T
15. F (It can cause excitation or ionization until all its kinetic energy has been spent.)
16. F (Attenuation is the reduction in the number of primary photons in the x-ray beam through absorption and scatter as the beam passes through the patient in its path.)
17. F (Characteristic radiation is also emitted from the atom when the outer-shell electron fills the inner-shell vacancy.)
18. F (The minimum energy required to produce an electron-positron pair is 1.022 MeV.)
19. F (The target in the x-ray tube is also known as the *anode*.)
20. T
21. T
22. T
23. F (The atomic number of tungsten is 74.)
24. T
25. T

Exercise 4: Fill in the Blank

1. manmade
2. electrons, photons
3. electrical voltage
4. degrade
5. image
6. coherent (classical, elastic, or unmodified)
7. small-angle scatter, backscatter, sidescatter
8. Compton, photoelectric
9. Auger
10. absorption
11. electrons, positively

199

12. energy, energy
13. one-third
14. intensity
15. Milliampere-seconds (mAs)
16. darker
17. increase
18. glass window
19. fluorescent
20. Coherent (classical, elastic, unmodified)
21. random
22. Pathologic
23. absorption
24. recoil
25. kinetic

Exercise 5: Labeling

A. **Primary, exit, and attenuated photons.**

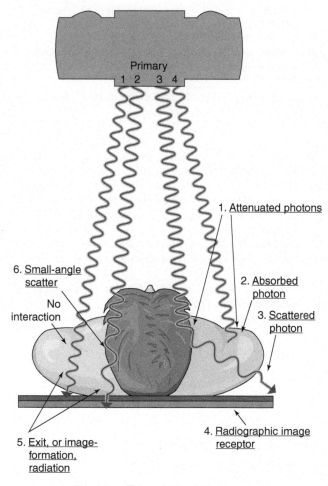

Primary − Exit = Attenuation

B. **Process of photoelectric absorption.**

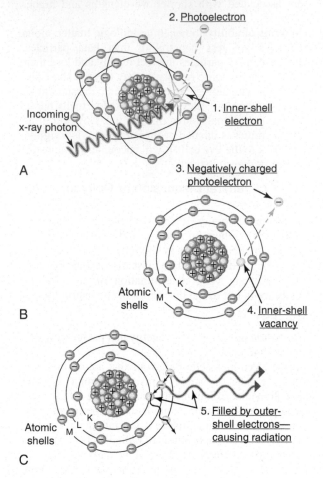

C. **Process of Compton scattering.**

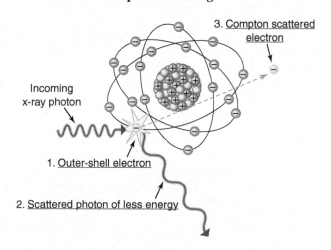

Exercise 6: Short Answer

1. Five types of interactions between x-radiation and matter are possible: (1) coherent (classical, elastic, or unmodified) scattering, (2) photoelectric absorption, (3) Compton (incoherent, inelastic, or modified) scattering, (4) pair production, and (5) photodisintegration.

2. Because the level of energy (beam quality) and the number of x-ray photons are controlled by technique factors selected by the radiographer, the radiographer is responsible for the radiation dose the patient receives during an imaging procedure. With a suitable understanding of these factors, radiographers will be able to select appropriate techniques that can minimize that dose to the patient while producing optimal-quality images.

3. Absorption and the differences in the absorption properties of various body structures make it possible to produce diagnostically useful images in which different anatomic structures can be perceived and distinguished.

4. Reducing the amount of tissue irradiated decreases the amount of fog that is produced by small-angle scatter. The radiographer can achieve this by confining, or collimating, the x-ray beam to include only the region of interest.

5. The energy of the electrons inside a diagnostic x-ray tube is generally specified in terms of the electrical voltage applied across the tube. In diagnostic radiology, this voltage is expressed in thousands of volts, or kilovolts (kV). Because the voltage across the tube fluctuates, it is characterized by kilovolt peak (kVp).

6. The minimum energy required to produce an electron-positron pair is 1.022 MeV.

7. Positive contrast media consist of solutions (e.g., barium or iodine based) containing elements having higher atomic numbers than surrounding tissue. These solutions are either swallowed or injected into the tissues or structures to be visually enhanced.

8. Three unstable nuclei used in positron emission tomography (PET) scanning are fluorine-18 (^{18}F), carbon-11 (^{11}C), and nitrogen-13 (^{13}N).

9. A photoelectron possesses kinetic energy equal to the energy of the incident photon minus the binding energy of the electron shell.

10. Scattered radiation may contribute to degradation of the radiographic image by creating an additional, unwanted exposure, known as *radiographic fog.*

11. During a fluoroscopic procedure, radiographers present in the x-ray room can protect themselves by wearing protective lead shielding.

12. During the process of coherent scattering, because the wavelengths of both incident and scattered waves are the same, no net energy has been absorbed by the atom.

13. Mass density is specified in grams per cubic centimeter.

14. Within the energy range of diagnostic radiology, the greater the difference in the amount of photoelectric absorption in body tissue, the greater the contrast in the radiographic image will be between adjacent structures of differing atomic numbers.

15. Annihilation radiation is used in positron emission tomography (PET).

Exercise 7: General Discussion or Opinion Questions

The questions in this exercise are intended to allow students to express their knowledge and understanding of the subject matter covered in this chapter. These questions may be used to stimulate class discussion. Because the answers may vary, determination of an answer's acceptability is left to the discretion of the instructor.

POST-TEST

1. photoelectric
2. Attenuation is the reduction in the number of primary photons in the x-ray beam through absorption and scatter as the beam passes through the patient in its path.
3. minimizes
4. personnel
5. partially
6. peak kilovoltage (kVp)
7. random
8. photodisintegration
9. Photoelectric absorption
10. C
11. A
12. B
13. A
14. D
15. A
16. 13.8
17. Absorbed dose
18. contrast
19. Compton
20. The term *fluorescent yield* refers to the number of x-rays emitted per inner-shell vacancy.

Chapter 4
Exercise 1: Matching

1. J	6. L	11. S	16. A	21. I
2. D	7. O	12. N	17. K	22. U
3. C	8. B	13. H	18. P	23. Q
4. G	9. Y	14. T	19. F	24. R
5. E	10. M	15. W	20. X	25. V

Exercise 2: Multiple Choice

1. C	6. D	11. B	16. B	21. D
2. A	7. C	12. D	17. A	22. B
3. D	8. C	13. C	18. D	23. D
4. C	9. A	14. D	19. D	24. D
5. D	10. D	15. A	20. C	25. A

Exercise 3: True or False

1. T
2. F (The paper was coated with a material compound of barium, platinum, and cyanide [barium platinocyanide].)
3. T
4. T

5. F (Maximum permissible dose [MPD] replaced tolerance dose.)
6. F (They were revised by the International Commission on Radiological Protection [ICRP], based on data from studies of the atomic bomb survivors.)
7. T
8. F (Louis Harold Gray)
9. T
10. F (Sievert is the SI unit that is used in the calculation of the radiation quantities EqD and EfD.)
11. F (Air kerma is replacing the traditional quantity, exposure.)
12. T
13. T
14. F (The number of electron-ion pairs also increases.)
15. T
16. F (Skin erythema dose was a crude and inaccurate way to measure radiation exposure because the amount of radiation required to produce an erythema reaction varied from one person to another.)
17. T
18. T
19. F (The higher the atomic number of a material, the more x-ray energy it absorbs.)
20. T
21. F (It may be determined and expressed in the SI unit sievert.)
22. T
23. F (Anatomic structures in the body possess different absorption properties.)
24. T
25. T

Exercise 4: Fill in the Blank

1. Wilhelm Conrad Roentgen
2. cancerous
3. energy
4. exposure
5. organs, organ systems
6. Absorbed dose
7. coulomb
8. biologic effect
9. 0.05, 0.001
10. risk, risk
11. metric
12. nonhazardous
13. measure
14. multiply
15. workable
16. ionized
17. 0.2, 0.1
18. roentgen
19. safety
20. Crookes tube

21. Louis Harold Gray
22. ionization chamber
23. μGy
24. ionization (charge)
25. pressure, temperature

Exercise 5: Labeling

A. **Standard or free air ionization chamber.**

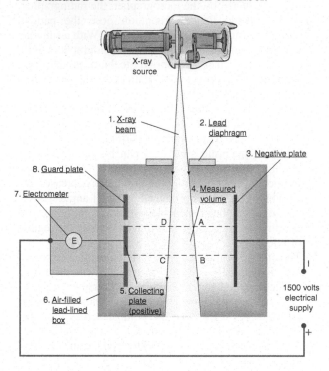

B. **Radiation weighting factors for different types and energies of ionizing radiation.**

Radiation Type and Energy Range	Radiation Weighting Factor (W_R)
X-ray and gamma ray photons, and electrons (every energy)	1. 1
Neutrons, energy <10 keV	2. 5
10 keV-100 keV	3. 10
>100 keV-2 MeV	4. 20
>2 MeV-20 MeV	5. 10
>20 MeV	6. 5
Protons	7. 2
Alpha particles	8. 20

C. Summary of radiation quantities and units.

Type of Radiation	Quantity	SI	Measuring Medium	Radiation Effect Measured
X-radiation or gamma	Exposure (X)	1. Coulomb per kilogram (C/kg)	Air	Ionization of air radiation
All ionizing radiations	2. Absorbed dose (D)	Gray (Gy)	Any object	Amount of energy per unit mass absorbed by object
All ionizing radiations	Equivalent dose (EqD)	3. Sievert (Sv)	Body tissue	Biologic effects
All ionizing radiations	4. Effective dose (EfD)	Sievert (Sv)	Body tissue	Biologic effects

Exercise 6: Short Answer

1. Thomas A. Edison discontinued his x-ray research because of the severe injuries and death of his friend, Clarence Dally, which were attributed to radiation-induced cancer.

2. Skin erythema dose was the unit used for measuring radiation exposure from 1900 to 1930.

3. Early tissue reactions of ionizing radiation are effects that appear within minutes, hours, days, or weeks of the time of radiation exposure. Late tissue reactions appear months or years after exposure to ionizing radiation.

4. Tolerance dose is a radiation dose to which occupationally exposed persons could be continuously subjected without any apparent harmful acute effects, such as erythema of the skin.

5. Maximum permissible dose (or MPD) replaced tolerance dose for radiation protection purposes in the 1950s.

6. In the late 1970s, dose limits were calculated and established to ensure that the risk from radiation exposure acquired on the job did not exceed risks encountered in "safe" occupations, such as clerical work, in which the risk is approximately 10^{-4} (one chance in 10,000) per year.[1]

7. The Bragg-Gray theory relates the ionization produced in a small cavity within an irradiated medium or object to the energy absorbed in that medium as a result of its radiation exposure. With the use of appropriate correction factors, the theory essentially links the determination of the absorbed radiation dose in a medium to a relatively simple measurement of ionization charge. The Bragg-Gray theory is the most important theory in all of radiation dosimetry.

8. When the human body is exposed to ionizing radiation, absorbed energy is responsible for any biologic damage to the tissues resulting from this exposure.

9. For precise measurement of radiation exposure in radiography, the total amount of ionization (charge) an x-ray beam produces in a known mass of air must be obtained. This type of direct measurement is accomplished in an accredited calibration laboratory using a standard, or free air, ionization chamber.

10. The radiation weighting factors are selected by national and international scientific advisory bodies (NCRP, ICRP) and are based on quality factors and linear energy transfer.

11. If absorbed dose is stated in the traditional unit rad, the SI equivalent number of gray may be determined by dividing the rad value by 100.

12. If the area of the irradiated surface is 100 cm^2, then the DAP will be 40 mGy $\times$ 100 cm^2 = 4000 mGy-cm^2.

13. Coulomb per kilogram (C/kg) is used for x-ray equipment calibration because x-ray output intensity is measured directly with an ionization chamber. It can also be used to calibrate radiation survey instruments. Air kerma can also be used to measure x-ray tube output and inputs to image receptors. A standard, or free air, ionization chamber is the instrument that can be calibrated to read air kerma.

14. If the radiation exposure is given in R, it can be converted to C/kg by multiplying the number of roentgens by 2.58 $\times$ 10^{-4}.

15. The radiation quantity *equivalent dose* uses radiation weighting factors (W_R) to adjust the value of the absorbed dose to reflect the different capacity for producing biologic harm by various types and energies of ionizing radiation. The quantity *effective dose* uses tissue weighting factors (W_T) to adjust the quantity *equivalent dose* to reflect the difference in harm to the person as a whole depending on the tissues and organs that have been irradiated. Therefore effective dose takes into account both the type of radiation and the part of the body irradiated.

Exercise 7: General Discussion or Opinion Questions

The questions in this exercise are intended to allow students to express their knowledge and understanding of the subject matter covered in this chapter. Because the answers may vary, determination of an answer's acceptability is left to the discretion of the instructor.

Exercise 8: Calculation Problems

A.

1. 8000 rad = 8000 ÷ 100 rad per Gy = 80 Gy
2. 8 rad = 8 ÷ 100 rad per Gy = 0.08 Gy
3. 450 rad = 450 ÷ 100 rad per Gy = 4.5 Gy
4. 4.5 rad = 4.5 ÷ 100 rad per Gy = 0.045 Gy
5. 375 rad = 375 ÷ 100 rad per Gy = 3.75 Gy
6. 7 Gy = 7 × 100 rad per Gy = 700 rad
7. 25 Gy = 25 × 100 rad per Gy = 2500 rad
8. 0.4 Gy = 0.4 × 100 rad per Gy = 40 rad
9. 0.087 Gy = 0.087 × 100 rad per Gy = 8.7 rad
10. 0.96 Gy = 0.96 × 100 rad per Gy = 96 rad

B.

1.

Radiation Type	D	×	W_R	=	EqD
X-radiation	0.6 Gy	×	1	=	0.6 Sv
Fast neutrons	0.25 Gy	×	20	=	5 Sv
Alpha particles	0.4 Gy	×	20	=	8 Sv
			Total EqD	=	13.6 Sv

2.

Radiation Type	D	×	W_R	=	EqD
X-radiation	0.3 Gy	×	1	=	0.3 Sv
Fast neutrons	0.28 Gy	×	20	=	5.6 Sv
Gamma rays	0.8 Gy	×	1	=	0.8 Sv
Protons	0.9 Gy	×	2	=	1.8 Sv
Alpha particles	0.4 Gy	×	20	=	8 Sv
			Total EqD	=	16.5 Sv

3.

Radiation Type	D	×	W_R	=	EqD
X-radiation	7 rad	×	1	=	7 rem
Fast neutrons	2 rad	×	20	=	40 rem
Alpha particles	5 rad	×	20	=	100 rem
			Total EqD	=	147 rem

4.

Radiation Type	D	×	W_R	=	EqD
X-radiation	3 rad	×	1	=	3 rem
Fast neutrons	0.35 rad	×	20	=	7 rem
Gamma rays	6 rad	×	1	=	6 rem
Protons	2.5 rad	×	2	=	5 rem
Alpha particles	8 rad	×	20	=	160 rem
			Total EqD	=	181 rem

5.

Radiation Type	D	×	W_R	=	EqD
X-radiation	0.6 Gy	×	1	=	0.6 Sv
Fast neutrons, energy <10 keV	0.2 Gy	×	5	=	1 Sv
Gamma rays	4 Gy	×	1	=	4 Sv
Protons	0.8 Gy	×	2	=	1.6 Sv
Alpha particles	6 Gy	×	20	=	120 Sv
			Total EqD	=	127.2 Sv

C.

	D	×	W_R	×	W_T	=	EfD
1.	0.5 Gy	×	20	×	0.05	=	0.5 Sv
2.	0.4 Gy	×	1	×	0.2	=	0.08 Sv
3.	6 rad	×	20	×	0.12	=	14.4 rem
4.	25 rad	×	1	×	0.05	=	1.25 rem
5.	0.9 Gy	×	1	×	0.12	=	0.108 Sv

D.

	Number	×	Average EfD (Sv)	=	ColEfD
1.	400	×	0.2	=	80 person-sievert
2.	300	×	0.17	=	51 person-sievert
3.	250	×	0.24	=	60 person-sievert
4.	1000	×	0.10	=	100 person-sievert
5.	100	×	0.30	=	30 person-sievert

E.

	Number of Gy	×	1000	=	Number of mGy
1.	0.020 Gy	×	1000	=	20 mGy
2.	0.200 Gy	×	1000	=	200 mGy

	Number of Sv	×	1000	=	Number of mSv
3.	0.030 Sv	×	1000	=	30 mSv
4.	0.300 Sv	×	1000	=	300 mSv

POST-TEST

1. Number exposed people × Average EfD (Sv) = ColEfD

   400 × 0.2 Sv = 80 person-sievert
2. Effective dose (EfD)
3. Linear energy transfer (LET)
4. Coulombs per kilogram (C/kg) and air kerma
5. Leukemia
6. Wilhelm Conrad Roentgen
7.

Radiation Type	D	×	W_R	=	EqD
X-radiation	5 Gy	×	1	=	5 Sv
Fast neutrons	0.3 Gy	×	20	=	6 Sv
Alpha particles	0.7 Gy	×	20	=	14 Sv
				Total EqD =	25 Sv

8. $D \times W_R \times W_T = EfD$

   $5 \text{ Gy} \times 1 \times 0.12 = 0.6 \text{ Sv}$
9. 800 mSv
10. $EqD = D \times W_R$
11. A
12. C
13. Skin erythema
14. Coulomb (C)
15. D
16. Total effective dose equivalent (TEDE)
17. Centigray (cGy)
18. cancerous
19. Radiation exposure received by radiation workers in the course of exercising their professional responsibilities.
20. The energy deposited in biologic tissue by ionizing radiation.

Chapter 5

Exercise 1: Matching

1. K	6. N	11. Y	16. Q	21. J
2. M	7. B	12. W	17. D	22. S
3. L	8. O	13. R	18. G	23. X
4. C	9. A	14. P	19. E	24. V
5. H	10. I	15. U	20. F	25. T

Exercise 2: Multiple Choice

1. D	6. B	11. A	16. A	21. A
2. D	7. C	12. D	17. C	22. C
3. A	8. C	13. D	18. D	23. A
4. C	9. B	14. D	19. A	24. D
5. C	10. A	15. A	20. A	25. B

Exercise 3: True or False

1. F (Personal dosimeters do not protect the wearer from ionizing radiation.)
2. T
3. T
4. F (Cost is a factor; personnel dosimeters selected for use must be cost-effective.)
5. F (The personnel digital ionization dosimeter does provide an instant readout of dose information when connected to a computer via a connector such as a USB.)
6. F (Exposure time is too short to allow the meter to appropriately respond.)
7. T
8. T
9. F (All radiation survey meters are not equally sensitive in the detection of ionizing radiation.)

10. T
11. F (Pocket dosimeters are usually used for a short duration.)
12. T
13. T
14. F (Filters in an optically stimulated luminescence [OSL] are made of aluminum, tin, and copper.)
15. T
16. T
17. F (An OSL dosimeter can be worn up to 1 year; it is commonly worn for 1 to 3 months.)
18. T
19. T
20. F (A thermoluminescent dosimeter [TLD] can be read only once because the reading destroys the stored information.)
21. T
22. T
23. T
24. T
25. T

Exercise 4: Fill in the Blank

1. thyroid, eyes
2. periodically
3. optically stimulated, ionization, thermoluminescent
4. inexpensive
5. lightweight
6. radiation-free
7. equivalent
8. trigger
9. charged, zero
10. Medical physicists, electrometers
11. sensitive
12. lost
13. radiation output
14. occupational
15. laser light
16. second, gestation
17. deep, shallow
18. reused, cost-effective
19. Control
20. usage, placement
21. employment
22. worn
23. physical
24. 5, 40
25. plastic

Exercise 5: Labeling

A. **Pocket ionization chamber (pocket dosimeter).**

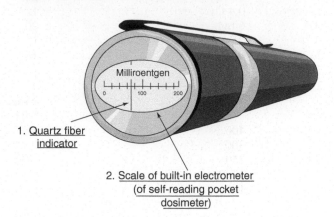

1. Quartz fiber indicator

2. Scale of built-in electrometer (of self-reading pocket dosimeter)

Exercise 6: Short Answer

1. By detecting and measuring the quantity of ionizing radiation to which the dosimeter has been exposed over time.
2. If the facility does not have an in-house reader, OSL dosimeters must be shipped to the monitoring company for reading and exposure determination. This task takes time.
3. An extremity dosimeter measures the approximate equivalent dose to the hands of the wearer of the dosimeter.
4. Fluoroscopy, surgery, and special radiographic procedures produce the highest occupational radiation exposure for diagnostic imaging personnel.
5. If a pregnant radiographer wears a second monitoring device at abdominal level, the monitor provides an estimate of the equivalent dose to the embryo-fetus.
6. Three radiation survey instruments used for area monitoring are the ionization chamber–type survey meter (cutie pie), the proportional counter, and the Geiger-Müller (GM) meter.
7. Proportional counters are generally used in a laboratory setting to detect alpha and beta radiation and small amounts of other types of low-level radioactive contamination.
8. Some disadvantages of the TLD are (1) the initial high cost; (2) the fact that it can be read only once because the readout process destroys the stored information; and (3) the fact that calibrated dosimeters must be prepared and read with each group of TLDs as they are processed.
9. The OSL dosimeter contains an aluminum oxide (Al_2O_3) detector (thin layer).
10. In addition to x-radiation and gamma radiation, if equipped with a suitable window, a cutie pie can also measure beta radiation.

206

11. Because a GM tube tends to lose its calibration over time, the instrument generally has a "check source" to verify its constancy daily.

12. When a protective lead apron is used during fluoroscopy or special procedures, the personnel dosimeter should be worn outside the apron at collar level on the anterior surface of the body because the unprotected head, neck, and lenses of the eyes receive 10 to 20 times more exposure than the protected body trunk. When the personnel dosimeter is located at collar level, it also provides a reading of the approximate equivalent dose to the thyroid gland and eyes of the occupationally exposed person.

13. The cumulative columns provide a continuous audit of actual absorbed radiation equivalent dose.

14. When the letter *M* appears under the current monitoring period or in the cumulative columns of a personnel monitoring report, it signifies that an equivalent dose below the minimum measurable radiation quantity was recorded during that time.

15. When changing employment, a radiation worker must convey the data pertinent to the accumulated permanent equivalent dose to the new employer so that this information can be placed on file.

Exercise 7: General Discussion or Opinion Questions

The questions in this exercise are intended to allow students to express their knowledge and understanding of the subject matter covered in this chapter. Because the answers may vary, determination of an answer's acceptability is left to the discretion of the instructor.

POST-TEST

1. effective

2. An OSL dosimeter is a device for monitoring personnel exposure. It contains an aluminum oxide detector. The dosimeter is read out by using laser light at selected frequencies. When such laser light is incident on the sensing material, it becomes luminescent in proportion to the amount of radiation exposure received.

3. The working habits and working conditions of diagnostic imaging personnel can be assessed over a designated period through the use of the personnel dosimeter.

4. results

5. Attached to the clothing on the front of the body at collar level.

6. A

7. D

8. In a health care facility, a radiographer's deep, eye, and shallow occupational exposure as measured by an exposed monitor may be found on the personnel monitoring report.

9. A GM meter

10. zero (0)

11. abdomen

12. The data pertinent to the accumulated permanent equivalent dose so that they may be placed on file with the new employer.

13. survey

14. employment

15. Radiation workers are required to wear personnel monitoring devices whenever they are likely to risk receiving 10% or more of the annual occupational EfD limit of 50 mSv (5 rem) in any single year as a consequence of their work-related activities.

16. primary

17. The radiation safety officer (RSO)

18. 1, 3

19. Ionization chamber connected to an electrometer

20. pregnant

Chapter 6
Exercise 1: Matching

1. D	6. C	11. E	16. J	21. Y
2. M	7. N	12. R	17. U	22. X
3. L	8. A	13. H	18. I	23. V
4. K	9. P	14. T	19. B	24. S
5. F	10. G	15. O	20. W	25. Q

Exercise 2: Multiple Choice

1. C	6. B	11. A	16. B	21. D
2. B	7. D	12. C	17. A	22. C
3. C	8. B	13. B	18. D	23. B
4. B	9. C	14. B	19. D	24. B
5. D	10. B	15. C	20. C	25. C

Exercise 3: True or False

1. T
2. F (Water normally accounts for 80% to 85% of protoplasm.)
3. T
4. F (The body's primary defense mechanism against infection and disease is the antibodies.)
5. T
6. F (Hydrogen bonds attach the nitrogenous bases to each other.)
7. T
8. T
9. F (All cellular metabolic functions occur in the cytoplasm.)
10. T
11. T
12. T
13. F (The cell membrane is a frail, semipermeable, and flexible structure.)
14. T
15. T
16. T
17. F (Radiation-induced damage to chromosomes may be evaluated during metaphase.)
18. T
19. T
20. F (Glucose is the primary energy source for the human cell.)

21. T
22. F (Cells are essential for life.)
23. T
24. F (Proteins contain the most carbon of all the organic compounds.)
25. F (Carbohydrates are most abundant in the liver and in muscle tissue.)

Exercise 4: Fill in the Blank

1. cell
2. homeostasis
3. 4
4. amino acids
5. repair enzymes
6. hormones
7. liver, muscle
8. DNA
9. osmotic
10. fraternal
11. DNA
12. high
13. water, fluid
14. Metabolism
15. metabolism
16. Ribosomes
17. catalytic, repair
18. macromolecules
19. nucleus
20. endoplasmic reticulum
21. replication
22. lysosomes
23. Oxidative
24. Salts
25. electrolytes

Exercise 5: Labeling

A. **Typical cell.**

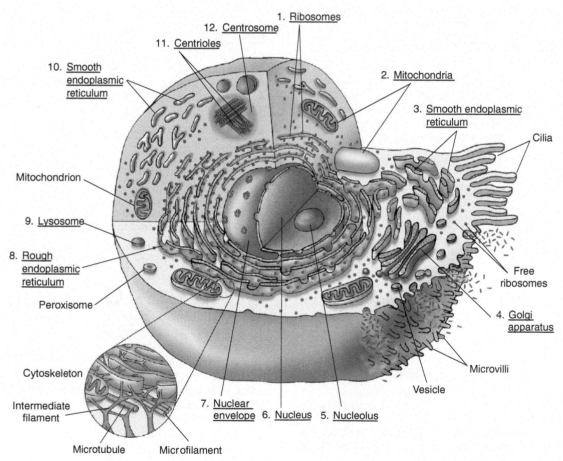

From Thibodeau A: *Anatomy and physiology,* ed 5, St. Louis, 2003, Mosby.

B. Cellular life cycle.

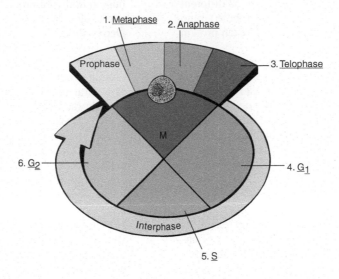

From Bushong SC: *Radiologic science for technologists: physics, biology, and protection,* ed 10, St. Louis, 2013, Mosby.

C. Summary of cell components.

Title	Site	Activity
1. Cell membrane	Cytoplasm	*Plastic storage bag*—Functions as a barricade to protect cellular contents from their environment and controls the passage of water and other materials into and out of the cell; performs many additional functions such as elimination of wastes and refining of material for energy through breakdown of the materials
2. Endoplasmic reticulum	Cytoplasm	*The highway*—Enables the cell to communicate with the extracellular environment and transfers food from one part of the cell to another
3. Golgi apparatus	Cytoplasm	*Freight hauling*—Unites large carbohydrate molecules and combines them with proteins to form glycoproteins and transports enzymes and hormones through the cell membrane so that they can exit the cell, enter the bloodstream, and be carried to areas of the body in which they are required
4. Mitochondria	Cytoplasm	*Power-generating stations*—Produce energy for cellular activity by breaking down nutrients through a process of oxidation
5. Lysosomes	Cytoplasm	*Garbage bags with poison pills*—Dispose of large particles such as bacteria and food as well as smaller particles; also contain hydrolytic enzymes that can break down and digest proteins, certain carbohydrates, and the cell itself if the lysosome's surrounding membrane breaks
6. Ribosomes	Cytoplasm	*Manufacturing facilities*—Manufacture the various proteins that cells require
7. Centrosomes	Cytoplasm	*Spindle weavers*—Believed to play some part in the formation of the mitotic spindle during cell division
8. Nucleus	Nucleus	*Information processing and administrative center of the cell*—Contains the genetic or hereditary material, DNA, and proteins. Also contains the nucleolus. The nucleus controls cell division and multiplication and the biochemical reactions that occur within the cell and also directs protein synthesis
9. DNA	Nucleus	*The blueprint*—Contains the genetic material; controls cell division and multiplication and also biochemical reactions that occur within the living cell
10. Nucleolus	Nucleus	*RNA copy center*—Holds a large amount of RNA and synthesizes ribosomes

Exercise 6: Short Answer

1. To ensure efficient cell operation, the body must provide food as a source of raw material for the release of energy, supply oxygen to help break down the food, and have enough water to transport inorganic substances such as calcium and sodium into and out of the cell.

2. Destructive metabolism, or catabolism, is the breakdown of large molecules into smaller ones.

3. Proteins are formed when organic compounds called amino acids combine into long, chainlike molecular complexes. In these complexes a chemical link, called

209

a *peptide bond,* connects each amino acid. Protein production, or *protein synthesis,* involves 22 different amino acids. The order of arrangement of these amino acids determines the precise function of each protein molecule.

4. Enzymatic proteins function as *organic catalysts*—that is, agents that affect the rate of speed of chemical reactions without being altered themselves. Enzymatic proteins moderate or control the cell's various physiologic activities. They can cause an increase in cellular activity that in turn causes biochemical reactions to occur more rapidly to meet the needs of the cell in stressful situations. Hence proper cell functioning depends on enzymes.

5. Lipids are substances such as fats or fatty acids that constitute approximately 2% of cell content. They perform many functions for the body; for example, they (1) act as reservoirs for long-term storage of energy; (2) insulate and guard the body against the environment; (3) support and protect organs such as the eyes and kidneys; (4) provide essential substances for growth and development; (5) lubricate the joints; and (6) assist in the digestive process.

6. Ribosomes function as protein factories for the cell; they manufacture (synthesize) the various proteins that cells require using the blueprints provided by messenger ribonucleic acid (mRNA).

7. Within the cell, water is indispensable for metabolic activity because it is the medium in which the chemical reactions that are the bases of these activities occur. It also acts as a solvent, keeping compounds dissolved so that they can more easily interact and their concentration can be regulated. Outside the cell, water functions as a transport vehicle for minerals the cell uses or eliminates. In addition, water is responsible for maintaining a constant body core temperature of 98.6°F (37°C) while at the same time serving to lubricate both the digestive system and the skeletal articulations (joints). Organs such as the brain and lungs are also protected by a cushion of compounds comprised primarily of water.

8. The nucleus controls cell division and multiplication and the biochemical reactions that occur within the cell. By directing protein synthesis, the nucleus plays an essential role in active transport, metabolism, growth, and heredity.

9. Four distinct phases of the cellular life cycle are identifiable: G_1 (pre-DNA synthesis phase), S (synthesis phase), G_2 (post-DNA synthesis phase), and M (mitosis phase).

10. Carbohydrates are referred to as *saccharides.* A monosaccharide is a simple sugar molecule (e.g., glucose). A disaccharide is made up of two units of a simple sugar linked together (e.g., sucrose [cane sugar] and lactose). A *polysaccharide* contains several or many molecules of a simple sugar. Plant starches and animal glycogen are the two most important polysaccharides. Through the process of metabolism, the body breaks these down into simpler sugars for energy.

11. The four major classes of organic compounds in the human body are proteins, carbohydrates, lipids (fats), and nucleic acids.

12. Deoxyribonucleic acid (DNA) is a type of nucleic acid that carries the genetic information necessary for cell replication and regulates all cellular activity to direct protein synthesis.

13. Structural proteins, such as those found in muscle, provide the body with its shape and form and are a source of heat and energy.

14. In the nucleus of a living cell, two nuclear components, DNA and protein, are arranged in long threads called *chromatin.* When a cell divides, this genetic-containing material contracts into tiny rod-shaped bodies called *chromosomes* that carry genes within their DNA.

15. Hormones are chemical secretions manufactured by various endocrine glands and carried by the bloodstream to influence the activities of other parts of the body. Hormones produced by the thyroid gland located in the neck control metabolism throughout the body. Hormones also regulate functions such as growth and development.

Exercise 7: General Discussion or Opinion Questions

The questions in this exercise are intended to allow students to express their knowledge and understanding of the subject matter covered in this chapter. Because the answers may vary, determination of an answer's acceptability is left to the discretion of the instructor.

POST-TEST

1. matter
2. organic
3. Repair enzymes
4. nitrogenous
5. water
6. The DNA macromolecule is composed of two long sugar-phosphate chains that twist around each other in a double-helix configuration and are linked by pairs of nitrogenous organic bases at the sugar molecules of the chain to form a tightly coiled structure resembling a twisted ladder or spiral staircase. The sugar-phosphate compounds are the side rails, and the pairs of nitrogenous bases, which consist of complementary chemicals, are the steps, or rungs, of the DNA ladder-like structure. Hydrogen bonds attach the bases to each other, joining the two side rails of the DNA ladder.
7. Mapping
8. C
9. C
10. During metaphase
11. Ribosomes synthesize the various proteins that cells require.
12. Approximately 30,000
13. The affected cells will function abnormally or die.
14. 22
15. A nucleotide

16. DNA
17. Cytoplasm
18. Interphase
19. Lipids
20. The cell membrane encases and surrounds the cell, functions as a barricade to protect cellular contents from the outside environment, and controls the passage of water and other materials in and out of the cell.

Chapter 7
Exercise 1: Matching

1. N	6. L	11. B	16. Y	21. S
2. O	7. A	12. G	17. P	22. Q
3. H	8. K	13. M	18. W	23. X
4. D	9. I	14. J	19. R	24. U
5. E	10. F	15. C	20. V	25. T

Exercise 2: Multiple Choice

1. B	6. D	11. C	16. B
2. B	7. D	12. A	17. C
3. A	8. C	13. A	18. A
4. D	9. D	14. A	19. A
5. A	10. A	15. B	20. C

Exercise 3: True or False

1. F (Most cells can be damaged by radiation.)
2. T
3. F (The characteristics of ionizing radiation vary among the different types of ionizing radiation.)
4. T
5. F (High-LET radiation is of greatest concern when internal contamination is possible.)
6. F (HOH⁺ and HOH⁻ are basically unstable.)
7. T
8. F (The embryo-fetus contains large numbers of immature, unspecialized cells and is therefore radiosensitive.)
9. T
10. T
11. F (Experimental data strongly indicate that deoxyribonucleic acid [DNA] is the irreplaceable master, or key molecule in the human cell.)
12. T
13. F (Ionizing radiation can adversely affect cell division.)
14. T
15. T
16. T
17. F (The presence of free radicals dramatically increases the amount of biologic damage produced.)
18. F (X-ray photons may interact with and ionize water molecules in the human body.)
19. T
20. T
21. F (The human body is composed of different types of cells and tissues, which vary in their degree of radiosensitivity.)
22. F (In radiation therapy the presence of oxygen plays a significant role in radiosensitivity.)
23. F (The more mature and specialized in performing functions a cell is, the less sensitive it is to radiation.)

24. T
25. T

Exercise 4: Fill in the Blank

1. cellular
2. energy
3. sublethal
4. mass, charge
5. internal
6. permanent
7. hydroxyl
8. Gene
9. Radiosensitivity
10. ionizing radiation
11. infection
12. platelets
13. Granulocytes
14. decrease
15. mitosis
16. radiosensitive
17. radiosensitive
18. microcephaly (small head circumference), intellectual disability
19. insensitive
20. radiosensitive
21. dies, restored
22. 2
23. 5, 6
24. immature, susceptible
25. 0.25

Exercise 5: Labeling
A. **Radiolysis of water.**

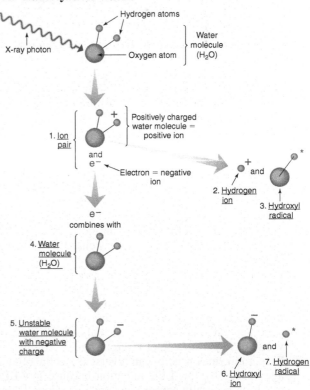

B. Indirect action of ionizing radiation on biologic molecules.

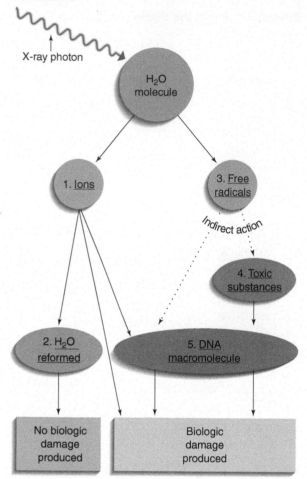

C. Examples of radiosensitive and radioinsensitive cells.

Radiosensitive Cells	Radioinsensitive Cells
1. Basal cells of the skin	4. Brain cells
2. Intestinal crypt cells	5. Muscle cells
3. Reproductive (germ) cells	6. Nerve cells

Exercise 6: Short Answer

1. High-energy charged particles (e.g., alpha and beta particles and protons) may ionize atoms by interacting electromagnetically with orbital electrons. The alpha particle, which is composed of two protons and two neutrons and therefore carries an electrical charge of $+2$, strongly attracts the negatively charged electron as it passes by.

2. Characteristics that vary (e.g., charge, mass, and energy) among the different types of radiations determine the extent to which different radiation modalities transfer energy into biologic tissue.

3. LET generally is described in units of kiloelectron volts (keV) per micron (1 micron [μm] $= 10^{-6}$ m).

4. Repair enzymes usually can reverse the cellular damage caused by low-LET radiation because low-LET radiation generally causes sublethal damage to DNA.

5. Free radicals are solitary atoms (e.g., a lone hydrogen atom [H]) or most often a combination of atoms that behave as single entities and are very chemically reactive as a result of the presence of unpaired valence electrons.

6. All cells in the body other than female and male germ cells are classified as somatic cells.

7. Oxygen enhances the effects of ionizing radiation on biologic tissue by increasing tissue radiosensitivity. If oxygen is present when a tissue is irradiated, more free radicals are formed in the tissue; this increases the indirect damage potential of the radiation.

8. Damage to the cell's nucleus from ionizing radiation reveals itself in one of the following ways: instant death; reproductive death; apoptosis, or programmed cell death (interphase death); mitotic, or genetic, death; mitotic delay; interference with function.

9. With *direct action,* biologic damage occurs as a result of ionization of atoms on essential molecules (e.g., DNA), produced by straight interaction with the incident radiation. *Indirect action* refers to a multistage process that first involves the production of free radicals that are created by the interaction of radiation with water (H_2O) molecules. These unstable agents are so highly reactive that they have the capability to substantially disrupt master molecules with resulting cell death.

10. If the nucleus in an adult nerve cell is destroyed by exposure to ionizing radiation, the cell dies and is never restored.

11. Even small doses of ionizing radiation (e.g., doses as low as 0.1 Gy$_t$) could cause menstrual irregularities, such as delay or suppression of menstruation.

12. Ionizing radiation interacts randomly with matter, giving up energy in the process. Consequently, because of this energy transfer, exposure to radiation can lead to the occurrence of deleterious changes in biologic tissue including the following in the cell nuclei: (1) a single-strand break in one chromosome; (2) a single-strand break in one chromatid; (3) a single-strand break in separate chromosomes; (4) a strand break in separate chromatids; (5) more than one break in the same chromosome; (6) more than one break in the same chromatid; and (7) chromosome stickiness, or clumping.

13. Radiation damage is observed on three levels: molecular, cellular, and organic systems.

14. Ionizing radiation causes complete chromosome breakage when two direct hits occur in the same rung of a DNA macromolecule.

15. In 1906 two French scientists, Jean A. Bergonié and Louis F. A. Tribondeau, observed the effects of ionizing radiation on testicular germ cells of rabbits they had exposed to x-rays. They established that radiosensitivity was a function of the metabolic state of the cell receiving the exposure. Their findings eventually became known as the Law of Bergonié and Tribondeau, which states that the radiosensitivity of cells is directly proportional to their reproductive activity and inversely proportional to their degree of differentiation.

212

Exercise 7: General Discussion or Opinion Questions

The questions in this exercise are intended to allow students to express their knowledge and understanding of the subject matter covered in this chapter. Because the answers may vary, determination of an answer's acceptability is left to the discretion of the instructor.

POST-TEST

1. The following formula is used:
   Dose in Gy_t from 250 kVp
   x-rays (reference radiation)
   = Relative biologic effectiveness (RBE)
   Dose in Gy_t of test radiation
   $21 \div 7 = 3$
   RBE = 3
2. Water
3. apoptosis
4. LET is the average energy deposited per unit length of track to an object by ionizing radiation during its passage through the object. It is described in units of kiloelectron volts per micron (keV/μm).
5. When irradiated in an oxygenated, or aerobic, state, biologic tissue is more sensitive to radiation than when it is exposed to radiation under anoxic (without oxygen) or hypoxic (low-oxygen) conditions. This is known as the oxygen effect. The oxygen enhancement ratio (OER) describes this effect numerically.[1,2]
6. direct
7. C
8. D
9. target
10. indirect
11. Lymphocytes
12. Law of Bergonié and Tribondeau
13. mutations
14. A cell survival curve is used to display the sensitivity of a particular type of cell to radiation, which helps determine the types of cancer cells that will respond to radiation therapy.
15. bond
16. Measurable hematologic depression
17. repopulate
18. blood count
19. intellectual disability
20. Ionizing radiation causes complete chromosome breakage when two direct hits occur in the same rung of the DNA macromolecule.

Chapter 8
Exercise 1: Matching

1. O	6. N	11. Y	16. F	21. U
2. E	7. D	12. H	17. Q	22. W
3. M	8. G	13. X	18. C	23. S
4. K	9. J	14. B	19. V	24. R
5. A	10. I	15. P	20. L	25. T

Exercise 2: Multiple Choice

1. A	6. D	11. C	16. D	21. D
2. A	7. C	12. C	17. C	22. B
3. C	8. D	13. D	18. C	23. B
4. D	9. D	14. D	19. D	24. A
5. D	10. A	15. D	20. A	25. C

Exercise 3: True or False

1. F (Current radiation protection programs do not rely on hematologic depression as a means for monitoring imaging personnel.)
2. F (The risk of hemorrhage increases.)
3. F (Chromosomal damage caused by radiation exposure can be evaluated during metaphase.)
4. T
5. T
6. F (Radiation exposure causes a decrease in the number of red cells, white cells, and platelets in the circulating blood.)
7. F (The lethal dose [LD] 50/30 for adult humans is estimated to be 3 to 4 Gy_t.)
8. T
9. T
10. F (Early tissue reactions occur within a short period after exposure to ionizing radiation.)
11. F (Ionizing radiation produces the greatest amount of biologic damage when a large dose of densely ionizing [high linear energy transfer (LET)] radiation is delivered to a large or radiosensitive area of the body.)
12. F (Acute radiation syndrome [ARS] is actually a collection of symptoms associated with high-LET radiation exposure.)
13. T
14. F (Radiation doses in this range produce a decrease in the number of bone marrow stem cells.)
15. T
16. F (Whole-body equivalent doses greater than 12 Gy_t are considered fatal regardless of medical treatment.)
17. T
18. T
19. F (Karyotyping is done during metaphase.)
20. T
21. T
22. F (LD 50/60 may be more accurate for humans than is LD 50/30.)
23. T
24. F (All layers of the skin and accessory structures are actively involved.)
25. T

Exercise 4: Fill in the Blank

1. substantial, dose, dose
2. 1
3. Radiation sickness
4. early, late
5. platelets
6. biologic criteria
7. death

213

8. repair, repopulation
9. functional
10. high
11. William Herbert Rollins
12. 2
13. 100, 200
14. radiosensitive
15. menstruation
16. atrophy

17. chromosomal abnormalities
18. 0.25
19. anemia
20. indirect action
21. photograph, photomicrograph
22. Grenz rays
23. ionizing radiation
24. neutrophils
25. impaired fertility

Exercise 5: Labeling

A. Overview of acute radiation lethality.

Stage	Dose Gy$_t$	Average Survival Time	Signs and Symptoms
1. Prodromal	1	—	Nausea, vomiting, diarrhea, fatigue, leukopenia
2. Latent	1-100	—	None
3. Hematopoietic	1-10	6-8 wk (doses > 2 Gy)	Nausea; vomiting; diarrhea; decrease in number of red blood cells, white blood cells, and platelets in the circulating blood; hemorrhage; infection
4. Gastrointestinal	6-10	3-10 days	Severe nausea, vomiting, diarrhea, fever, fatigue, loss of appetite, lethargy, anemia, leukopenia, hemorrhage, infection, electrolytic imbalance, and emaciation
5. Cerebrovascular	≥50	Several hours to 2 or 3 days	Same as hematopoietic and gastrointestinal, excessive nervousness, confusion, lack of coordination, loss of vision, a burning sensation of the skin, loss of consciousness, disorientation, shock, periods of agitation alternating with stupor, edema, loss of equilibrium, meningitis, prostration, respiratory distress, vasculitis, coma

B. Development of the germ cell from stem cell phase to the mature cell.

Male:

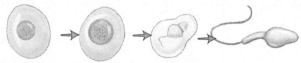

1. Spermatogonia 2. Spermatocyte 3. Spermatid 4. Sperm

Female:

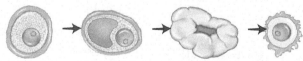

1. Primordial follicle 2. Mature follicle 3. Corpus luteum 4. Ovum

C. **Progressive development of various cells from a single pluripotential stem cell.**

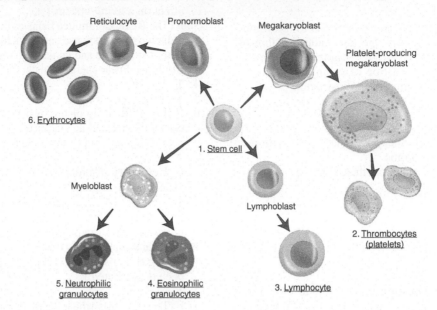

Reticulocyte   Pronormoblast   Megakaryoblast

Platelet-producing megakaryoblast

6. Erythrocytes

1. Stem cell

Myeloblast

Lymphoblast

2. Thrombocytes (platelets)

5. Neutrophilic granulocytes   4. Eosinophilic granulocytes   3. Lymphocyte

Exercise 6: Short Answer

1. Numerous laboratory animal studies and data from observation of some irradiated human populations provide substantial evidence of the consequences of high-dose radiation exposure.
2. During the explosion, several tons of burning graphite, uranium dioxide fuel, and other contaminants such as cesium-137, iodine-131, and plutonium-239 were ejected upward into the atmosphere in a 3-mile-high radioactive plume of intense heat.
3. ARS presents in four major response stages: prodromal, latent period, manifest illness, and recovery or death.
4. The three separate dose-related syndromes that occur as part of the total-body syndrome are hematopoietic syndrome (bone marrow syndrome), gastrointestinal syndrome, and cerebrovascular syndrome.
5. When bone marrow cells are being destroyed by exposure to radiation, the body becomes more susceptible to infection (from its own intestinal bacteria) and more prone to hemorrhage.
6. A bone marrow transplant is not an absolute cure for patients with hematopoietic syndrome because many individuals undergoing bone marrow transplant die of burns or other radiation-induced damage they sustained before the transplanted stem cells have had a chance to support recovery.
7. Some of the symptoms of the cerebrovascular syndrome are excessive nervousness, confusion, severe nausea, vomiting, diarrhea, loss of vision, a burning sensation of the skin, and loss of consciousness.
8. The techniques used to study and observe the chromosomes of each human cell have greatly contributed to advancing genetic analysis and the understanding of influence of radiation on genetics.
9. The term *somatic* comes from the Greek *soma,* meaning "body."
10. If both oxygenated and hypoxic cells receive a comparable dose of low-LET radiation, the oxygenated cells are more severely damaged, but those that survive repair themselves and recover from the injury. Even though they are less severely damaged, the hypoxic cells do not repair and recover as efficiently.
11. The radiation dose required to cause a particular syndrome and the average survival time are the most important measures used to quantify human radiation lethality.
12. When the number of lymphocytes in the blood are decreased by exposure to ionizing radiation, the body becomes vulnerable to infection by foreign invaders.
13. When shedding of the outer layer of skin occurs after reception of higher radiation doses, it generally manifests first as moist desquamation, and then dry desquamation may develop.
14. The overall goal of radiation therapeutic treatment was to deposit the radiant energy at a planned location within a specified treatment volume enclosing the tumor while sparing as much healthy surrounding tissue as possible.
15. Most lethal dose data represent an estimate of the role played by radiation in fatalities in which other factors were present. Specifications of lethal effects are further complicated by the medical treatment that the patient may receive during the prodromal and latent stages, before many of the symptoms of ARS appear. When medical treatment is given promptly, the patient is supported through initial symptoms, and so answering the question of long-term survival may simply be delayed. For this reason LD 50/60 for humans is probably a more accurate measure for human survival than is any shorter period.

Answer Key

Exercise 7: General Discussion or Opinion Questions

The questions in this exercise are intended to allow students to express their knowledge and understanding of the subject matter covered in this chapter. Because the answers may vary, determination of an answer's acceptability is left to the discretion of the instructor.

POST-TEST

1. early effects
2. Hematopoietic syndrome, gastrointestinal syndrome, cerebrovascular syndrome
3. prodromal, latent period, manifest illness, recovery, or death
4. B
5. LD 50/30
6. cumulative
7. D
8. C
9. C
10. Early tissue reactions are early somatic effects on organs or organ systems that result from high doses of radiation. These reactions may appear within minutes, hours, days, or weeks after such an exposure.
11. Metaphase
12. Without effective physical monitoring devices, biologic criteria such as the occurrence of nausea and excessive vomiting played an important role in the identification of radiation casualties in the first 2 days after the 1986 accident at the Chernobyl nuclear power plant.
13. gastrointestinal
14. 3 to 4 Gy_t
15. karyotype
16. 0.1, 2, 5, 6
17. 0.1
18. Cells of the hematopoietic system all develop from a single precursor cell, the pluripotential stem cell.
19. 50
20. bone marrow syndrome

Chapter 9

Exercise 1: Matching

1. L	6. N	11. U	16. F	21. B
2. E	7. D	12. H	17. Q	22. W
3. S	8. G	13. O	18. X	23. C
4. K	9. J	14. Y	19. P	24. R
5. A	10. I	15. V	20. T	25. M

Exercise 2: Multiple Choice

1. A	6. D	11. A	16. D	21. D
2. B	7. D	12. C	17. A	22. D
3. B	8. D	13. A	18. D	23. A
4. C	9. D	14. C	19. B	24. B
5. B	10. C	15. C	20. A	25. A

Exercise 3: True or False

1. T
2. F (If a nonthreshold relationship exists between a radiation dose and a biologic response, even the smallest dose of ionizing radiation will have some biologic effect on a living system.)
3. F (The BEIR Committee believes that the nonthreshold radiation dose-response curve is a more accurate reflection of stochastic and genetic effects at low-dose levels from low–linear energy transfer [LET] radiation.)
4. T
5. T
6. F (It is difficult to distinguish radiation-induced cancer by its physical appearance because it does not appear different from cancers initiated by other agents.)
7. T
8. F (Hereditary disorders are present in approximately 10% of all living newborns in the United States.)
9. T
10. F (Radium watch dial painters of the 1920s and 1930s provide proof of radiation carcinogenesis.)
11. F (Many cases of radiation-induced skin cancer among early radiation workers in the early 1900s have been documented.)
12. T
13. F (Technologists who entered the medical radiation industry before 1950 have demonstrated a somewhat higher risk of dying from leukemia compared with individuals who entered the workforce in 1950 or later.)
14. F (No conclusive proof exists that low-level ionizing radiation doses below 0.1 Gy cause a significant increase in the risk of malignancy.)
15. T
16. T
17. T
18. T
19. F (Follow-up studies of Japanese atomic bomb survivors have demonstrated late tissue reactions and stochastic effects of ionizing radiation.)
20. T
21. T
22. F (The lens of the eye contains transparent fibers that transmit light.)
23. F (Cancer is the most important late stochastic somatic effect caused by exposure to ionizing radiation.)
24. T
25. T

Exercise 4: Fill in the Blank

1. somatic, hereditary (genetic)
2. linear, threshold
3. overestimate, underestimate
4. natural, irradiated
5. risk, low
6. months, years
7. cancers
8. calcium
9. cellular
10. breast
11. 1.56
12. Thorotrast, reticuloendothelial
13. malignancy
14. thyroid
15. 4:1, 10:1

16. leukemia
17. cancer-causing
18. follow-up studies
19. thyroid, iodine
20. time

21. leukemia
22. lens
23. radiosensitive, damaged
24. first, stem
25. death

Exercise 5: Labeling

A. **Radiation dose-response curves.**

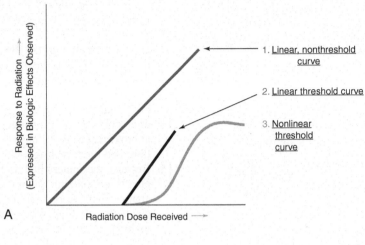

1. Linear, nonthreshold curve
2. Linear threshold curve
3. Nonlinear threshold curve

A

Response to Radiation (Expressed in Biologic Effects Observed)

Radiation Dose Received

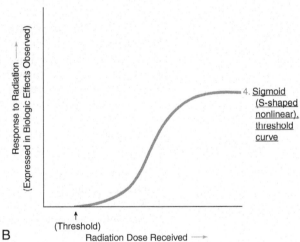

4. Sigmoid (S-shaped nonlinear), threshold curve

B

Response to Radiation (Expressed in Biologic Effects Observed)

(Threshold)

Radiation Dose Received

B. **Dose-response curve.**

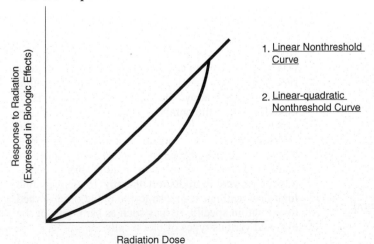

1. Linear Nonthreshold Curve

2. Linear-quadratic Nonthreshold Curve

Response to Radiation (Expressed in Biologic Effects)

Radiation Dose

C. **Late somatic effects.**

Late Tissue Reactions
1. Cataract formation
2. Fibrosis
3. Organ atrophy
4. Loss of parenchymal cells
5. Reduced fertility
6. Sterility

Stochastic Effects
1. Cancer
2. Genetic (hereditary) effects

Exercise 6: Short Answer

1. With reference to ionizing radiation, if a threshold exists between the radiation dose and a biologic response, this means that below a certain radiation level or dose, no biologic effects are observed. Biologic effects are observed only when the threshold level or dose is reached. A nonthreshold relationship means that any radiation dose will produce a biologic effect. No radiation dose is believed to be absolutely safe.

2. Laboratory experiments on animals and data from human populations observed after acute high doses of radiation provided the foundation for a linear threshold curve of radiation dose-response.

3. Epidemiologic studies consist of observation and statistical analysis of data, such as the incidence of disease within groups of people. The latter studies include the risk of radiation-induced cancer. The incident rates at which these irradiation malignancies occur are determined by comparing the natural incidence of cancer occurring in a human population with the incidence of cancer occurring in an irradiated population. Risk factors are then determined for the general human population.

4. To minimize the possibility of genetic effects in those persons engaged in the practice of medical imaging, and in patients, gonadal shielding must be effectively used, and all radiation exposure must be maintained as low as reasonably achievable (ALARA).

5. Using all data available on high radiation exposure, members of the scientific and medical communities have concluded that three categories of health consequences also require study at low dose levels: cancer induction, damage to the unborn from irradiation in utero, and genetic effects.

6. The three major types of late effects are carcinogenesis, cataractogenesis, and embryologic effects (birth defects). Of these, carcinogenesis and embryologic effects are considered stochastic events, and cataractogenesis is regarded as a late tissue reaction.

7. Evidence of human radiation cataractogenesis comes from observation of small groups of people who accidentally received substantial doses to the eyes. These groups include Japanese atomic bomb survivors, nuclear physicists working with cyclotrons between 1932 and 1960, and patients undergoing radiation therapy who received significant exposures to the eyes during treatment.

8. Fetal radiosensitivity decreases as gestation progresses. Hence, during the second and third trimesters of pregnancy when lesser numbers of cells are differentiating, the developing fetus is less sensitive to ionizing radiation exposure. However, even in these later trimesters, congenital abnormalities and functional disorders such as sterility may be caused by radiation exposure. Leukemia also may be induced by exposure to radiation during the second and third trimesters.

9. Mutagens, such as ionizing radiation, can increase the incidence of mutations that occur as part of the natural order of events.

10. Researchers commonly use two models for extrapolation of risk from high-dose to low-dose data. These are the linear and linear-quadratic models.

11. The only evidence that ionizing radiation causes genetic effects comes from extensive experiments with fruit flies and mice at high radiation doses.

12. Point mutations (genetic mutations at the molecular level) may be either dominant (probably expressed in the offspring) or recessive (probably not expressed for several generations). Radiation is thought to cause primarily recessive mutations, if any.

13. Animal studies of radiation-induced hereditary changes have led to the development of the doubling dose concept. This dose measures the effectiveness of ionizing radiation in causing mutations.

14. Gestation in humans is divided into three stages: preimplantation, which corresponds to 0 to 9 days after conception; organogenesis, which corresponds approximately to 10 days to 12 weeks after conception; and the fetal stage, which corresponds to term.

15. Because the miners had no knowledge of the adverse effects of ionizing radiation, they did not promptly change their work clothing on returning home. Because the clothing was contaminated by radioactive material, the miners' immediate families were extremely vulnerable to radiation-induced cancers.

Exercise 7: General Discussion or Opinion Questions

The questions in this exercise are intended to allow students to express their knowledge and understanding of the subject matter covered in this chapter. Because the answers may vary, determination of an answer's acceptability is left to the discretion of the instructor.

POST-TEST

1. Organogenesis
2. Cancer
3. During the embryonic stage of development
4. 8
5. Absolute risk model
6. Late tissue reactions are late effects that can be directly related to the dose the body receives and occur months or years after a high-level radiation exposure.
7. Linear nonthreshold curve
8. C
9. D
10. Risk estimates to predict cancer incidence in a population may be given in terms of absolute risk or relative risk caused by a specific exposure to ionizing radiation (over and above background exposure). Both models forecast the number of excess cancers, or cancers that would not have occurred in the population in question without the exposure to ionizing radiation.
11. The sigmoid, or S-shaped (nonlinear), threshold curve of the radiation dose-response relationship is generally employed in radiation therapy to demonstrate high-dose cellular response to the radiation absorbed doses within specific tissues such as skin, lens of the eye, and various types of blood cells.

12. Mutant genes cannot properly govern the cell's normal chemical reactions or properly control the sequence of amino acids in the formation of specific proteins. These incapacities result in various genetic diseases.
13. Thyroid cancer
14. The term *linear-quadratic* implies that the equation that best fits the data has components that depend on dose to the first power (linear or straightline behavior) and also dose squared (quadratic or curved behavior).
15. Ionizing radiation can induce genetic damage by altering the essential base coding sequence of DNA.
16. Spontaneous mutations
17. greatest
18. With reference to ionizing radiation, the term *threshold* means that below a certain absorbed radiation dose no biologic effects are observed. Biologic effects are observed only when the threshold level, or dose, is reached.
19. 2
20. Thyroid cancer is considered the most pronounced health consequence of the radiation accident at the Chernobyl nuclear power plant.

Chapter 10
Exercise 1: Matching

1. X	6. J	11. C	16. U	21. Y
2. N	7. Q	12. S	17. O	22. F
3. T	8. P	13. M	18. V	23. A
4. G	9. B	14. D	19. E	24. L
5. R	10. I	15. K	20. H	25. W

Exercise 2: Multiple Choice

1. B	6. D	11. C	16. A	21. A
2. D	7. A	12. B	17. C	22. D
3. B	8. A	13. A	18. B	23. D
4. D	9. D	14. C	19. D	24. B
5. A	10. A	15. B	20. D	25. B

Exercise 3: True or False
1. F (The International Commission on Radiologic Protection [ICRP] does not function as an enforcement agency for radiation protection purposes.)
2. T
3. T
4. F (The Nuclear Regulatory Commission [NRC] does not regulate and inspect x-ray imaging facilities.)
5. T
6. F (Health care facilities that provide imaging services do need to have an effective radiation safety program.)
7. T
8. T
9. F (The Center for Devices and Radiologic Health [CDRH] is not responsible for credentialing radiographers; it conducts an ongoing electronic product radiation control program.)
10. T
11. T
12. T
13. F (The Food and Drug Administration [FDA] does not facilitate the development and enforcement of regulations pertaining to the control of radiation in the environment; the Environmental Protection Agency [EPA] does.)
14. T
15. T
16. T
17. F (The embryo-fetus is particularly sensitive to radiation exposure.)
18. F (Effective dose [EfD] limits do not include background radiation or exposure acquired when a worker undergoes medical imaging procedures.)
19. T
20. F (The NRC does require the name of the radiation safety officer [RSO] on a health care facility's radioactive materials license to ensure that licensee management has always identified a responsible, qualified person, who can directly interact with the NRC during inspections and also concerning any inquiries about the facility's program.)
21. T
22. F (The Right-to-Know Act requires employers to evaluate their workplace for hazardous agents and provide training and written information to their employees.)
23. T
24. T
25. T

Exercise 4: Fill in the Blank
1. previous, existing, new
2. dose limits
3. nongovernmental, nonprofit
4. biologic, risk
5. radon
6. radioactive
7. radiation safety
8. dose limits
9. optimization
10. stochastic
11. 1
12. risk
13. random
14. mutations
15. linear, linear-quadratic
16. risk
17. greater
18. 0.4
19. 8, 15
20. cancer, hereditary
21. whole body
22. nonoccupationally
23. same
24. external, internal
25. 50, 10

Exercise 5: Labeling

A. Summary of radiation protection standards organizations.

Organization	Function
1. ICRP	Evaluates information on biologic effects of radiation and provides radiation protection guidance through general recommendations on occupational and public dose limits
2. NCRP	Reviews regulations formulated by the ICRP and decides ways to include those recommendations in U.S. radiation protection criteria
3. UNSCEAR	Evaluates human and environmental ionizing radiation exposure and derives radiation risk assessments from epidemiologic data and research conclusions; provides information to organizations such as the ICRP for evaluation
4. NAS/NRC-BEIR	Reviews studies of biologic effects of ionizing radiation and risk assessment and provides the information to organizations such as the ICRP for evaluation

B. Summary of U.S. regulatory agencies.

Agency	Function
1. NRC	Oversees the nuclear energy industry, enforces radiation protection standards, publishes its rules and regulations in Title 10 of the *U.S. Code of Federal Regulations,* and enters into written agreements with state governments that permit the state to license and regulate the use of radioisotopes and certain other material within that state
2. Agreement states	Enforces radiation protection regulations through their respective health departments
3. EPA	Facilitates the development and enforcement of regulations pertaining to the control of radiation in the environment
4. FDA	Conducts an ongoing product radiation control program, regulating the design and manufacture of electronic products, including x-ray equipment
5. OSHA	Functions as a monitoring agency in places of employment, predominantly in industry

C. Summary of the National Council on Radiation Protection and Measurements (NCRP) recommendations*† (NCRP Report No. 116).

A. Occupational exposures‡
  1. Effective dose limits
    a. Annual   1. 50 mSv
    b. Cumulative   2. 10 mSv × age
  2. Equivalent dose annual limits for tissues and organs
    a. Lens of eye   3. 150 mSv
    b. Localized areas of the skin, hands, and feet   4. 500 mSv
B. Guidance for emergency occupational exposure‡ (see Section 14, NCRP Report No. 116)
C. Public exposures (annual)
  1. Effective dose limit, continuous or frequent exposure‡   5. 1 mSv
  2. Effective dose limit, infrequent exposure‡   6. 5 mSv
  3. Equivalent dose limits for tissues and organs‡
    a. Lens of eye   7. 15 mSv
    b. Localized areas of the skin, hands, and feet   8. 50 mSv
  4. Remedial action for natural sources
    a. Effective dose (excluding radon)   9. >5 mSv
    b. Exposure to radon and its decay products§   10. >26 J/(sm^{-3})‖

> D. Education and training exposures (annual)‡
>   1. Effective dose limit   11. 1 mSv
>   2. Equivalent dose limit for tissues and organs
>   a. Lens of eye   12. 15 mSv
>   b. Localized areas of the skin, hands, and feet   13. 50 mSv
> E. Embryo-fetus exposures‡
>   1. Equivalent dose limit
>   a. Monthly   14. 0.5 mSv
>   b. Entire gestation   15. 5 mSv
> F. Negligible individual dose (annual)‡   16. 0.01 mSv

Exercise 6: Short Answer

1. Exposure of the general public, patients, and radiation workers to ionizing radiation must be limited to minimize the risk of harmful biologic effects. To this end, scientists have developed occupational and nonoccupational effective dose (EfD) limits and equivalent dose (EqD) limits for tissues and organs such as the lens of the eye, skin, hands, and feet.

2. Medical imaging professionals must be familiar with previous, existing, and new guidelines because they share the responsibility for patient safety from radiation exposure and are subject themselves to such exposure in the performance of their duties. By keeping informed, they will be more conscious of good radiation safety practices.

3. Four major organizations that are responsible for evaluating the relationship between radiation equivalent dose (EqD) and induced biologic effects are the International Commission on Radiological Protection (ICRP), the National Council on Radiation Protection and Measurements (NCRP), the United Nations Scientific Committee on the Effects of Atomic Radiation (UNSCEAR), and the National Academy of Sciences/National Research Council Committee on the Biological Effects of Ionizing Radiation (NAS/NRC-BEIR).

4. Five U.S. regulatory agencies are responsible for enforcing radiation protection standards for the protection of the general public, patients, and occupationally exposed personnel: the Nuclear Regulatory Commission (NRC); states that have signed an NRC agreement; the Environmental Protection Agency (EPA); the Food and Drug Administration (FDA); and the Occupational Safety and Health Administration (OSHA).

5. The NRC mandates that a radiation safety committee (RSC) be established for the health care facility. This committee provides guidance for the program and facilitates its ongoing operation.

6. The necessary training and experience for a radiation safety officer (RSO) are described in §10 CFR 35.50 and §10 CFR 35.900 of the *Code of Federal Regulations*. Three training pathways are specified: (1) certification by one of the professional boards approved by the NRC; (2) didactic and work experience as described in detail in the regulations; and (3) identification as an authorized user, authorized medical physicist, or authorized nuclear physicist on the license, with experience in the types of use for which the individual has RSO responsibility.

7. To define *ALARA,* health care facilities usually adopt investigation levels, defined as level I and level II. In the United States these levels traditionally are one-tenth to three-tenths the applicable regulatory limits.

8. In practice, "keep occupational and nonoccupational dose limits ALARA" means keeping EfD and EqD well below maximum allowable levels.

9. Occupational risk associated with radiation exposure may be equated with occupational risk in other industries that are generally considered reasonably safe. The risk generally is estimated to be a 2.5% chance of a fatal accident over an entire career.

10. The Consumer-Patient Radiation Health and Safety Act of 1981 carries no legal penalty for noncompliance; therefore several states simply have not responded with appropriate legislation.

11. The term that has replaced the older terms *nonstochastic* and *deterministic* is *tissue reactions*.

12. In the interest of safety, risk of injury should be overestimated rather than underestimated.

13. The purpose of the Consumer-Patient Radiation Health and Safety Act of 1981 is to ensure that standard medical and dental radiologic practices adhere to rigorous safety precautions and standards.

14. The EPA was established on December 2, 1970, to bring several departments under one organization that would be responsible for protecting the health of humans and for safeguarding the natural environment.

15. Exposure linearity is defined as the ratio of the difference in mR/mAs values between two successive generator stations to the sum of those mR/mAs values. It must be less than 0.1.

Exercise 7: General Discussion or Opinion Questions

The questions in this exercise are intended to allow students to express their knowledge and understanding of the subject matter covered in this chapter. Because the answers may vary, determination of an answer's acceptability is left to the discretion of the instructor.

Exercise 8: Calculation Problems

1. EqD = 10 mSv × Age (in years)
   EqD = 10 mSv × 54
   EqD = 540 mSv
2. EqD = 10 mSv × Age (in years)
   EqD = 10 mSv × 46
   EqD = 460 mSv
3. EqD = 10 mSv × Age (in years)
   EqD = 10 mSv × 33
   EqD = 330 mSv
4. EqD = 10 mSv × Age (in years)
   EqD = 10 mSv × 25
   EqD = 250 mSv
5. EqD = 10 mSv × Age (in years)
   EqD = 10 mSv × 18
   EqD = 180 mSv

POST-TEST

1. Risk to a radiographer from radiation exposure may be equated with occupational risk in other industries that are generally considered to be reasonably safe.
2. national security
3. Occupational Safety and Health Administration (OSHA)
4. The radiation safety officer (RSO)
5. EqD = 10 mSv × Age (in years)
   EqD = 10 mSv × 39
   EqD = 390 mSv
6. Effective dose limit is the upper boundary dose of ionizing radiation that results in a negligible risk of body injury and hereditary damage.
7. Effective dose-limiting system
8. ALARA is the acronym for *as low as reasonably achievable.*
9. B
10. C
11. 0.5 mSv
12. linear nonthreshold
13. The greatest risk for radiation-induced intellectual disability occurs from 8 to 15 weeks after conception.
14. The essential concept underlying radiation protection is that any organ in the human body is vulnerable to damage from exposure to ionizing radiation.
15. The NCRP now recommends an equivalent dose limit of 5 mSv during the entire period of gestation after declaration of pregnancy.
16. 50 mSv
17. Tissue weighting factors are significant because various tissues and organs do not have the same degree of sensitivity.
18. effective
19. Radiation hormesis is a beneficial aspect or result to groups of individuals from continuing exposure to small amounts of radiation.

20. Internal action limits are established by health care facilities to trigger an investigation to uncover the reasons for any abnormal exposures received by individual staff members.

Chapter 11
Exercise 1: Matching

1. N	6. O	11. U	16. A	21. V
2. I	7. Y	12. C	17. T	22. D
3. L	8. F	13. S	18. G	23. X
4. J	9. P	14. H	19. Q	24. B
5. K	10. E	15. W	20. M	25. R

Exercise 2: Multiple Choice

1. D	6. A	11. B	16. D	21. A
2. B	7. A	12. C	17. A	22. B
3. A	8. D	13. C	18. B	23. B
4. A	9. D	14. A	19. C	24. A
5. C	10. A	15. B	20. C	25. D

Exercise 3: True or False

1. T
2. F (During a routine radiographic examination, the radiographer must ensure that collimation is adequate by collimating the radiographic beam so that it is no larger than the size of the image receptor being used for the examination.)
3. F (Radiographic cones are earlier x-ray beam limitation devices.)
4. T
5. F (Inherent filtration in an x-ray tube used for routine radiography amounts to 0.5-mm aluminum equivalent.)
6. T
7. F (Every radiographic x-ray tube must have a device in place to ensure accurate beam alignment.)
8. F (Because filtration absorbs some of the photons in a radiographic beam, it decreases the overall intensity of the incident radiation.)
9. T
10. T
11. F (Europium-activated barium fluorohalide is the most commonly used photostimulable phosphor in computed radiography imaging plates.)
12. T
13. F (In standard image intensification fluoroscopy, an x-ray beam half-value layer [HVL] of 3- to 4.5-mm aluminum is considered acceptable when kVp ranges from 80 to 100.)
14. F (The patient dose increases as grid ratio increases.)
15. F (It is not acceptable to overexpose a patient initially to avoid the possibility of a repeat examination.)
16. F (In computed radiography [CR] imaging the practice of overexposing patients to possibly avoid repeat radiographic exposures is unethical and unacceptable.)
17. T

18. T
19. T
20. F (The coincidence requirements between the radiographic beam and the localizing light are known as *alignment* and *congruence*.)
21. T
22. F (The effective metric equivalent of 40 inches is 100 cm.)
23. F (A primary protective barrier of 2-mm lead equivalent is required for a fluoroscopic unit.)
24. T
25. T

Exercise 4: Fill in the Blank

1. manufacturers, federal
2. limitation
3. under
4. dead-man, incapacitated
5. decreases
6. latitude, less
7. center
8. Technique
9. wedge
10. electronic
11. same
12. distance
13. image matrix
14. mAs
15. quality
16. collimator
17. filtration
18. Resolution
19. brightness
20. Fluoroscopy
21. mispositioning
22. dose reduction
23. multifield
24. entrance, exit
25. energized

Exercise 5: Labeling

A. **X-ray tube, collimator, and image receptor.**

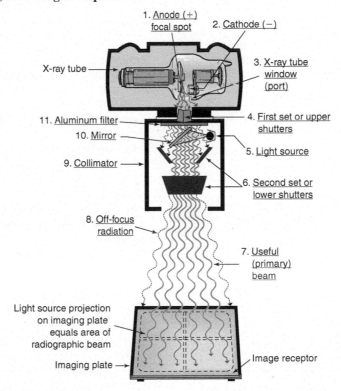

1. Anode (+) focal spot
2. Cathode (−)
3. X-ray tube window (port)
4. First set or upper shutters
5. Light source
6. Second set or lower shutters
7. Useful (primary) beam
8. Off-focus radiation
9. Collimator
10. Mirror
11. Aluminum filter

X-ray tube

Light source projection on imaging plate equals area of radiographic beam

Imaging plate

Image receptor

B. **Image intensification fluoroscopic unit.**

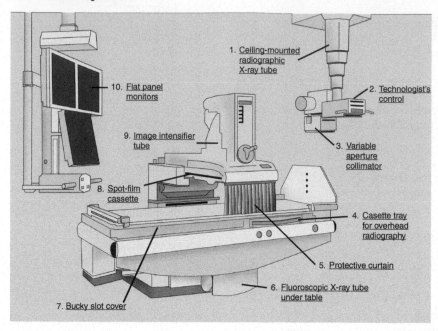

1. Ceiling-mounted radiographic X-ray tube
2. Technologist's control
3. Variable aperture collimator
4. Casette tray for overhead radiography
5. Protective curtain
6. Fluoroscopic X-ray tube under table
7. Bucky slot cover
8. Spot-film cassette
9. Image intensifier tube
10. Flat panel monitors

From Bushong SC: *Radiologic science for technologists: physics, biology and protection*, ed 10, St. Louis, 2013, Elsevier.

C. **HVL required by the Radiation Control for Health and Safety Act of 1968 and detailed by the Bureau of Radiological Health* in 1980.**

Peak Kilovoltage	Minimum Required HVL in Millimeters of Aluminum
30	1. 0.3
40	2. 0.4
50	3. 1.2
60	4. 1.3
70	5. 1.5
80	6. 2.3
90	7. 2.5
100	8. 2.7
110	9. 3.0
120	10. 3.2

*The Bureau of Radiological Health changed its name to the Center for Devices and Radiological Health in 1982.

Exercise 6: Short Answer

1. If adequate filtration were not present, very-low-energy photons (20 keV or less) would enter the patient and be almost totally absorbed in the body, thus increasing the patient's radiation dose, especially near or at the surface, but contributing nothing to the image process.
2. The first set of shutters in the collimator, the set of upper shutters, is mounted as close as possible to the x-ray tube window to reduce the amount of x-rays emitted from parts of the tube other than the focal spot, coming from the primary beam and exiting at various angles from the x-ray tube window. This off-focus radiation can never be completely eliminated because the metal shutters cannot be placed immediately beneath the actual focal spot of the x-ray tube. However, by placing the first set, or upper shutters, as close as possible to the tube window, this off-focus radiation can be reduced significantly, thereby decreasing the patient's exposure.
3. In general diagnostic radiology, aluminum (atomic number 13) is the metal most widely selected as a filter material because it effectively removes low-energy (soft) x-rays from a polyenergetic (heterogeneous) x-ray beam without severely decreasing the x-ray beam intensity. In addition, aluminum is lightweight, sturdy, relatively inexpensive, and readily available.
4. Because HVL is a measure of beam quality, or effective energy of the x-ray beam, a certain minimal HVL is required at a given kVp.
5. Either each image should be monitored by an independent quality control technologist at a separate monitor or a quality control system should be used whereby for each technologist the number of images per examination is compared with the number ordered.
6. The purpose of a protective x-ray tube housing is to keep radiation leakage from getting through any portion of the housing; serve as a shield against the high voltage entering the x-ray tube, thereby preventing electric shock; and facilitate cooling of the x-ray tube.
7. Inherent filtration includes the glass envelope encasing the x-ray tube, the insulating oil surrounding the tube, and the glass window in the x-ray tube housing.

8. Two reasons for high radiation exposure to personnel during interventional procedures that are performed by a nonradiologist physician are (1) operating the fluoroscopic tube for longer periods in continuous mode in place of pulsed mode; and (2) failure to use the protective curtain, or floating shields, on the stationary fluoroscopic equipment's image intensifier as a means of protection.

9. The Food and Drug Administration (FDA) has recommended that a notation be placed in the patient's record if skin dose in the range of 1 to 2 Gy_t is received.

10. The use of a pulsed progressive system for digital fluoroscopy results in decreased patient dose.

11. Because filtration absorbs some of the photons in the radiographic beam, it decreases the overall intensity (amount or quantity) of incident radiation. The remaining photons, however, are as a whole more penetrating and therefore less likely to be absorbed in body tissue.

12. Added filtration is located outside the glass window of the x-ray tube housing, above the collimator shutters.

13. The housing enclosing the x-ray tube must be constructed so that the leakage radiation measured at a distance of 1 m from the x-ray source does not exceed 1 mGy_a/hr (100 mR/hr) when the tube is operated at its highest voltage at the highest current that allows continuous operation.

14. The control panel must be located behind a suitable protective barrier that has a radiation-absorbent window that permits observation of the patient during any procedure.

15. The thickness of a radiographic examination tabletop must be uniform, and for under-table x-ray tubes as used in fluoroscopy, the patient support surface also should be as radiolucent as possible, thereby reducing the patient's radiation dose.

16. It is also known as a *trough filter.*

17. Eleven procedures involving extended fluoroscopic time are (1) percutaneous transluminal angioplasty, (2) radiofrequency cardiac catheter ablation, (3) vascular embolization, (4) stent and filter placement, (5) thrombolytic and fibrinolytic procedures, (6) percutaneous transhepatic cholangiography, (7) endoscopic retrograde cholangiopancreatography, (8) transjugular intrahepatic portosystemic shunt, (9) percutaneous nephrostomy, (10) biliary drainage, and (11) urinary or biliary stone removal.

18. The resettable cumulative timing device on fluoroscopic equipment measures the x-ray beam-on time and sounds an audible alarm or in some cases temporarily interrupts the exposure after the fluoroscope has been activated for 5 minutes. It serves to make the radiologist aware of how long the patient has been receiving x-ray exposure for each fluoroscopic examination.

19. For dose reduction purposes, whenever possible, it is best to position the C-arm so that the x-ray tube is under the patient. Scatter radiation is less intense with the x-ray tube in this position. When the tube is positioned over the patient, scatter radiation becomes more intense and the patient dose increases accordingly.

20. Scattered radiation is all the radiation that arises from the interaction of an x-ray beam with the atoms of a patient or any other object in the path of the beam.

Exercise 7: General Discussion or Opinion Questions

The questions in this exercise are intended to allow students to express their knowledge and understanding of the subject matter covered in this chapter. Because the answers may vary, determination of an answer's acceptability is left to the discretion of the instructor.

POST-TEST

1. HVL is defined as the thickness of a designated absorber (customarily a metal such as aluminum) required to decrease the intensity of the primary beam by 50% of its initial value.
2. Carbon fiber
3. protective, control
4. Light-localizing variable-aperture rectangular collimator
5. Scattered radiation is all the radiation that arises from the interaction of an x-ray beam with the atoms of a patient or any object in the path of the beam.
6. Use of a radiographic grid results in an increase in the patient dose.
7. digital, image matrix
8. D
9. B
10. integral dose
11. Positive beam limitation (PBL), size
12. Interventional
13. source–to–skin distance (SSD), exposure
14. The radiologist should use the practice of pulsed, or intermittent, fluoroscopy to reduce the overall length of exposure.
15. D
16. Patient–image intensifier distance should be as short as possible.
17. pixels
18. Radiographic equipment must have a source–to–image receptor distance (SID) indicator.
19. D
20. unethical, unacceptable

Chapter 12
Exercise 1: Matching

1. N	6. O	11. X	16. A	21. V
2. J	7. W	12. D	17. U	22. R
3. L	8. K	13. S	18. C	23. I
4. Y	9. P	14. H	19. Q	24. B
5. M	10. E	15. G	20. F	25. T

Exercise 2: Multiple Choice

1. D	6. A	11. D	16. B	21. B
2. B	7. D	12. D	17. D	22. A
3. B	8. D	13. D	18. A	23. C
4. A	9. D	14. A	19. C	24. C
5. C	10. A	15. C	20. D	25. D

Exercise 3: True or False

1. T
2. F (Patients do need to be given the opportunity to ask questions before any radiation procedure.)
3. F (Shadow shields are suspended from above the radiographic beam-defining system.)
4. T
5. F (An air gap technique removes scatter radiation by using an increased object–to–image receptor distance.)
6. T
7. F (During a diagnostic radiographic examination, the lens of the eye, breasts, thyroid gland, and reproductive organs do need to be selectively shielded.)
8. F (Primary beam exposure for male patients may be reduced as much as 90% to 95% when covered with a contact shield containing 1 mm lead.)
9. T
10. T
11. F (Use of higher kVp and lower mAs reduces patient exposure.)
12. T
13. F (A gonadal shield should be a secondary protective measure, not a substitute for an adequately collimated beam.)
14. F (The entrance skin exposure [ESE] dose levels set in regulations cannot be exceeded.)
15. F (When performing any radiographic procedure, it is not an acceptable practice to overexpose a patient initially. This is an unethical and unacceptable practice.)
16. F (The radiation dose to the breast of a young patient may be further reduced by performing the scoliosis examination with the x-ray beam entering the posterior surface of the patient's body instead of the anterior surface.)
17. T
18. T
19. T
20. F (If a patient moves during a radiographic exposure, the radiographic image will be blurred, resulting in a repeat examination and an increase in patient dose. Proper body or body part immobilization and the use of motion reduction techniques can eliminate or at least minimize patient motion, resulting in a better quality image. Therefore adequate immobilization is of significant value and is necessary.)
21. T
22. F (Motion controlled by a patient's will is classified as voluntary motion.)
23. F (Every imaging department should establish a written shielding protocol for each of its radiologic procedures. Ultimately, this practice reduces the cumulative population gonad dose.)
24. T
25. T

Exercise 4: Fill in the Blank

1. reduction, protective, minimize
2. Holistic, effective
3. cooperate
4. poor
5. reproductive
6. female, male
7. reduces
8. symphysis pubis
9. remote, over
10. beam-defining
11. milliampere-seconds
12. compromised
13. protocol
14. clinical interest
15. 0.20
16. smaller
17. primary
18. minimal
19. 50
20. additional
21. less
22. mean marrow
23. leukemia
24. benefits, risks
25. pregnancy, menstrual period

Exercise 5: Labeling

A. **Technical exposure factor considerations.**

1. Mass per unit volume of tissue of the area of clinical interest
2. Effective atomic numbers and electron densities of the tissues involved
3. Type of image receptor
4. Source–to–image receptor distance (SID)
5. Type and quantity of filtration employed
6. Type of x-ray generator used
7. Balance of radiographic brightness and contrast required

B. **Lead filter with breast and gonad shielding device.**

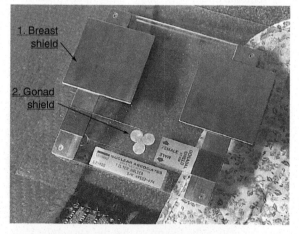

Courtesy Fluke Biomedical. Everett, WA.

C. **Reasons for unacceptable images.**
1. Patient mispositioning
2. Incorrect centering of the radiographic beam
3. Patient motion during the radiographic exposure
4. Incorrect collimation of the radiographic beam
5. Presence of external foreign bodies
6. Postprocessing artifacts

Exercise 6: Short Answer

1. During a diagnostic x-ray procedure, radiographers must limit the patient's exposure to ionizing radiation by employing appropriate radiation reduction techniques and by using protective devices that minimize radiation exposure. Patient exposure can be substantially reduced by using proper body or part immobilization, motion reduction techniques, appropriate beam limitation devices, adequate filtration of the x-ray beam, and gonadal or other specific area shielding. Selection of suitable technical exposure factors used in conjunction with computer-generated digital images, use of appropriate digital image processing, and the elimination of repeat radiographic exposures can also contribute significantly to limiting patient exposure.

2. The radiographer must achieve a balance in technical radiographic exposure factors to ensure the presence of adequate information in the recorded image and minimize patient dose.

3. The four basic types of gonadal shielding devices that can be used during a diagnostic x-ray procedure are flat contact shields, shadow shields, shaped contact shields, and clear lead shields.

4. To minimize or possibly eliminate patient motion, the radiographer must employ very short exposure times by selecting a high-mA station and also make use of effective immobilization techniques.

5. Protective shielding is a structure or device made of certain materials (e.g., concrete, lead, or lead-impregnated material) that will adequately attenuate ionizing radiation.

6. To perform an air gap technique, the image receptor is placed 10 to 15 cm (4 to 6 inches) from the patient and the x-ray tube is placed approximately 300 to 366 cm (10 to 12 feet) away from the image receptor. The scattered x-rays from the patient are disseminated in many directions at acute angles to the primary beam when the radiographic exposure is made. Because of the increased distance between the anatomic structures being imaged and the image receptor, a higher percentage of the scattered x-rays produced is then less likely to strike the image receptor. This air gap method effectively produces an adequate grid-type scatter cleanup effect. In general, the use of an air gap technique requires the selection of technical exposure factors that are comparable to those used with an 8:1 ratio grid. Therefore, when patient dose is compared with a nongrid technique, it is higher, but compared with the patient dose resulting from the use of a midratio grid (8:1), the dose from an air gap technique is about the same.

7. Before ordering a radiologic examination, the referring physician must determine whether the benefit to the patient in terms of medical information gained sufficiently justifies subjecting the patient to the risk of the absorbed radiation resulting from the procedure.

8. An accurate determination of a patient's skin, or surface, dose can be made with a thermoluminescent dosimeter (TLD) because the sensing material in the TLD responds in a manner similar to human tissue when exposed to ionizing radiation.

9. Three ways to specify the amount of radiation a patient receives from a diagnostic imaging procedure are entrance skin exposure (ESE) (includes skin and glandular), bone marrow dose, and gonadal dose.

10. The selection of scientifically correct technical exposure factors for each examination ensures patients a useful diagnostic image with minimal patient dose.

11. Members in a population who cannot bear children (e.g., those who are beyond reproductive years) have no genetic impact and would not be included in genetically significant dose considerations.

12. It is strongly recommended that the result of a pregnancy test be obtained before the pelvis is irradiated.

13. Four types of gonadal shielding devices that can be used during diagnostic procedures are flat contact shields, shadow shields, shaped contact shields, and clear lead shields.

14. This creates a sense of trust between the patient and the radiographer and encourages further communication.

15. Six x-ray procedures now considered nonessential are (1) a chest x-ray examination automatically scheduled on admission to the hospital; (2) a chest x-ray examination as part of a preemployment physical; (3) a lumbar spine examination as part of a preemployment physical; (4) chest x-ray studies or other unjustified x-ray examinations as part of a routine health checkup; (5) a chest x-ray examination for mass screening for tuberculosis; and (6) a whole-body computed tomography (CT) screening.

16. A clear lead shield contains approximately 30% lead by weight.

17. A contact type shield is always used for the lens of the eye and positioned directly on the patient.

18. Protection of the reproductive organs is of particular concern in diagnostic radiology because genetic effects may result from exposure to ionizing radiation.

19. $0.50 \times 0.6 = 0.3 \text{ mGy}_t$

20. A small, relatively thin pack of TLDs is secured to the patient's skin in the middle of the clinical area of interest and exposed during a radiographic procedure. Because lithium fluoride (LiF), the sensing material in the TLD, responds in a manner similar to human tissue when exposed to ionizing radiation, an accurate determination of surface dose can be made.

227

Exercise 7: General Discussion or Opinion Questions

The questions in this exercise are intended to allow students to express their knowledge and understanding of the subject matter covered in this chapter. Because the answers may vary, determination of an answer's acceptability is left to the discretion of the instructor.

POST-TEST

1. Radiographers and imaging facilities can "pledge" to Image Gently and then follow through by fulfilling the pledge in the clinical setting of their own imaging departments.
2. F. B. Reynold stated the official position of the American College of Radiology at a press conference on October 20, 1976: "Abdominal radiologic examinations that have been requested after full consideration of the clinical status of a patient, including the possibility of pregnancy, need not be postponed or selectively scheduled."
3. double dose
4. Patients with the potential to reproduce should have gonadal protection during x-ray procedures whenever the diagnostic value of the examination is not compromised.
5. The genetically significant dose (GSD) is the equivalent dose to the reproductive organs that, if received by every human, would be expected to bring about an identical gross genetic injury to the total population, as does the sum of the actual doses received by exposed individual members of the population.
6. To safeguard the ovaries of a female patient, the ovarian shield should be placed approximately 2.5 cm (1 inch) medial to each palpable anterior superior iliac spine.
7. Fluoroscopically guided positioning (FGP) is viewed as an unacceptable and unethical practice by the American Society of Radiologic Technologists (ASRT).
8. D
9. D
10. collimated
11. posterior, anterior
12. The referring physician
13. 50
14. About 0.20 millisievert (mSv)
15. D
16. A calculated estimate of the approximate equivalent dose to the embryo-fetus as a result of the examination should be obtained.
17. three
18. The symphysis pubis can be used to guide shield placement over the testes.
19. B
20. Adequately collimating the x-ray beam to include only the clinical area of interest should always be the first step for the radiographer to provide gonadal protection for patients.

Chapter 13

Exercise 1: Matching

1. U	6. Y	11. Q	16. H	21. J
2. F	7. V	12. W	17. K	22. L
3. S	8. M	13. C	18. I	23. X
4. O	9. G	14. D	19. P	24. R
5. T	10. A	15. E	20. N	25. B

Exercise 2: Multiple Choice

1. C	6. D	11. A	16. A	21. D
2. A	7. B	12. C	17. D	22. B
3. B	8. C	13. B	18. A	23. C
4. D	9. D	14. C	19. B	24. A
5. A	10. A	15. C	20. C	25. D

Exercise 3: True or False

1. F (The *A* stands for *axial*.)
2. T
3. F (Dose throughout a computed tomography [CT] slice is more uniform than it is for an area imaged in radiography.)
4. T
5. F (Contact shields are generally not recommended for CT because, if contact shields were in the field of view, automatic exposure control [AEC] would then adjust the dose inappropriately. Angular AEC can be used for dose sparing on some scanners. Dose to regions outside the field of view do not receive significant amounts of scatter.)
6. T
7. F (Pitch equals CT dose index volume [$CTDI_{VOL}$] times dose length product [DLP].)
8. F (Angular tube current modulation [TCM] or AEC may be used to lower patient dose on one side of the patient.)
9. F (Contact shields of any kind are generally not recommended for CT because, if contact shields were in the field of view, AEC would then adjust dose inappropriately. Angular AEC can be used for dose sparing on some scanners. Dose to regions outside of the field of view do not receive significant amounts of scatter.)
10. T
11. T
12. T
13. F (If the patient is placed closer to the x-ray tube when the scout view [radiographic] image is obtained, then the image of the patient is magnified, causing the TCM system or AEC to increase the tube current, thereby overdosing the patient.)
14. T
15. F (The factors that convert DLP to effective dose are scan-region dependent. Different factors are used when different body parts are in the field of view.)
16. T
17. F ($CTDI_{VOL}$ is equal to weighted CTDI [$CTDI_W$] divided by the pitch.)

18. T
19. T
20. T
21. F (The increased density of the breasts of younger women tends to reduce radiographic contrast, and therefore conventional screen-film mammography is often less sensitive in the average younger woman than in the average older woman. Studies that look at populations of women who began screening decades ago reflect this difference. Modern digital mammography units, however, which can enhance contrast with image gray-level manipulation, offer substantial improvement for patients with dense breasts.)
22. F (Digital tomosynthesis systems allow the same views as conventional systems at comparable doses; in addition, they can provide three-dimensional information about the breast.)
23. F (Mammography x-ray tubes use targets that emit a range of photon energies up to the maximum kVp used.)
24. F (Beryllium takes the place of glass in the window of the low kVp mammographic unit)
25. T

Exercise 4: Fill in the Blank

1. spiral, or helical
2. greater than
3. collimated
4. overlap of margins, interslice scatter
5. internal
6. pitch
7. "scout view" or "radiographic mode"
8. tube current modulation
9. automatic exposure control
10. filtered
11. iterative
12. dose
13. effective
14. acrylic
15. 16, 32
16. Dose length product
17. low
18. best, an acceptable
19. yearly
20. false-positive
21. dense
22. 40, 49
23. craniocaudal, mediolateral
24. tungsten, molybdenum, rhodium
25. rhodium, silver

Exercise 5: Labeling

A. **List four dose reduction methods that lead to optimization of patient dose in CT.**

1. Tube current modulation (longitudinal, angular)
2. Iterative reconstruction
3. Optimization of tube voltage and other scan parameters
4. Correct patient centering

B. **Fill in the typical effective dose values for the CT examinations listed in the following table.**

Examination	Effective dose (mSv)
Head	1-2
Chest	2-6
Abdomen	5-8
Pelvis	3-6
Coronary artery calcification	0.1-3
Coronary angiography	1-18

Exercise 6: Short Answer

1. Two concerns related to patient dose in CT scanning are skin dose and dose distribution.
2. The use of multiple views from many angles reduces the need for any one view to acquire enough x-ray exposure to achieve an acceptable image.
3. A small overlap of the margins of the x-ray beam occurs when each tomographic section is made. When a series of adjacent slices is obtained, some radiation will also scatter from the slice being made into the adjacent slices.
4. Because of the rotational nature of the exposure, a shield is no more effective than the collimators that already exist on the device.
5. The greater the pitch, the lower the patient dose.
6. Tube current modulation or automatic exposure control.
7. Two methods for image reconstruction in CT are filtered back projection and iterative reconstruction.
8. Patient dose increases.
9. Four CT dose parameters are CT dose index (CTDI), $CTDI_W$, $CTDI_{VOL}$, and dose length product (DLP).
10. Scan region–specific conversion factor.
11. The maximum allowed dose for Food and Drug Administration (FDA)–approved screening mammography is 3 mGy.
12. The technique that allows the radiologist to get a three-dimensional view of the breast is digital tomosynthesis.
13. Craniocaudal and mediolateral projections of the breast are typically used for screening mammography to maintain acceptable low radiation dose.
14. Target materials other than tungsten are sometimes used in mammography to make use of their energy characteristic x-ray emissions.
15. Rhenium is used as a filter for most breasts, and silver is used as a filter for thicker breasts when tungsten targets are used for digital mammography.

Exercise 7: General Discussion or Opinion Questions

The questions in this exercise are intended to allow students to express their knowledge and understanding of the subject matter covered in this chapter. Because the answers may vary, determination of an answer's acceptability is left to the discretion of the instructor.

229

POST-TEST

1. more
2. C
3. A
4. couch increment
5. B
6. D
7. tube current compensation
8. Angular-based
9. filtered, iterative
10. increases
11. greater
12. A
13. data channels
14. dose length product
15. 50
16. dose length product
17. 4.5
18. D
19. tungsten
20. B

Chapter 14
Exercise 1: Matching

1. C	6. U	11. J	16. V	21. E
2. P	7. I	12. T	17. B	22. Y
3. F	8. O	13. A	18. N	23. H
4. S	9. Q	14. G	19. X	24. D
5. K	10. L	15. R	20. M	25. W

Exercise 2: Multiple Choice

1. A	6. D	11. C	16. D	21. D
2. D	7. D	12. D	17. C	22. D
3. D	8. D	13. C	18. D	23. A
4. D	9. A	14. B	19. C	24. A
5. B	10. B	15. D	20. D	25. D

Exercise 3: True or False

1. T
2. F (Personal medical and natural background radiation exposures are not included in a radiographer's annual occupational effective dose [EfD].)
3. T
4. T
5. F (The intensity of radiation is inversely proportional to the square of the distance from the source.)
6. F (Radiographic and fluoroscopic exposures should only be made when room doors are closed.)
7. F (If the peak energy of an x-ray beam is 100 kVp, a protective lead [Pb] apron must be equivalent to at least 0.25-mm thickness of lead.)
8. T
9. F (The Bucky slot shielding device protects the radiologist and radiographer at the gonadal level.)
10. T
11. F (The physical configuration of the C-arm fluoroscopic unit limits the methods that the operator can use to achieve protection from scattered radiation.)
12. T

13. F (A radiographer should never stand in the useful beam to restrain a patient during a radiographic exposure.)
14. T
15. T
16. F (Filtration primarily benefits the patient.)
17. F (During a diagnostic x-ray procedure, the patient becomes a source of scattered radiation as a consequence of the Compton scattering process.)
18. T
19. T
20. F (Diagnostic imaging department staff members who are pregnant should be able to continue performing their duties without interruption of employment, if they follow established radiation safety practices.)
21. F (The amount of radiation a worker receives at a particular location is directly proportional to the length of time the individual is exposed to ionizing radiation.)
22. T
23. T
24. T
25. F (During fluoroscopic examinations, the radiographer should always wear a protective apron when he or she is in the x-ray room during a procedure.)

Exercise 4: Fill in the Blank

1. equivalent dose
2. Scattered
3. safety
4. safety, embryo-fetus
5. direct
6. Shortening
7. distance
8. shielding
9. aprons, gloves, thyroid shields
10. housing, high-tension
11. Compton scatter, Compton scatter
12. 0.5 mSv, 5.0 mSv
13. 0.5 mm lead, 1.0 mm lead
14. time, distance, shielding
15. four, 4
16. perpendicular
17. 1.6 mm lead, 2.1 meters
18. 0.8 mm lead
19. 0.5 mm lead
20. scattered, patient, assistance
21. 0.25 mm lead
22. magnify
23. wraparound
24. right angles, 90, least
25. routine

Exercise 5: Labeling
A. **Relationship between distance and intensity.**
   1. $^1/_4$ intensity
   2. $^1/_9$ intensity
   3. $^1/_{16}$ intensity

B. Protective barriers.

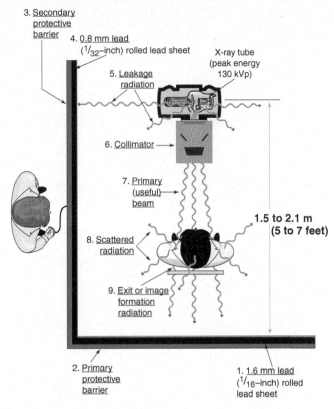

3. Secondary protective barrier
4. 0.8 mm lead ($^1/_{32}$–inch) rolled lead sheet
X-ray tube (peak energy 130 kVp)
5. Leakage radiation
6. Collimator
7. Primary (useful) beam
1.5 to 2.1 m (5 to 7 feet)
8. Scattered radiation
9. Exit or image formation radiation
2. Primary protective barrier
1. 1.6 mm lead ($^1/_{16}$–inch) rolled lead sheet

C. Standing at right angles to the scattering object.

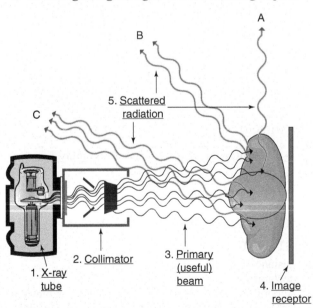

A
B
C
5. Scattered radiation
2. Collimator
1. X-ray tube
3. Primary (useful) beam
4. Image receptor

Exercise 6: Short Answer

1. The annual limit for occupational personnel only includes occupational dose. It does not include personal medical exposure that an employee may receive or background exposure that all people receive.
2. Lead aprons are designed to provide protection from secondary (leakage and scatter) radiation.

3. Radiation warning signs are required to be magenta or purple or black on a yellow background.
4. Most health care facilities have policies for protecting pregnant personnel from radiation. Under these policies, an imaging professional who becomes pregnant first informs her supervisor. After this voluntary "declaration" has been made, the health care facility officially recognizes the pregnancy. The facility, through its radiation safety officer, provides essential counseling and furnishes an appropriate additional monitor that should be worn at waist level during all radiation procedures.
5. The three basic principles of radiation protection are time, distance, and shielding.
6. A qualified medical physicist should determine the exact protection requirements for a particular imaging facility.
7. Protective aprons, gloves, and thyroid shields are made of lead-impregnated vinyl.
8. Diagnostic imaging personnel can substantially reduce scatter radiation to the lens of the eye by wearing protective eyeglasses with optically clear lenses that contain a minimal lead equivalent protection of 0.35 mm. Side shields on the glasses are also available for procedures that require turning of the head. A wraparound frame containing optically clear lenses with a 0.5-mm lead equivalency is also available.
9. A lead-lined, metal, diagnostic-type protective tube housing protects both the radiographer and the patient from off-focus, or leakage, radiation by restricting the emission of x-rays to the area of the useful, or primary, beam.
10. Remote control fluoroscopic systems provide the best radiation protection for imaging personnel. These systems permit the radiologist and assisting radiographer to remain outside the fluoroscopy room at a control console located behind a protective barrier until needed. This increases imaging personnel safety because distance is used as a means of increased protection. With remote equipment, the radiologist and assisting radiographer can view the patient directly through clear protective shielding and will enter the x-ray room only when absolutely necessary to provide essential patient care or perform procedural functions.
11. Positioning of a C-arm fluoroscope with the x-ray tube over the table and the image intensifier underneath the table results in higher patient exposure and increased scatter radiation. As scatter increases, radiation exposure of all personnel in the immediate vicinity of the C-arm also increases. Therefore from the perspective of increased radiation safety, it is best to reverse the C-arm to place the x-ray tube under the table and the image intensifier over the table.
12. Exposure of personnel is caused by scatter radiation from the patient. During operating room procedures in which cross-table exposures are made with a mobile C-arm fluoroscope, an understanding of the patterns of x-ray scatter is particularly useful. The exposure rate caused by scatter near the entrance surface of the

231

patient (the x-ray tube side) exceeds the exposure rate caused by scatter near the exit surface of the patient (the image intensifier side). The difference in the amount of scatter, typically a factor of 2 or 3, is caused by the higher radiation intensity at the entrance surface of the patient. Thus the location of the lower potential scatter dose is on the side of the patient away from the x-ray tube (i.e., the image intensifier side).

13. The radiologist or other interventional physician can reduce radiation exposure during a high-level-control interventional procedure by the following means: decreasing the duration of the procedure, thereby reducing fluoroscopic beam-on time; taking fewer digital images; reducing the use of continuous fluoroscopic mode in relation to pulsed mode of operation; retaining the protective curtain, if available, on the image intensifier or keeping the scatter shield in place during a procedure; and regularly using the last-image-hold feature to view the most recent fluoroscopic image. These practices will substantially decrease exposure not only to all participating personnel but to the patient as well.

14. Because the hands and forearms of physicians performing interventional procedures can be subject to large radiation exposures if the safety protocol is not carefully followed—and sometimes this may not be possible—it is important that extremities be monitored. Physicians need to be aware of the recommended dose limits that have been established for the extremities. The National Council on Radiation Protection and Measurements (NCRP) currently recommends an annual equivalent dose limit to localized areas of the skin and hands of 500 mSv. To avoid even remotely approaching this quite large limit and consequently increasing the possibility of future adverse effects, protective gloves should be worn whenever feasible by any physician whose hands will, of necessity, often be close to the fluoroscopic beam.

15. Eight radiation-absorbent barrier design considerations are (1) the mean energy of the x-ray beam that will strike the barrier, (2) whether the barrier is of a primary or secondary nature, (3) the distance from the x-ray source to a position of occupancy 0.3 m from the barrier, (4) the workload of the unit, (5) the use factor of the unit, (6) the occupancy factor behind the barrier, (7) the intrinsic shielding (e.g., tube housing attenuation) of the x-ray unit, and (8) whether the area beyond the barrier is controlled or uncontrolled.

Exercise 7: General Discussion or Opinion Questions

The questions in this exercise are intended to allow students to express their knowledge and understanding of the subject matter covered in this chapter. Because the answers may vary, determination of an answer's acceptability is left to the discretion of the instructor.

Exercise 8: Calculation Problems

1. $\dfrac{I_1}{I_2} = \dfrac{(d_2)^2}{(d_1)^2}$

$\dfrac{9}{I_2} = \dfrac{(6)^2}{(3)^2}$

$\dfrac{9}{I_2} = \dfrac{36}{9}$ (cross-multiply)

$36 I_2 = 81$

$I_2 = 2.25$ mGY$_a$/hr

2. $\dfrac{I_1}{I_2} = \dfrac{(d_2)^2}{(d_1)^2}$

$\dfrac{5}{I_2} = \dfrac{(4)^2}{(2)^2}$

$\dfrac{5}{I_2} = \dfrac{16}{4}$ (cross-multiply)

$16 I_2 = 20$

$I_2 = 1.25$ mGY$_a$/hr

3. $\dfrac{I_1}{I_2} = \dfrac{(d_2)^2}{(d_1)^2}$

$\dfrac{4}{I_2} = \dfrac{(10)^2}{(5)^2}$

$\dfrac{4}{I_2} = \dfrac{100}{25}$ (cross-multiply)

$100 I_2 = 100$

$I_2 = 1$ mGy$_a$/hr

4. $\dfrac{I_1}{I_2} = \dfrac{(d_2)^2}{(d_1)^2}$

$\dfrac{7}{I_2} = \dfrac{(2)^2}{(1)^2}$

$\dfrac{7}{I_2} = \dfrac{4}{1}$ (cross-multiply)

$4 I_2 = 7$

$I_2 = 1.75$ mGy$_a$/hr

5. $\dfrac{I_1}{I_2} = \dfrac{(d_2)^2}{(d_1)^2}$

$\dfrac{6}{I_2} = \dfrac{(12)^2}{(6)^2}$

$\dfrac{6}{I_2} = \dfrac{144}{36}$ (cross-multiply)

$144 I_2 = 216$

$I_2 = 1.5$ mGy$_a$/hr

6. $\dfrac{I_1}{I_2} = \dfrac{(d_2)^2}{(d_1)^2}$

$\dfrac{6}{I_2} = \dfrac{(6)^2}{(2)^2}$

$\dfrac{6}{I_2} = \dfrac{36}{24}$ (cross-multiply)

$36 I_2 = 24$

$I_2 = 0.666$ mGy$_a$/hr

7. $(10/5)^2$ $10 \div 5 = 2$ $2 \times 2 = 4$
8. $(12/4)^2$ $12 \div 4 = 3$ $3 \times 3 = 9$
9. $(4/1)^2$ $4 \div 1 = 4$ $4 \times 4 = 16$
10. $(8/2)^2$ $8 \div 2 = 4$ $4 \times 4 = 16$

POST-TEST

1. Distance
2. declaration
3. According to as low as reasonably achievable (ALARA) guidelines, radiographers' work schedules should be designed to distribute radiation exposure risk evenly to all employees.
4. Scattered radiation

5. gonadal
6. "The intensity of radiation is inversely proportional to the square of the distance from the source."
7. restrain
8. Time, distance, and shielding
9. D
10. B
11. B
12. records
13. thickness
14. scattered
15. $\dfrac{I_1}{I_2} = \dfrac{(d_2)^2}{(d_1)^2}$

   $I = 2.5\ Gy_a$

   $\dfrac{10}{I_2} = \dfrac{36}{9}$ (cross-multiply)

   $36I_2 = 90$
16. Secondary protective barrier
17. patient
18. 500 mSv
19. radiographer
20. 0.5, 5.0

Chapter 15
Exercise 1: Matching

1. S	6. T	11. A	16. F	21. R
2. V	7. H	12. E	17. C	22. Q
3. K	8. O	13. Y	18. X	23. G
4. J	9. N	14. L	19. P	24. I
5. M	10. W	15. D	20. U	25. B

Exercise 2: Multiple Choice

1. C	6. D	11. C	16. D	21. C
2. C	7. A	12. B	17. B	22. C
3. D	8. C	13. D	18. C	23. C
4. C	9. B	14. B	19. D	24. D
5. C	10. A	15. C	20. B	25. C

Exercise 3: True or False
1. F (^{125}I is an unstable isotope.)
2. T
3. T
4. F (In a positron emission tomography [PET] device, annihilation radiation is initiated by the decay of an unstable atom.)
5. F (The nucleus of ^{18}F has nine neutrons.)
6. F (The possible use of radiation as a terrorist weapon is of concern to the general population.)
7. T
8. T
9. F (The same procedures that control infection are useful for preventing the spread of radioactive contamination.)
10. F (Diagnostic techniques in nuclear medicine typically make use of short-lived radioisotopes as radioactive tracers.)
11. F (No, technetium-99m is the radioisotope most often used in nuclear medicine.)
12. T
13. T
14. T
15. F (Geiger counters are most often used to monitor radioactive contamination.)
16. F (Radiation therapy uses ionizing radiation for the treatment of disease—namely, cancer.)
17. T
18. F (A positron is a form of antimatter.)
19. T
20. T
21. F (These 511-keV photons cannot be shielded by an ordinary lead apron.)
22. T
23. T
24. T
25. T

Exercise 4: Fill in the Blank
1. 90, adjacent
2. cancer spread
3. 6, nucleus
4. Positron
5. prep
6. radiation
7. dirty bomb
8. radiosensitive
9. beta
10. electron capture
11. patient
12. unstable
13. annihilation
14. metabolic
15. Geiger
16. vary
17. plastic container
18. pregnant, 6
19. decay
20. residual, sparing
21. isolated, minimize
22. radiotracer
23. 9
24. full
25. Monitoring

Exercise 5: Labeling

A. Dose-effect relation after acute whole-body radiation from gamma rays or x-rays.

Whole-Body Absorbed Dose	Effect
0.05 Gy$_t$	No symptoms
1. <u>0.15 Gy$_t$</u>	No symptoms, but possible chromosomal aberrations in cultured peripheral blood lymphocytes
2. <u>0.5 Gy$_t$</u>	No symptoms (minor decreases in white blood cell and platelet counts in a few persons)
3. <u>1 Gy$_t$</u>	Nausea and vomiting in approximately 10% of patients within 48 hr after exposure
4. <u>2 Gy$_t$</u>	Nausea and vomiting in approximately 50% of persons within 24 hr, with marked decreases in white blood cell and platelet counts
5. <u>4 Gy$_t$</u>	Nausea and vomiting in 90% of persons within 12 hr, and diarrhea in 10% within 8 hr; 50% mortality in the absence of medical treatment
6. <u>6 Gy$_t$</u>	100% mortality within 30 days because of bone marrow failure in the absence of medical treatment
7. <u>10 Gy$_t$</u>	Approximate dose that is survivable with the best medical therapy available
8. <u>≥10-30 Gy$_t$</u>	Nausea and vomiting in all persons in less than 5 min; severe gastrointestinal damage; death likely in 2-3 wk in the absence of treatment
9. <u>≥30 Gy$_t$</u>	Cardiovascular collapse and central nervous system damage, with death in 24-72 hr

From Gusev I, Guskova AK, Mettler FA Jr, eds: *Medical management of radiation accidents*, ed 2, Boca Raton, Fla, 2001, CRC Press.

Exercise 6: Short Answer

1. Therapeutic isotopes may be characterized by relatively long half-lives that are measured in terms of multiple days or multiple years and, with the exception of a few of them, by relatively high-energy radiation emissions. The radiation may be in the form of gamma rays or fast electrons (beta radiation).

2. Electron capture occurs when an inner-shell electron is captured by one of the nuclear protons, followed directly by the two combining to produce a neutron.

3. In beta decay, a neutron transforms itself into a combination of a proton and an energetic electron (called a *beta particle*). There is also emission of another particle called a *neutrino*. The electron exits the nucleus and interacts with surrounding atoms.

4. Diagnostic techniques in nuclear medicine typically make use of short-lived radioisotopes as radioactive tracers. These radionuclides have been attached to biologically active substances or chemicals and form radioactive compounds that predominantly diffuse into certain regions or organs where it is medically desired to scrutinize particular physiologic processes.

5. Positron emission tomography (PET) is an important imaging modality because it can examine metabolic processes within the body. This is particularly relevant to the proliferation of cancer cells.

6. Fluorodeoxyglucose (FDG) is a radioactive tracer that is very similar in chemical behavior to ordinary glucose, and so it is readily taken up or metabolized by cancerous cells. As such it reveals the locations of these cells through its positron emission decay and subsequent generation of oppositely traveling annihilation photons. These annihilation event sites are physically localizable through the PET scanner's patient-surrounding ring of coincidence detectors.

7. If a PET scanner is mechanically joined in a tandem configuration with a computed tomography (CT) scanner to produce a single joint imaging device, then in essence a facility gains not only the ability to detect the presence of abnormally high regions of glucose metabolism, yielding evidence of cancer spread (metastasis) into other body areas but also, at the same time, the means to obtain detailed information about the anatomic location and extent of these lesions or growths.

8. After the attack on the World Trade Center by hijacked airplanes on September 11, 2001, use of other possible terrorist weapons, such as radiation, became a public health concern.

9. The Environmental Protection Agency (EPA) sets limits for radioactive contamination that assume that a 1 in 10,000 risk of causing a fatal cancer is unacceptable. This type of regulation requires hospitals, educational facilities, and industries to control accidental exposures so that the health of the population cannot be measurably affected. It also assumes many other carcinogens are present and that all are regulated to a similarly low level.

10. Personnel should wear gowns, masks, and gloves when working with a patient who has surface radioactive contamination.
11. The health care facility's radiation safety officer.
12. Normal badge limits do not apply during a radiation emergency. Other special limits have been established for radiation emergency situations.
13. Medical management during the first 48 hours of acute radiation syndrome (ARS) involves simply treating the symptoms (e.g., nausea and vomiting) and trying to prevent dehydration.
14. Annihilation radiation is initiated by the radioactive decay of the nucleus of an unstable isotope. It is radiation in the form of two oppositely moving, 511-keV photons generated as the result of mutual annihilation of matter and antimatter (i.e., an electron and a positron).
15. A radioactive dispersal device, or dirty bomb, is a radioactive source mixed with conventional explosives. When it explodes, this device is intended to contaminate an area with radioactive material and thereby cause panic.

Exercise 7: General Discussion or Opinion Questions

The questions in this exercise are intended to allow students to express their knowledge and understanding of the subject matter covered in this chapter. Because the answers may vary, determination of an answer's acceptability is left to the discretion of the instructor.

POST-TEST

1. The EPA.
2. A radioactive dispersal device, or dirty bomb, is a radioactive source mixed with conventional explosives.

When it explodes, this device is intended to contaminate an area with radioactive material and thereby cause panic.
3. Therapeutic radioisotopes may be characterized by their relatively long half-lives, which are measured in terms of multiple days or multiple years and, with the exception of a few of them, by relatively high-energy radiation emissions. The radiation may be in the form of gamma rays or fast electrons (beta radiation).
4. B
5. neutrons
6. Rapidly
7. A neutrino is a particle that has no charge and an almost negligible mass, but its energy of motion balances the energy of the reaction.
8. After a dirty bomb explodes, externally contaminated individuals can be decontaminated by removal of contaminated clothing and immersion in a shower to cleanse the skin.
9. Annihilation radiation
10. 2
11. FDG
12. short-lived
13. 250 mSv
14. Electron capture is a process wherein an inner-shell electron is captured by one of the nuclear protons followed directly by the two combining to produce a neutron.
15. Positron emitters result in the production of high-energy radiation.
16. A Geiger-Müller (GM) detector (Geiger counter).
17. Technetium-99 m.
18. Radiation emergency plan and trained personnel.
19. high-energy
20. beta

Reference

1. National Council on Radiation Protection and Measurements (NCRP): Limitation of exposure to ionizing radiation, Report No. 116, Bethesda, MD, 1993, NCRP.